1985

An Introduction to

HUMAN SERVICES
MANAGEMENT

Social Administration: The Management of the Social Services, Second Edition
Volume I: An Introduction to Human Services Management
Volume II: Managing Finances, Personnel, and Information in Human Services

Simon Slavin is Professor of Social Administration and founding Dean Emeritus, Temple University. He established the School of Social Administration in 1968 and served as its Dean for ten years. Prior to that, he was Professor of Social Work at the Columbia University School of Social Work, where he headed the work in community organization and chaired the doctoral program. Among other responsibilities, Dr. Slavin was Executive Director of the Educational Alliance and the Mt. Vernon YM and YWHA. Currently, he is Editor-in-Chief of the quarterly journal *Administration in Social Work*, and Adjunct Professor at the Hunter College School of Social Work. He has authored many articles in the professional literature, edited *Applying Computers in Social Service and Mental Health Agencies*, and coedited, with Felice D. Perlmutter, *Leadership in Social Administration*.

Much of his time is now spent playing violin in several chamber music groups.

An Introduction to

HUMAN SERVICES MANAGEMENT

Volume I of
SOCIAL ADMINISTRATION:
The Management of the
Social Services, *second edition*

Edited by
SIMON SLAVIN

THE HAWORTH PRESS
NEW YORK • LONDON

Social Administration: The Management of the Social Services,
first edition, was published jointly in 1978 by The Haworth Press
and the Council on Social Work Education.

The Haworth Press, Inc.   EUROSPAN/Haworth
28 East 22 Street   3 Henrietta Street
New York, New York   10010   London WC2E 8LU England

Book design by Trudy Raschkind Steinfeld

Printed in the United States of America

Library of Congress Cataloging in Publication Data

Main entry under title:

Social administration.

   Includes bibliographies and indexes.
   Contents: v. 1. An introduction to human services management—
v. 2. Managing finances, personnel, and information in human services.
   1. Social work administration—Addresses, essays, lectures—Collected
works. I. Slavin, Simon.
HV41.S618   1985   361'.068   84-29049
ISBN 0-86656-347-4 (set)
ISBN 0-86656-348-2 (soft : set)
ISBN 0-86656-343-1 (v. 1)
ISBN 0-86656-344-X (soft : v. 1)
ISBN 0-86656-345-8 (v. 2)
ISBN 0-86656-346-6 (soft : v. 2)

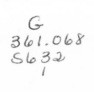

Contents

PART III: The Structure and Uses of Authority

A. Governing Boards

B. Executive Authority

C. Board-Executive Relationships

D. Minority and Female Executives

E. Participation in Executive Management

PART IV: Organizational Conflict and Change

PART V: Trends and Context in Administering Human Services

Contributors

DAVID M. AUSTIN, Professor of social work, School of Social Work, University of Texas at Austin.

WILLIAM E. BERG, Associate Professor, School of Social Welfare, University of Wisconsin-Milwaukee.

CHERYL BLACKBURN, Director of Emergency Services, Dede Wallace Center, Nashville, Tennessee, at the time this paper was written.

GEORGE BRAGER, D.S.W., Dean, School of Social Work, Columbia University, New York, New York.

ROSLYN H. CHERNESKY, D.S.W., Professor, Graduate School of Social Service at Lincoln Center, Fordham University, New York.

KENNETH P. FALLON, JR., M.S.W., Psychotherapist, Langdon Clinic, Anchorage, Alaska.

CHARLES A. GLISSON, Ph.D., Associate Professor, School of Social Work, University of Hawaii at Manoa, Honolulu.

RICHARD M. GRINNELL, JR., Ph.D., Chairman, Department of Social Work, and Associate Dean, School of Behavioural Sciences, La Trobe University at Bundoora, Victoria, Australia.

YEHESKEL HASENFELD, Ph.D., Associate Dean, School of Social Work, University of Michigan, Ann Arbor, Michigan.

ADAM W. HERBERT, Ph.D., Director of Research, Joint Center for Political Studies, Washington, D.C.

STEPHEN HOLLOWAY, D.S.W., Associate Professor, School of Social Work, Columbia University, New York, New York.

CHRISTOPHER B. KEYS, Ph.D., associate professor, Psychology Department, University of Illinois at Chicago Circle.

LOUIS E. KOPOLOW, M.D., Chief, Patient Rights and Advocacy Program, Mental Health Services Development Branch, Division of Mental Health Service Programs, National Institute of Mental Health, Rockville, Maryland. The views expressed in Chapter 20 are those of the author and do not necessarily represent those of the National Institute of Mental Health.

JOEL KOTIN, M.D., Assistant Adjunct Professor, Department of Psychiatry and Human Behavior, University of California at Irvine, Irvine, California, and in the private practice of psychiatry in Orange, California.

MICHAEL W. LANKFORD, M.S.S.W., Program Manager in Family and Children Services, Texas Department of Human Resources, Austin.

HERMAN LEVIN, deceased, was Professor, School of Social Work, University of Pennsylvania, Philadelphia.

HAROLD LEWIS, D.S.W., A.C.S.W., Dean, School of Social Work, Hunter College, City University of New York, New York.

PATRICIA YANCEY MARTIN, Ph.D., Professor of Social Work and Affiliated Professor of Sociology, School of Social Work, The Florida State University, Tallahassee.

DARYL G. MITTON, B.Ch.E., M.B.A., Ph.D., Professor of Management, San Diego State University, San Diego, California.

SCOTT MULLIS, Ph.D., Director of Corporate Development. Servio Logic Corporation, Portland, Oregon.

RINO J. PATTI, D.S.W., Professor, School of Social Work, University of Washington, Seattle, Washington.

ERMINIA LOPEZ RINCON, M.S., School Psychologist, Northwest Indiana Special Education Cooperative, Crown Point, Indiana.

ARTHUR J. ROBINS, Ph.D., Professor, Department of Psychiatry, University of Missouri-Columbia, Columbia, Missouri.

PAMELA A. RUSSELL, M.S.S.W., individual and family counselor, and doctoral student in marriage and family therapy at East Texas State University, Commerce.

ROSEMARY C. SARRI, Professor, School of Social Work, University of Michigan, Ann Arbor, Michigan.

MYRON R. SHARAF, Ph.D., Lecturer, Department of Psychiatry, Harvard Medical School, Harvard University, Cambridge, Massachusetts.

SIMON SLAVIN, Ed.D., Dean, School of Social Administration, Temple University, Philadelphia, Pennsylvania.

HERMAN D. STEIN, D.S.W., New York School of Social Work, Columbia University, New York.

MORTON I. TEICHER, Ph.D., Professor, School of Social Work, University of North Carolina, Chapel Hill.

RICHARD A. WEATHERLEY, Ph.D., Associate Professor, School of Social Work, University of Washington, Seattle, and visiting at The Florence Heller Graduate School for Advanced Studies in Social Welfare, Brandeis University, Waltham, Massachusetts.

Acknowledgments

PART I

Lewis, H. Management in the Nonprofit Social Service Organization.
Reprinted with permission of the author and the Child Welfare League of America, Inc., from Child Welfare, Vol. LIV, No. 9, November 1975, pp. 615–623.

Austin, D. M. Administrative Practice in Human Services: Future Directions for Curriculum Development.
Reprinted with permission of JAI Press, Inc. from The Journal of Applied Behavioral Science, Vol. 19, No. 2, 1983, pp. 141–152. Copyright © 1983 by JAI Press, Inc.

Patti, R. J. Patterns of Management Activity in Social Welfare Agencies.
Reprinted with permission of The Haworth Press, Inc. from Administration in Social Work, Vol. 1, No. 1, Spring 1977, pp. 5–18. Copyright © 1977 by the Haworth Press, Inc.

Teicher, M. I. Who Should Manage a Social Agency?
Reprinted with permission of The Haworth Press, Inc. from Administration in Social Work, Vol. 4, No. 1, Spring 1980, pp. 99–103. Copyright © 1980 by The Haworth Press, Inc.

PART II

Slavin, S. A Framework for Selecting Content for Teaching About Social Administration.
Reprinted with permission of The Haworth Press, Inc. from Administration in Social Work, Vol. 1, No. 3, Fall 1977, pp. 245–257. Copyright © 1978 by The Haworth Press, Inc.

Martin, P. Y. Multiple Constituencies, Dominant Societal Values, and the Human Service Administrator: Implications for Service Delivery.
Reprinted with permission of The Haworth Press, Inc. from Administration in Social Work, Vol. 4, No. 2, Summer 1980, pp. 15–27. Copyright © 1980 by The Haworth Press, Inc.

Mullis, S. Management Applications to the Welfare System.
  Reprinted with permission of the author and the American Public Welfare
  Association from Public Welfare, Vol. 33, No. 4, Fall 1975, pp. 31–34.
  Copyright © 1975 by the American Public Welfare Association.

Glisson, C. A. A Contingency Model of Social Welfare Administration.
  Reprinted with permission of The Haworth Press, Inc. from Administration
  in Social Work, Vol. 5, No. 1, Spring 1981, pp. 15–29. Copyright © 1981
  by The Haworth Press, Inc.

PART III

Mitton, D. G. Utilizing the Board of Trustees: A Unique Structural Design.
  Reprinted with permission of the author and the Child Welfare League of
  America, Inc. from Child Welfare, Vol. LIII, No. 6, June 1974, pp.
  345–351.

Robins, A. J., and Blackburn, C. Governing Boards in Mental Health: Roles and
  Training Needs.
  Reprinted with permission of the senior author from Administration in
  Public Health, Summer 1974, pp. 37–45.

Berg, W. E. Evolution of Leadership Style in Social Agencies: A Theoretical
  Analysis.
  Reprinted with permission of Family Service Association of America from
  Social Casework: The Journal of Contemporary Social Work, Vol. 61, No. 1,
  Jan. 1980, pp. 22–28. Copyright © 1980 by Family Service Association of
  America.

Russell, P. A., Lankford, M. W., and Grinnell, R. M., Jr. Administrative Styles of
  Social Work Supervisors in a Human Service Agency.
  Reprinted with permission of The Haworth Press, Inc. from Administration
  in Social Work, Vol. 8, No. 1, Spring 1984, pp. 1–16. Copyright © 1984
  by The Haworth Press, Inc.

Kotin, J., and Sharaf, M. R. Management Succession and Administrative Style.
  Copyright © 1967 by the William Alanson White Psychiatric Foundation,
  Inc. Reprinted with permission of the senior author and by special permission of the copyright holder, The William Alanson White Psychiatric Foundation, Inc. from Psychiatry, Vol. 30, 1967, pp. 237–248.

Stein, H. D. Board, Executive, and Staff.
  Reprinted with permission of the author and the publishers from The So-
  cial Welfare Forum, 1962. Copyright © 1962 by National Conference on
  Social Welfare. New York: Columbia University Press, 1962, pp. 215–230.

Levin, H. The Board-Executive Relationship Revisited.
Reprinted with permission of Family Service Association of America from Social Casework: The Journal of Contemporary Social Work, Vol. 61, No. 2, Feb. 1980, pp. 114–117. Copyright © 1980 by Family Service Association of America.

Herbert, A. W. The Minority Administrator: Problems, Prospects, and Challenges.
Reprinted with permission of the author and the American Society of Public Administration from Public Administration Review, November/December 1974, pp. 556–563.

Chernesky, R. H. The Sex Dimension of Organization Processes: Its Impact on Women Managers.
Reprinted with permission of The Haworth Press, Inc. from Administration in Social Work, Vol. 7, Nos. 3/4, Fall/Winter 1983, pp. 133–143. Copyright © 1983 by The Haworth Press, Inc.

Rincon, E. L., and Keys, C. B. The Latina Social Service Administrator: Developmental Tasks and Management Concerns.
Reprinted with permission of The Haworth Press, Inc. from Administration in Social Work, Vol. 6, No. 1, Spring 1982, pp. 47–58. Copyright © 1982 by The Haworth Press, Inc.

Fallon, K. P., Jr. Participatory Management: An Alternative in Human Service Delivery Systems.
Reprinted with permission of the author and the Child Welfare League of America, Inc. from Child Welfare, Vol. LIII, No. 9, November 1974, pp. 555–562.

Kopolow, L. E. Client Participation in Mental Health Service Delivery.
Reprinted with permission of Human Sciences Press from Community Mental Health Journal, Vol. 17, No. 1, Spring 1981, pp. 46–53. Copyright © 1981 by Human Sciences Press.

Weatherley, R. A. Participatory Management in Public Welfare: What Are the Prospects?
Reprinted with permission of The Haworth Press, Inc. from Administration in Social Work, Vol. 7, No. 1, Spring 1983, pp. 39–49. Copyright © 1983 by The Haworth Press, Inc.

PART IV

Slavin, S. Concepts of Social Conflict: Use in Social Work Curriculum.
Reprinted with permission of the Council on Social Work Education from Journal of Education for Social Work, Vol. 5, No. 2, Fall 1969, pp. 47–60.

Holloway, S., and Brager, G. Some Considerations in Planning Organizational Change.
Reprinted with permission of The Haworth Press, Inc. from Administration in Social Work, Vol. 1, No. 4, Winter 1977, pp. 349–357. Copyright © 1978 by The Haworth Press, Inc. This chapter is a partial and revised version of chapter one from Changing Human Services Organizations: Politics and Practice by George Brager and Stephen Holloway (New York: Free Press, 1978).

Patti, R. J. Organizational Resistance and Change: The View from Below.
Reprinted with permission of the author and the copyright holder from Social Service Review, Vol. 8, No. 3, September 1974, pp. 367–383. Copyright © 1974 by The University of Chicago Press.

PART V

Sarri, R. C. Management Trends in the Human Services in the 1980s.
Reprinted with permission of The Haworth Press, Inc. from Administration in Social Work, Vol. 6, Nos. 2/3, Summer/Fall 1982, pp. 19–30. Copyright © 1982 by The Haworth Press, Inc.

Hasenfeld, Y. The Changing Context of Human Services Administration: Implications for the Future.
Paper prepared for the Symposium on Administration and Community Organization, Council on Social Work Education, 1983 Annual Program Meeting, Fort Worth, Texas. Reprinted with permission of The National Association of Social Workers from Social Work (in press). Copyright © 1984 by National Association of Social Workers.

Preface

Seven years have passed since *Social Administration: The Management of the Social Services* first appeared. Much has happened in the intervening years affecting the administration and management of the human-social services. More books have been published in this period than in the preceding three decades. The emergence of the quarterly journal *Administration in Social Work* in 1977 provided a forum for scholarly writing, producing more periodical literature than had appeared in the preceding years.

All this is a reflection of the social, political, and economic environment that social agencies faced, as well as the process of maturation of thought and experience of those responsible for organizational development and for teaching social agency management. A restrictive economic circumstance and its concomitant conservative social ethos focused attention on the postulated need for examining the efficiency with which social programs were managed. Public policy and resources looked with favor on educational institutions that directed their attention to developing managerial skills and knowledge. In the social services, time-honored concern with clinical preoccupations began to shift interest to organizational issues. Programs in schools of social work placed increasing emphasis on the organizational and institutional context of clinical practice. One after another, these schools incorporated concentrations in "macro practice"—social policy, planning, and administration. The schools that have no offerings in administration are now the exception rather than the rule.

The response to the appearance of *Social Administration* reflected this growing interest, and it rapidly became adopted in administration courses in schools of social work. The widespread use of the volume has encouraged the preparation of an updated revision, responding to the growing sophistication of the field and the greater availability of materials. The original volume reflected the then-current state of the art. This edition similarly reflects a more fully developed state of theoretical and practical insight and awareness. Most of the selections are new to this volume. More attention is given to delineating what it is that administrators do and to some current perspectives on administrative thought. Greater emphasis is also given to the analysis of executive behavior, managerial styles, and approaches to participation in the administrative process. A new section on current trends, issues, and context concludes the volume.

Throughout this book the terms "administration" and "management" are used interchangeably. They refer to the same distinctive organizational function in social agencies—the responsibility for organizing and overseeing social service delivery. Business texts generally use the term "management"; in the fields of education and health, "administration" is the preferred term. The use of one label or the other grows out of historical tradition and consensus. In the social work community there is some ambivalence on this score. For example, the current *Encyclopedia of Social Work* (National Association of Social Workers, 1977) includes separate entries on "Management of Human Service Organizations" (Alexander, 1977) and on "Administration in Social Welfare" (Sarri, 1977) without any indication of the criteria used to differentiate their boundaries or content. They both appear to be describing the same phenomenon. More recently, "management" has been creeping into the social service lexicon. Of the recent books on this subject, use of the two terms has been about equally divided. This is likely a consequence of the sociopolitical environment within which social agencies in general find themselves. In a period of financial stringency and social policy regression, "management" seems to conjure an image of fiscal and social responsibility.

A word about the terms used to identify the organizational context of the social programs discussed in this book: although used variously by the contributing authors, "social agency," "social service agency," "social service organization," "social welfare agency," and "human service organization" all refer essentially to the same social structure—an organization whose function is the delivery of social services.

These human service organizations bear a special relationship to a variety of organizational systems with which they share some common organizational boundaries. In some respects human service organizations are like *all* organizations, "social units which are predominantly oriented to the attainment of specific goals" (Etzioni, 1969, p. 155). The study of organizations as such casts some light on understanding social service organizations, but fails to illuminate those aspects that differentiate them both in form and substance from all other organizations.

In some ways these organizations are similar to *market-based* organizations. Much that goes on internally within the organization, between organization members and consumers, and between the internal and external organizations contains elements of analysis that have similar meaning for business and social service organizations. It is clear, however, that in significant ways they differ markedly, most especially in pursuing a profit rather than a service ethic. And, as Drucker observes, "the service institution is in a fundamentally different 'business' from business. It is different in its purpose. It has different values. It needs different objectives. And it makes a different contribution to society" (Drucker, 1973, p. 45). Yet there is much to learn from studies and research of business organizations: management information systems, financial accounting systems, and marketing concepts, as well as selected aspects of research on human relations in industry, personnel management, executive styles, and the like.

Social service organizations also find common ground with a variety of *nonprofit* organizations. Both differ from business organizations to the extent that they use a nonprofit calculus for evaluating organizational effectiveness. This characteristic has significant meaning for canons of financial management and accountability. Thus, recent literature on accounting and financial reporting for nonprofit organizations (Gross & Jablonsky, 1979) speaks in direct ways to these and other nonprofit organizations.

There is, finally, a range of other *human service organizations* whose boundaries more or less overlap. These include educational institutions, hospitals, and mental health facilities, all of which deal with a "human" service. The social services, which are our main concern in these pages, although sharing many common characteristics, deal with a somewhat unique set of social functions, have a distinctive history, and have developed a characteristic culture and outlook.

This special and distinctive character grows out of several attributes, which in toto differentiate them from these other organizations. They are concerned with an organizational product that is responsive to social needs resulting from individual and group vulnerability, as well as social action directed at confronting harmful social circumstances. The interventive skills and expertise applied to these objectives grow out of the practice wisdom and professional behaviors honed from decades of experience in working with this clientele—people who find it difficult to manage their social relations and affairs unaided and who seek to enhance the quality of their social living.

Social administration or the management of the human-social services is concerned with that aspect of professional practice in the social agency that organizes the means to make such a service possible (Reynolds, 1942, p. 41). According to Reynolds, "Skill in administration consists not only in building organizational machinery which is adapted to the work to be done, but also in so dealing with the human parts of the machine that they will work at their individual and collective best" (pp. 35–36). If administration is "organization to get something done" (p. 207), then that "something" in social administration is the delivery of a social service. The processes that organize and monitor the social service delivery in an agency do so in the light of an explicit or implicit social policy that provides direction and purpose for the service system.

The practice detailed in the body of this book is a professional pursuit, calling upon skills, knowledge, values, and philosophical orientation that provide a creative dimension to organizational development. It has its technical and scientific aspects, but it is also in part an art, enlightened by practice wisdom, disciplined role performance, and balanced judgment.

A basic assumption underlies the organization and content of all that follows: social administration is an identifiable field of practice, more or less bounded and distinct from other administrative pursuits and rooted in the organization of the social services. Aspects of its work have parallels elsewhere, but as a constellation of skills, knowledge, and values it is sufficiently unique to warrant special study, application, and training. Although interdisciplinary in many ways, it relies heavily on the accumulated and recorded experience of the core profession, social work.

THE PLAN OF THE BOOK

Part I provides an overview of the administration of the social services. It introduces the reader to considerations concerning the nature of the administrative enterprise, to the vexing questions about boundaries, and to conceptual overlaps with cognate disciplines. Specific patterns of work entailed in social agency managerial practice are delineated.

Part II examines some theoretical issues explored in the literature. It provides perspectives for looking at social administration, and indicates some multidisciplinary contributions that can be readily incorporated in theory building. Some distinctive philosophical and technical characteristics are indicated, and suggestions are made for the integration of practice and theory in educational programs.

Part III explores in considerable detail one of the essential characteristics of administration—the structure and uses of authority. In part, it is concerned with the dilemma recently posed by John Gardner—how to advance organizational participation without eroding administrative authority. The parallel systems of authority in social agency governance, lay and professional, are described and their internal processes developed. The roles of trustees in decision making and of executives in providing professional leadership are stressed. The essential relationships between the two are elaborated.

Two neglected aspects of social agency administration (as well as of other institutional systems) are reviewed—the special problems of racism and sexism. The issues confronted by minority and female administrators are set forth, as is the need to understand and deal with the existent patterns of discrimination on both policy and operational levels.

The sharing of authority in human service systems has recently been highlighted in the literature, and concludes this section.

The perennial issues and problems of organizational conflict and change are presented in Part IV. Concepts and strategies in their management are identified, and the inevitable difficulties and constraints encountered by practitioners located variously in the organizational hierarchy are elaborated.

Finally, Part V reviews some trends in the management of the human services and looks at the context in which these trends are developing.

This book is intended for use in schools of social work and other educational enterprises that deal with human services management. It can be used in undergraduate courses on administration as an introduction to the field, and in graduate courses both as an overview and as the beginning of a sequence of courses geared to the preparation of social administrators.

Administrators of social agencies will also find the combination of theoretical and practical material relevant to their preoccupation with day-to-day managerial concerns.

The material included in this volume reflects significant developments of the past decade, during which the bulk of the selections were written. I am indebted to my students in graduate classes in administration at the School of Social Administration, Temple University, and those in the advance program at the Hunter College School of Social Work for their stimulation, encouragement, and response to the activity that resulted in the production of this volume.

REFERENCES

Alexander, Chauncy A. Management of human service organizations. *Encyclopedia of social work*. Washington, D.C.: National Association of Social Workers, 1977, 844–849.

Drucker, Peter F. Managing the public service institution. *The Public Interest*, #33, Fall, 1973, 43–60.

Etzioni, Amitai. *A sociological reader on complex organizations*. New York: Holt, Rinehart and Winston, 1969.

Gross, Malvern J., Jr., and Jablonsky, Stephen F. *Principles of accounting and financial reporting for nonprofit organizations*. New York: John Wiley and Sons, 1979.

National Association of Social Workers. *Encyclopedia of social work*. Washington, D.C.: NASW, 1977.

Reynolds, Bertha C. *Learning and teaching in the practice of social work*. New York: Rhinehardt and Co., 1942.

Sarri, Rosemary C. Administration in social welfare. *Encyclopedia of social work*. Washington, D.C.: NASW, 1977, pp. 42–51.

PART I

Introduction— Mapping the Territory

Editor's Introduction

Although administration is among the oldest of the methods of social practice—the first social agency had to be administered—there remains a series of unresolved issues in determining its conceptual and practical territory. The delineation of the social services given in the Preface suggests their functional boundaries, but leaves unanswered questions concerning the relationship between the several systems of administration. The historical connection between social administration and the development and evaluation of the social services suggests that there is a core professional discipline that organizes the essential skill, technique, knowledge, values, and objectives required for effective service delivery. In like manner, medicine remains the core discipline that organizes health and hospital administration, and education is the profession that directs the public schools.

Yet, these disciplines, with their distinctive traditions and areas of expertise, are not fully bounded or discrete. There are aspects of each that draw on the same research and that utilize similar procedures. Such overlap of interest often includes structural considerations. Thus social administration of governmental services is part of public administration, social service departments in hospitals are part of health administration, school social work and counseling part of educational administration. As social administrators deal with planning, allocation and control of financial resources, institutional maintenance functions, personnel management, and the like, it is difficult to distinguish some of these organizational behaviors from those of business administration and management.

Thus, there are common and overlapping aspects that inhere in any administered system, at the same time that each system has its own set of preoccupations—of values, techniques, goals, policy dimensions, consumer targets, intervention modes, and knowledge constellations. Both general (G) and specific (S) elements require explication for an adequate understanding of each of the respective administrative disciplines. Social and behavioral research informs all administrative action, and organizational theory and perspectives provide especially significant insight into administrative behavior.

Paralleling these external conceptual and organizational relationships of social administration are somewhat similar considerations re-

3

specting social policy and social planning, processes internal to social work practice. The literature and practice both support the observation that administration incorporates at its core the development and implementation of policy, and that planning processes are integral to its operation. Here, too, we see both common (G) and distinctive (S) features. The development of policy, if it is not to be moribund, implies implementation (administration is essentially the implementation of policy), while administration defines its operations in the light of either explicit or implicit policy.

A look at models of practice of administrators and policy developers suggests that at the extremes there is an essential differentiation. Perhaps the critical variable is the closeness of such practitioners to the actual delivery of client services. The administrator of a family service agency or an institution for the retarded spends a significant part of his or her time dealing with problems that are quite different from those of, say, a regional official in a state department of welfare or a policy analyst in a consultant firm. One is in close touch with clients, providers of service, and supervisors; the other with developing, monitoring, and evaluating programs, grant proposals, and transmission of guidelines. Schools of social work divide in their teaching of administration between those that organize their curricula to differentiate social policy-planning from administration in both classroom instruction and in field work placements, and those that have a single, integrated concentration.

Studies of administrative practice suggest the broad dimensions of knowledge and skill required for managerial competence in organizing resources and delivering relevant and needed social services. As these services have grown, diverse professional interests have challenged their historic connection with social work. In recent years, public social policy, unsympathetic to the needs of the populations served by social agencies, has encouraged such forays into this professional territory. Questions concerning the relation between technical processes of administration and substantive content thus become highlighted. What an appropriate curriculum for preparing administrators should be, and which auspices can best provide that training, are part of the current debate.

The selections in this section deal, in part, with the issues suggested above. Lewis reviews some of the distinctive characteristics of social service organizations and discusses the cultural differences between them and business organizations. Special stress is placed on the meaning of nonmarket mechanisms for service evaluation. He analyzes such common managerial concepts as accountability, efficiency, and effectiveness, and suggests the importance of considering political and economic factors that bear upon managerial decision making. Balancing considerations of unit costs with client satisfaction, effect with effectiveness, and, especially, knowledge and value, is seen as an important aspect of professional managerial practice.

Austin continues the discussion of the distinctive character of the human service program. He takes into account the common factors that inhere in a variety of organizations, and elaborates the specific factors that differentiate human service administration from the business and public administrative domain. Conclusions drawn from this analysis lead to a specification of some of the requirements of a specialized curriculum directed at the preparation of human service managers. An integral place in such a curriculum is reserved for a political economy perspective that includes analysis of the broad social context, the internal organizational relationships, and the interorganizational structure of these social programs.

Patti presents the result of a study that examined how social agency managers allocated their time in a typical workweek, including a review of activities they considered most significant for the effective performance of their jobs. The extent to which patterns of management activity varied by agency auspice and administrative level are also revealed. This empirical study provides a current review of the essential functions of administration and their weighted significance in executive and subexecutive action. Patti goes on to discuss the implications of these findings for management education, and makes the case for the importance of graduate training as well as continuing education and in-service training, stressing the different emphases each should employ. The very complexity of knowledge and skill required for competent practice suggests that managerial learning needs to be both intensive and long term.

Teicher elaborates the view that administrators require an intimacy of knowledge about the nature of the enterprise, the needs of its clientele, the requirements of a staff competent to provide appropriate service, and above all, the humane purposes for which the organization is established. He contrasts this with the view of the professional manager who is technically equipped to deal with the organization's needs but who may lack a knowledge base and identification with ethics and values conducive to delivering quality client service.

1

Management in the Nonprofit Social Service Organization

HAROLD LEWIS

The late 1950s and early 1960s in social service organizations were bullish years for innovators. The mid-1960s to the end of the decade saw "problem solvers" come into their own. Today, as resources contract and demand expands, the call is out for managers. Is it only by chance that this cycle, often repeated in social welfare history, appears to coincide with periods of major social unrest, liberalization and reaction? Coincidence or not, the fact is that managers now enter center stage, as economic distress and political reaction threaten social services in all fields. In the eyes of professionals who must deliver the service, talk of budget cuts, personnel freezes, program retrenchment, and organizational rigidity linked to demands for accountability, is managerial talk. Managers in such trying circumstances find themselves speaking of efficiency, when the professionals—in daily practice—speak of insufficiency. Managers had best be strong and wise people, for theirs is an unenviable lot.

The need for intelligent and concerned management of nonprofit social service organizations has never been greater. There are more of these organizations, they are involved in increasingly complex and costly operations, they now influence the lives and livelihoods of millions. But

This paper was presented at the Seminar on Education for Management of Social Sciences, at the University of Pennsylvania, January 5, 1975. The seminar was made possible by a grant from the U.S. Department of Health, Education and Welfare.

The writer is indebted to Albert O. Hirschman, author of *Exit, Voice and Loyalty: Responses to Decline in Firms, Organizations and States* (Cambridge, Mass.: Harvard University Press, 1970), for a number of analogs used in this paper.

greater need does not necessarily attract better or greater resources. Administrators have always been there, minding the store in social service agencies. But apparently in the eyes of managers who can judge, these administrators are not very good managers.

Among social service administrators, there are many who accept this evaluation, readily expressing their own feelings of inadequacy. The upsurge in management courses and concentrations in schools of social work, the experiments in joint programs with schools of business administration and public administration, and seminars on management, all testify to a degree of agreement between the outside evaluators and those evaluated. On the assumptions that such agreement exists and that it is the social work managers who seek to learn more about management from the business school managers, and not the other way around, this discussion takes the perspective of a client seeking the service of managerial specialists.

DIFFERENT CULTURES

It is important to clarify the situation of social service administrators; what it is we want help with, and what factors in our circumstances condition the use we can make of help that may be provided. We come from a culture very different from that of the business manager. We operate nonprofit organizations and can, with little effort, spend for good purposes more than we have, thereby incurring a deficit, but no loss in profit. When our consumers no longer need our services, an optimistic interpretation is that success has been achieved; this is hardly the case in business when customers stop buying a firm's product. In the social service organization concern for fairness often takes precedence over efficiency. The service ethic considers unequal advantage justified only if it raises the expectations of the least advantaged. Since the most disadvantaged are also more likely to experience difficulty in making appropriate use of opportunities, special and costly effort may be required to reach out to them. This, despite the fact that other claimants who do not need this special effort are sufficient in number to absorb totally the available resources. What business would spend resources to attract the most difficult to serve and usually most deprived customer when there are more than enough cooperative and affluent customers prepared to buy all it has to sell?

In business, when competition doesn't bring efficiency, adversity will. In social service, rarely does competition compel efficiency, and adversity is not likely to be the result of a client taking his business elsewhere. Given our lack of resources, selective inefficiency may be a necessity for organizational survival. In one city I know well, if the society to protect children from neglect and abuse systematically and efficiently reached out and informed the total community of its charge and the services it was expected to provide, not only would it be overwhelmed with needy cases, but its overload would swamp the courts, public assistance agencies, and children's institutions. In our field, where need—our definition of demand—far exceeds allocated resources, a certain amount of selected inefficiency appears essential for survival. Organizational cultures differ in important respects from that of business, and unless we understand these differences, it may be difficult to play an appropriate service role.

DIFFICULT DAYS AHEAD

The clamor for our services that will increase with rising unemployment and inflation is not, of course, evidence of a healthy demand. Success measured in terms of basic human needs met and social problems overcome is increasingly unlikely in these difficult times. We have more than once experienced times when our clients increased in number as the means for meeting their needs declined. We on the firing line know our consumers are restless. They take seriously the promise of justice and fairness. They will not accept an efficient operation that leaves their needs unattended. We may be devoted to our tasks, but we are also human. Managerial help, to be useful, should provide supplements to our courage and convictions, to prepare us to suffer the anger and distrust that will be heaped on our heads not for our failings, though they be many, but for the failings of our profit-oriented political and economic institutions.

An important characteristic of social service organizations is their monopoly over the type of resource they offer their clientele. Usually, as noted earlier, there are no competitive services that offer the consumer options. Moreover, since the cost is rarely carried by consumer payments, the threat of nonpayment or withdrawal by individual recipients may be irritating, but rarely fatal. Unlike the private monopoly that public policies regulate to protect the consumer from exploitation and profiteering, the nonprofit social service organization can hardly be accused of exercising these negative options for its own gain. The critic of these organizations must look elsewhere to find fault, and this leads to the traditional charges that have always hounded the managers of social service programs: laxity, antiquated methods, ineffective and inefficient operations. What ill serves the consumer, our critics assume, must be because of mismanagement, since motives seem to be absent. How the agency offers service, the service offered and the lack of responsiveness of the program to changing conditions are the key targets.

Another characteristic of social service organizations is the use of unit service cost, in the absence of profit, as a measure of efficiency. When goals are displaced as functions, this also serves as one measure of success. Those who recall the Ormsby-Hill Family Agency cost studies and their followups will remember how cost measures were used in these ways. Thus, while the nonprofit organization and the profit organization both want to maximize client-consumer satisfaction and minimize client-consumer ill will, the former would achieve this purpose at the minimum cost per unit service, while the latter would achieve it without threatening maximum profits. That the social service organization can incur deficits without a loss of profit suggests the role of service costs as an equivalent to profit as an indicator of managerial achievement.

PROMOTING TRUST

Client satisfaction in the nonprofit social service agency is in part dependent on the quality of service and in part on the quality of the processes and procedures through which the service is provided. Since much of the service entails intimate human contact between the worker and client, these two elements—what is being provided and how it is being provided—are not readily separable. For close helping relationships to serve successfully as vehicles for service, mutual trust is crucial. Trust is evident in the ability, willingness and opportunity to share one's self with another. A client seeking social service help more often than not chooses an agency, not a particular worker. Thus, trusting the agency is a major requisite for instilling trust in the worker-client relationship. Good management should, therefore, embody in the agency's organization work those elements that promote trust. Developing trust must have a high priority in any procedure instituted to assure accountability.

Returning to the unit cost and satisfaction functions, it is apparent that good management should seek an appropriate mix of both, normally somewhere between the minimum of the former and the maximum of the latter. An effective manager would provide guidance in approaching this ideal blend. An unwise manager would focus on one element to the exclusion of the other. What social service managers need help with is the body of established principles of practice in approaching this blend.

Costs per unit in the condition of excessive demand and fixed income that typically confronts the social service organization can be altered by changing worker productivity, operational efficiency, quality of service and characteristics of clients. The options to increase the price and extend the market are not usually available. Managers, then, face limited internal choices in seeking to lower unit costs without courting client ill will. They can hire less costly staff, require more productivity of staff, limit waste, give less to each client, choose only the clients who need less. If none of these options works, the manager can control intake in order to manage with available resources, but this would not necessarily control unit costs.

PRIVACY AND ANONYMITY

A third characteristic of the social service organization is that it must respect the privacy of the client, while distinguishing privacy from anonymity. To develop trust, opportunity must be provided to demonstrate its presence. Both the client and worker must have something they are free to share with the other. Where there is no privacy, there can be no free choice to share, and trust is hardly likely to infuse the relationship. Privacy, therefore, requires sufficient personal contact to permit recognition of differences and idiosyncratic attributes. It requires a feeling and knowing human interface between client and agency. Anonymity masks client differences and seeks to assure uniform treatment. It minimizes worker judgments. The destructive result of failure to appreciate the difference between privacy and anonymity has been amply demonstrated in the New York City experience with the separation of income maintenance and service in the Department of Social Services. The clientele of this agency lost trust in the agency's program.

EFFECT AND EFFECTIVENESS

Two popular terms in the language of managers, "effect" and "effectiveness," should not be confused with issues of efficiency and accountability. Effectiveness measures are based on criterion variables intended to judge achievement of goals associated with terminal values. Effect, on the other hand, is measured in relation to criteria derived from purposes associated with instrumental values. The former helps in judging a program's success; the latter provides the basis for judging the achievements of a practice. Those who base managerial decisions solely on effect measures risk the tyranny of small decisions. On the other hand, those who base managerial decisions solely on effectiveness measures risk remaining in doubt as to what, in fact, did or did not help. An appropriate mix of both types of outcome measures provides a basis for choices to be informed by functional and goal achievements. For example, at the functional level it is important in a child neglect situation to determine if the help given did provide supervision previously absent. This is a measure of effect. On the other hand, it is important to know that as a result of such improved supervision, the child attended school regularly, experienced less interruption in expected routines because of illness, imprisonment, etc. The latter measure shows whether the social purpose of the program was achieved. With the foregoing discussion as background, it is possible to address specific issues of efficiency and accountability, areas in which those who manage nonprofit social service organizations need most assistance.

EFFICIENCY

Consider the following not uncommon experience in social service agency personnel management. The agency proposes to upgrade the educational preparation of its staff to improve the quality and efficiency of its services. In addition to setting up an inservice training program, it proposes to underwrite, by released time or scholarship, the costs of employees attending graduate programs in areas useful to the agency. It selects the best candidates available on its staff; they attend the program, return after graduation for an obligated period, and leave the agency.

The worker who received the education has increased his economic options. The new competence brings a wider range of job choices, and greater maneuverability. The worker seeks out the best agency, not necessarily the one that invested in the worker. But the agency may still want to pursue this policy. It can be rationalized as preparing personnel for the profession, thus assuring the presence of competent practitioners in other programs to which this agency often must turn for help with its clients. Theoretically, if all agencies followed the same route, the general level of practice would improve, and the market would ultimately distribute appropriately the various talents needed. There may, however, be another reason for maintaining this policy.

Suppose the agency, as much as the talented worker, recognizes the low level of its practice, but has a locked-in senior staff, with little likelihood of turnover. Also assume the agency has a relative monopoly on employment opportunities for a particular skill. In these circumstances staff at the lower level in the agency program have no place to go, in the agency or elsewhere. Discontent is inevitable, and the politics of organizational practice can be brutal. The more talented, frustrated employees may use their ability to highlight, for client and community alike, the limitations of the quality of service, and may organize the staff to "Fanshen" (to turn over)—as the Chinese say. Faced with this possibility, the organization's leadership can opt for education as an effective tool to defuse the powderkeg, decapitating the potential leadership through a process that provides the more able with the options to go elsewhere.

This hypothetical case points up the need to examine both the political and economic factors that influence managerial decisions. Failures to do so may be the major inefficiency in social service organizations. Discussions of technology, of rational decision mechanisms based on up-to-date information retrieval, of sound management of fiscal resources, of control and planning systems, of quality control, of organizational statesmanship, of personnel administration, of goal-directed practice —all make for interesting and useful dialogues, but still one encounters the cases of the Pennsylvania Railroad, Lockheed, the Pan Am syndrome. In social service organizations with access to the more sophisticated technological hardware and software—such as large public welfare departments—the same syndrome is evident. Obviously, help is needed in formulating principles of managerial practice to guide political and economic judgments. Such principles will at least promote a principled practice, using the best available technologies to achieve goals and purposes.

ACCOUNTABILITY

The issue most in need of attention in relation to accountability is posed by the question: Accountability to whom? Lacking the choice to go elsewhere, social service consumers form a natural base for a political pressure group with considerable sustaining energies.

But there is also accountability to the funding source, to the community, to the profession, to one's superior and, last but not least, to oneself. Which of all these accountabilities deserves the highest priority? Mechanisms and techniques for assuring accountability differ in accordance with the interests of those for whom the results are intended. Obviously, groups that can exercise the major influence will demand and get the major attention. If the funding source threatens to cut off payment, its interest will be attended to, and soon. In a review of the clout likely to be available to the different populations to whom one can be accountable, the weakest group may well be the least organized. A unionized staff or an organized profession can make a more telling demand than individual persons. A board, a single or major funding source, or collaborating funding sources can speak in a more commanding voice when united than when disagreements produce no clear message. Weakest of all is the unorganized client whose problems bring him to the agency, and whose personal inability to manage seriously limits his energies and other resources needed to command accountability. The major help social service managers need with the problem of accountability is a set of guiding principles to inform the use of technologies in a manner that would assure a just and fair, not merely a convenient, response to requests for accountability. This may require, at times, that we assist in organizing future trouble makers. In the short run, it is unlikely that managers will promote a source of power that can be used to restrict their choices. In the long run, failure to do so may not only restrict choices, but eliminate choice entirely.

THE PRACTICE SCIENCE OF MANAGEMENT

I agree with those management experts who recognize a distinction between theoretical science and practice science. Although we need the former to tell us where to look and what to look for, the latter provides us with the "how." Practice science is formulated in terms of principles and rules, not laws. And since practice sciences intend consequences, they are never value-free. This paper was intended to emphasize the linkage of knowledge and value in professional managerial practice.

SUMMARY

I have noted the following areas where assistance would serve both our immediate and long-term concerns. We need to know principles of management that:

1. will communicate in the organizational work of the agency those elements that promote trust and concurrently respect privacy;
2. will help us approach an appropriate mix of unit-cost and client satisfaction functions;
3. can provide a basis of choosing an appropriate mix of effect and effectiveness measures to inform managerial decisions;
4. will guide us in making appropriate political and economic judgments affecting organizational efficiency; and
5. will inform our use of technologies in a manner that will assist us in assuring a just and fair, not merely a convenient, response to requests for accountability.

2

Administrative Practice in Human Services: Future Directions for Curriculum Development

DAVID M. AUSTIN

The hows and whys of the preparation of administrators for human service programs have been debated at length. This chapter argues that education for administrative practice in the human services requires a distinctive curriculum based on a conceptual framework that takes into account the specific characteristics of human service programs. The paper deals with a limited number of core concepts, illustrative of the distinctive aspects of such a curriculum. Furthermore, the paper argues that schools of social work may be the appropriate context for developing such a distinctive curriculum rather than schools of business administration or schools of public administration.

Some initial assumptions about these issues underlie this discussion. The first assumption is that social work is a major profession and that the professional domain includes attention to the organizational and policy context within which direct services are provided. Professional education for administration is an appropriate element in professional social work education. I believe that it is both desirable and feasible to de-

This chapter is an adaptation of a paper prepared for the University of Chicago-Columbia University Conference on Political Aspects of Human Services Management, April 1981, Chicago, Illinois.

velop a significant administrative practice curriculum within social work. There is need for both an entry-level curriculum and an advanced or executive-level curriculum. The research-oriented Ph.D. or D.S.W. curriculum is not the appropriate vehicle for the executive-level program.

The second assumption is that practical experience is not a sufficient base for competent administrative practice, whether that experience is in social work, public administration, or business administration. Administrative practice in the human services involves mastery of analytic concepts as well as performance skills.

A third assumption is that human services administrative practice has its own theoretical framework. It requires a distinctive curriculum, rather than a curriculum borrowed from other disciplines. Some concepts of administrative practice from business administration or from public administration are relevant, but they are not sufficient for a curriculum dealing with administrative practice in the human services. This chapter deals with some of the concepts that are of central importance in such a curriculum.

IS HUMAN SERVICES ADMINISTRATION BUSINESS ADMINISTRATION?

Much of the discussion about the similarity, or difference, between business administration and human services administration has focused on the issue of profit, both as a motivating factor in administrative practice and as a criterion for assessing organizational performance. Such discussion has distracted attention from some important distinctions. Indeed, the fiscal constraints of human service administration operating within fixed annual budgetary allocations are more severe, rather than less severe, than those of business organizations in which losses can be carried forward, or charged back, as a tax credit, and in which financial reserves can be established to buffer against fluctuations in income.

The fundamental difference between administrative practice in human services and administrative practice in business is the greater complexity of administrative practice in the human services. Among the key elements of complexity are the following:

1. simultaneous accountability to multiple policy centers (for example, policy mandates from multiple governmental funding sources, regulatory agencies, and the organizational policy body);
2. multiple and diffuse accountability for program outcomes to funding sources, legislative bodies, special interest groups, client constituencies, court mandates, and professional and accrediting organizations;
3. coproduction of organizational outputs with active participation of

the service user required in the actual production of most human service program outputs;

4. organizational outcomes primarily in the form of changes in the conditions or behaviors of individual human beings, outcomes that are
ambiguous and difficult to define or measure and difficult to attribute to a single causative factor; and

5. organizational outcomes that are achievable only through interactions with other groups and organizations that are interdependent elements in program "implementation structures" over which the organization has no authoritative control.

These characteristics of the complexity of human service administration highlight the degree to which human service organizations are
dependent on, and controlled by, political economy elements in the environment within which they operate. The process of dealing with this political economy environment is one of the most distinctive aspects of human service administrative practice and requires the development of
distinctive curriculum content. The practice concepts and understandings dealing with this area from business administration and public administration are inadequate and often totally inappropriate.

THE NATURE OF HUMAN
SERVICE ADMINISTRATION

An analysis of political economy concepts relevant to the development
of an administrative practice curriculum starts with several general assumptions (Hasenfeld & English, 1974; Sarri & Hasenfeld, 1978; Vinter,
1974; Stein, 1981). The first is that voluntary, philanthropic organizations and governmental organizations constitute two of the four basic societal frameworks for the provision of helping services among human
beings. The other two are primary groups such as the family and the
marketplace. A second assumption is that the administrative function in
human service organizations involves two major objectives: the provision
of effective and efficient services and the maintenance and development
of the organization as an essential instrument for service provision. A
third assumption is that the key function in administrative practice is decision making, including decisions dealing with the process of service
provision, decisions dealing with the internal operations of the organization, and decisions dealing with the relation of the organization to its environment. Administrative decision making is sometimes an individual
action; sometimes it is a broadly inclusive process. But the administrator
has the ultimate responsibility. The decision process must be guided
by the fundamental values that underlie professional practice, but they

must also be based on a realistic analysis of the underlying political economy dynamics.

The study of the dynamics underlying administrative practice can be thought of as dealing with both organizational dynamics and environmental dynamics (Thompson, 1967). The distinction between the organization and its environment, however, is primarily an analytic distinction since the interplay between organizational dynamics and environmental dynamics in an open system is constant and complex. The boundary between the two, which is easy to discuss in theory, is extremely difficult to define in a real situation. The distinction, however, is one that can be used to identify significant elements of theory in a curriculum design.

THE POLITICAL ECONOMY OF THE EXTERNAL ENVIRONMENT

This chapter focuses specifically on three elements of the political economy of the organizational environment (Austin, 1981; Benson, 1975; Gamson, 1968; Walmsley & Zald, 1973):

1. the macro, or societal political economy;
2. the immediate, or operational political economy; and
3. the political economy of the interorganizational implementation structure on which the organization is dependent.

In reality, all three political economy segments are highly interrelated. But they involve different considerations in the development of curriculum and can be analyzed independently.

1. The societal environment includes the broad pattern of political/ economic forces, and the nature and pace of change in those forces, which are the fundamental framework for any organization in the human services and for the other organizations with which it interacts. This is the environment over which administrators in individual organizations have little or no control (although representatives from a number of organizations acting together may have a significant degree of control). The curriculum emphasis here is on developing an awareness of key elements in the political economy environment and the dynamics of change underway rather than on methods of intervention. Moreover, in the administrative practice curriculum, the specific emphasis is on understanding current reality, rather than on developing normative models of ideal or preferred societies.
2. The operational environment includes the political economy context

within which the individual organization deals with immediate issues of legitimation and resource acquisition. The immediate environment may have both vertical and horizontal dimensions—that is, a locality or community dimension—and a field of service or categorical dimension with local, state, national, and international components (Warren, 1963). This is the environment with which personnel in the organization directly interact and over which the organization has some degree of control. It is the environment that the organization may be able to modify. The curriculum emphasis here is on understanding the political/economy context that affects specific environment/agency transactions, the role of the administrator in those relationships, and methods of intervening to achieve change.

3. The implementation structure environment involves the network of organizations and groups with which any single organization must interact to carry out its mission and to achieve program objectives (Hjern & Porter, 1981). Here, too, there is a complex set of relationships that involves the definition of respective organizational domains, the carrying out of legitimation and regulatory processes, and provisions for access to and control over essential resources. The curriculum emphasis here is on developing an ability to define and analyze implementation structures, developing an understanding of the content of administrative practice in the interorganizational context (as contrasted to the intraorganizational context), and on the role of administrative practice in improving the performance of implementation systems.

The Societal Context

Although this chapter deals primarily with curriculum concepts related to the operational environment and the implementation structure environment, both of which the organizational administrator interacts with directly, it is essential to give consideration to the dynamics of the societal context. There are five aspects of change that appear to be critical elements of the present societal/political economy as it affects human service organizations.

1. The elaboration of interest group politics, at the expense of political party alignments, as the major element of political structure (Janowitz, 1978). This results in a limited commitment to concepts of national unity, or to national political objectives. National policy decisions are primarily shaped by interest-group coalitions that are by nature transitory. This also increases the tendency toward only negotiated and incremental changes in existing policies since extreme proposals by any single coalition on any one issue leads to the mobili-

zation and energizing of opposing and often counterbalancing coalitions. This puts major political power in the hands of power brokers and coalition builders, at the expense of highly visible, issue-oriented political leaders, except as such leaders can build and dominate a stable coalition through the impact of their personalities.

2. The emergence of an increasing number of new interest-group elements based in the women's movement, ethnic minority movements, and the "moral majority." These groups are unlikely to achieve the highly visible and fundamental policy changes they seek, but they are likely to have significant impact on the organizational/bureaucratic framework of human services by systematically influencing program decisions, selection of personnel, and allocation of resources. There is a strong likelihood that these and other special interest groups will increasingly seek to advance their objectives through efforts to assert veto-power control over administrative decision making at all levels of society.

3. A long-term increase in constraints on the economic growth of the United States. Given an increasing dependency on raw materials from outside the United States, the rate of economic growth, compared to other sectors of the international economy, will decrease. The overall economic "pie" to be shared within the United States will have little real increase. There will be a sense of comparative decline in economic status vis-à-vis other "developed" nations, and there will be a reluctance to support "redistributive" programs either internationally or domestically.

4. A continued weakening of the influence of the federal government in domestic policy, vis-à-vis states and localities, particularly in the area of redistributive and regulatory social policies and programs. In a federal system, in the absence of public conviction that there is a compelling social crisis, or military crisis, power to determine domestic social policy becomes increasingly decentralized. Both restrictions on the role of the federal government as the open-ended funding source for domestic programs and the crippling of federal administrative staff capabilities through recurrent cutbacks and frequent reorganizations contribute to the relative decline of federal authority. This, in turn, reduces the importance of the executive and legislative branches of the federal government as the focal point for efforts to achieve significant social change.

5. An intraregional and interregional shift of political and economic power within the United States. This has resulted in a reduced national political influence for the following: the industrially based labor movement; urban, ethnic-group-based political party structures; the East Coast intellectual and political establishment of all persuasions; the East Coast financial and business leadership structure; and

traditional social welfare coalitions built around East Coast leadership. Concurrent with this shift has been a major cultural confrontation between the urban, secular, ethnically diverse, sexuality-oriented culture that emerged in the 1960s and 1970s as the pervasive culture of the United States and a male, white, Anglo-Saxon, Protestant, traditional religion-based culture that has been the majority culture in the Midwest outside the industrial cities and in the South (the areas in which the Populist movement was strongest 100 years ago).

These critical elements of change in the societal context are not described here as having either positive or negative consequences for the administration of human service programs. The full range of consequences, in fact, cannot be predicted, and the assessments of the meaning of these possible changes will vary widely. This is the type of environment, however, that Emery and Trist (1965) have described as turbulent, that is, as having a pattern of both rapid and interrelated changes that threaten to disrupt established patterns of operation in existing organizations.

The Operational Context

The operational context involves that environment with which the administrator and other members of the organizational staff interact directly. It includes the immediate sources of legitimation and regulation and essential resources. At this level the political economy involves specific individuals and organizational units that make the decisions that affect the individual service organization. Administrative practice that deals with the operational context involves assessment of the political economy, planning action to deal with environmental uncertainty and to protect the organization (either through intervening in the environment to change it or buffering the organization against its impact), and implementation of the procedures outlined in such plans. Moreover, it is essential that this aspect of the curriculum have a firm base in a realistic analysis of the nature of the political economy specific to human service organizations.

The initial emphasis in dealing with the operational political economy is on methods of descriptive assessment, that is, the systematic analysis of the sources of legitimation, regulation, and financing that define the major constraints within which the organization functions, and that provide potential sources of control over other organizations. The description of the organizational political economy, however, is only an initial step. The most critical aspect of assessment is the analysis of the dynamics that are likely to affect the behavior of individuals and decision units that control the legitimation of the organization and the resources on which it depends. In carrying out such an analysis, there is often a tendency to use an implicit analogy based on a model borrowed from business management of the relation of business organizations to the marketplace. There is a marketplace demand for a particular product, and there is an organization with the productive capacity to respond to that demand. If demand goes up, the organization expands its production operations; if demand goes down, the organization contracts its activities.

In the case of human service programs, it is often assumed that evidence of the existence of a particular type of human need (children in need of an alternative home) is equal to a demand for services from a particular organization (child welfare agency). The actual relation between conditions of human need and the collective decision processes involved in legitimating and regulating services, and in resource allocation—in both governmental and voluntary arenas—is considerably more complex than this demand-supply response model suggests.

There are several distinctive, conceptual elements in the dynamics of the political economy of human service programs that distinguish it from the marketplace political economy of business organizations. First, the existence of human need does not necessarily constitute a demand for a specific organizational service. Second, the translation of need into an allocation of resources to support organizational services does not take place through a marketplace demand-supply response process, but through processes of collective decision making. Third, the processes of collective decision making deal primarily with the character of the "public good" to be provided through the allocation of either governmental or contributed resources, rather than with the "private good" benefit to the individual service user (Austin, 1981; Musgrave, 1959). Fourth, the "public good" may be a "universal" public good, a "redistributive" public good, a "social-control" public good, or a mixture of these, and the decision dynamics of each are different. Fifth, collective decisions about allocating resources to provide a "public good" are influenced by a number of other considerations besides the direct evidence of human need, or evidence that a particular program can meet that need.

The vast majority of all types of human need are met through primary relationships, that is, through services provided by members of a family, friends, or neighbors. In a "developed" society, however, primary relationships are not a sufficient resource. There may be no source of primary relationship assistance. Available primary relationship resources may not work—members of a family may dislike each other. Or the primary relationship resources may be insufficient.

A collective decision to establish either a voluntary/philanthrophic, or governmental, service organization, or to expand such an organization, involves a prior decision that there is a need that cannot be met either through primary relationships or through the marketplace. The collective decision to establish an organizational service program, or to allocate resources to it, also involves a decision about the "public good" to be created through such a program, that is, the nature of the benefit to the larger society that justifies the levying of taxes or the solicitation of contributions to support a particular service. As indicated above, the public good to be created through an organizationally provided service can take several forms. And it is essential in a human services administration curriculum to develop an awareness of how public-good dynamics differ from marketplace dynamics. First, the public good may take the form of a "universal" benefit with everyone sharing the cost and everyone benefiting. Such universal public goods may be nondivisible —national defense and clear air—or divisible—the provision of clean water in measureable quantities to individual homes through a water system built and owned collectively by the citizens of a municipality.

Second, the public good may take the form of a "redistributive" benefit with one group of individuals providing the financial support for the provision of organizational services to meet the needs of another group. The public good is created by providing "private goods" or benefits through an organizational program to a particular set of persons in need, persons who cannot meet those needs through their own resources (for example, the victims of a natural catastrophe). The provision of "redistributive" benefits is motivated by feelings of communal responsibility for other individuals who are defined as part of a common social unit—family, community, national society.

Human service programs are also established in response to a third concept of "public good" that takes the form of a "social control" or "behavior change" benefit. In this instance, one group of persons within a society decides that there is a "need" for a particular type of behavior-changing or behavior-controlling service to be provided for another group of individuals or households. One example is the decision, by past community leaders, that children of immigrant families "needed" to go to school to learn to read, write, and speak English, regardless of the preferences of either the children or their parents. The objective in the provision of such "social control" services is to create a public benefit through controlling, or changing, the behaviors of a "target" service population, in addition to the private benefits that accrue to the particular individuals who use the service for their own reasons.

Since the actual service users in a social control/behavior change service program do not value the services that are provided as highly as do those persons who decide to initiate the services, they are unlikely to seek equivalent services through primary relationships, or through the marketplace. Therefore, some form of collective action is necessary to initiate the potential service and to make provisions for sharing most or all of the costs among those persons who may be expected to share the "public good" benefit that results from such services.

If the members of the "target group" are to participate voluntarily in such "social control" services, they must be persuaded that the "private good" benefits they receive offset the costs or constraints attached to such services. Since, however, such "merit good" benefits are shaped primarily by the preferences of those who initiate them rather than by the users, there is always some element of compulsion or authority attached to such services to ensure participation. When the benefits are perceived by the users as very minimal, the degree of compulsion may be very high, for example, in the instance of the commitment of felony offenders to a maximum security prison to ensure their participation in "rehabilitation."

The dynamics of collective decision making involving public goods are different for each type of public good. In the instance of a service that is expected to provide a "universal" public good, the decision to initiate the service requires a collective determination that there is a need shared by all, or a substantial majority of, the persons within a given constituency. The specific characteristics of the service are likely to reflect the preferences of those individuals or groups most active in initiating the service and in influencing public attitudes about the service.

The basis of redistributive services is a collective decision that there is an obligation to help individuals who are recognized as part of a common social unit. The public good that is created through the support of such services is the collective sense of satisfaction in having fulfilled such an obligation. The level of support provided for a redistributive service is likely to reflect the intensity of feeling of obligation, that is, the degree of "in-group identification" with the service users. In any case, support is likely to be at the minimum level at which the sense of personal obligation is fulfilled for the majority of individuals supporting the collective decision.

Social control/behavior change services are established when a substantial majority of citizens, or a smaller group—if they are willing to meet the costs among themselves—fear the behavior of others or feel that their self-interests are threatened by the behavior or potential behavior of others. The level of support is likely to reflect the intensity of such feelings.

The Interorganizational Context

The interorganizational network of which the service organization is a part is the third major element in the external political environment that should be dealt with in the curriculum. The implementation of human service programs increasingly involves a series of specialized program components in a number of different administrative organizations, linked together operationally, although not structurally, as an "implementation structure." The implementation of a human resources services program includes a registration unit, job referral units, educational components, vocational and personal counseling, apprenticeship training, vocational rehabilitation, job development projects, aptitude testing, and so forth. These program components may be all within a single administrative structure, but that is unlikely.

The move away from creating large, inclusive, centrally administered governmental agencies and toward increasing decentralization of program administration makes multiorganization implementation structures increasingly important as the operating framework of service provision. In the early 1970s, the "services integration" effort attempted to address these issues. The focus then, however, was primarily on one-time, structural solutions and on the "integration" of complete organizations (Austin, 1978; Kahn & Kammerman, 1978). The implementation structure concept focuses on understanding existing processes, rather than on the design of freestanding innovations, and on operational relations among program components, rather than among complete organizations (Hjern & Porter, 1981).

Administrative practice in the context of implementation structures becomes critical when organizational viability depends on evidence of program accomplishments, and program accomplishments depend heavily on the performance of individuals and program components in other organizational settings over whom the administrator has no authoritative control. The situation of the administrator vis-à-vis the implementation structure is markedly different from the position of such a person in relation to other personnel within the same organization. The existence of implementation structures is often reflected in the development of a matrix structure within the service organization and a dual pattern of organizational and programmatic administration. Organizational administrators carry fundamental responsibility for organizational performance and organizational maintenance; program-unit administrators carry responsibility for program effectiveness, which often means not only responsibility for specialized operations within the agency but also for linkages with other essential elements in the implementation structure.

The political economy of the implementation structure involves a number of potential difficulties: conflicting domain assertions, interdependence among organizations that are also competitors for resources, professional and ideological disagreements, and a lack of legal and administrative precedents to serve as guidelines for administrators. Differences in public-goods goals in alignments with organized professions, even in diagnostic definitions, all add to the complexities.

Although administrative practice in dealing with the societal environment and the operational environment is primarily reactive—that is, coping with environmental pressures and changes in environmental factors—administrative practice in the implementation structure context can be proactive. This can include actively initiating interactions with program components in other organizations, developing formal and informal working agreements, establishing referral procedures, and negotiating purchase of service contracts and information-sharing procedures. It also means initiating efforts to develop information systems that can account for program outcomes across organizational lines and accounting systems that can identify actual service costs on a program-wide basis.

But an even more critical aspect of administrative practice in the implementation structure is the development of conflict-resolution procedures and skills. Although the difficulties that normally exist among organizations that are part of an implementation structure resemble a political battlefield, political-contest procedures are largely irrelevant in resolving the difficulties. Majority votes, or the exercise of dominant political power, seldom resolve interorganizational operational problems, particularly when different units of government are involved. The absence of an ultimate authority mechanism to resolve conflicts in interorganizational relationships requires attention to formal, conflict-resolution procedures, including solution-oriented task forces, and third-party mediation and arbitration procedures.

The curriculum approach to developing an understanding of the implementation-structure context includes as a starting point using an analytic process, similar to that used in the operational context. The analysis of implementation structures includes the identification of interrelated program components, the identification of the resource/regulatory framework of each component, and the characteristics of the network, including program gaps and problems in interorganizational linkages. A more complex step includes the design and evaluation of alternative mechanisms for improving the functioning of implementation structures. But the most fundamental curriculum issue is the development of an understanding of the essential importance of both the administrative functions within an organization and the administrative functions in critical interorganizational processes.

The Development of an Administrative Practice Curriculum

Political conditions are severe; pressures on administrators are increasing. The issue is, given impossible conditions, how should the preparation of administrators proceed? This chapter has dealt with three organizing concepts that illustrate the distinctive understandings that must be part of any human services administration curriculum and that make such a curriculum different from a business administration curriculum. There are also other essential concepts such as the relation of administration to professional practice and the impact of administration on the coproduction of services. A full consideration of curriculum development would also require attention to such issues as the relation between theoretical constructs and practice wisdom and the role of research in defining curriculum content.

The fundamental issue, however, is the decision to deal with human service administration as a distinctive, major task in contemporary society, one requiring high degrees of personal commitment and skill in human relationships and a distinctive set of conceptual understandings. Of equal importance is a realistic understanding of the dynamics of the political economy in an open, competitive, pluralistic, and politicized society. Indeed, the effective implementation of public policy, particularly as it affects human services, has become a central issue in the public credibility of democratic government. The proposal to define all program policy decisions as marketplace decisions is an effort to avoid critical issues, rather than to resolve them; the administrative practice issues will be much the same under public administration or private contract. The challenge is to find appropriate methods for implementing collective democratic decisions in a highly interdependent but diverse society.

REFERENCES

Austin, D. M. The political economy of social benefit organizations: Redistributive services and merit goods. In Stein, H. D. (Ed.), *Organization and the human services: Cross disciplinary reflections*. Philadelphia: Temple University Press, 1981. 37–88.

Austin, D. M. The politics and organization of services: Consolidation and integration. *Public Welfare*, 1978, *36*, 20–28.

Benson, J. K. The interorganizational network as a political economy. *Administrative Science Quarterly*, 1975, *20*, 229–249.

Emery, F. E., & Trist, E. L. The causal texture of organizational environments. *Human Relations*, 1965, *18*, 21–31.

Gamson, W. A. *Power and discontent*. Homewood, Ill.: Dorsey Press, 1968.

Hasenfeld, Y., & English, R. A. (Eds.), *Human service organizations*. Ann Arbor: The University of Michigan Press, 1974.

Hjern, B., & Porter, D. O. Implementation structures: A new unit of administrative analysis. *Organization Studies*, 1981, *2*(3), 211–227.

Janowitz, M. *The last fifty years: Societal change and politics in the United States*. Chicago: The University of Chicago Press, 1978.

Kahn, A. J., & Kammerman, S. B. The politics and organization of services: The course of 'personal social services.' *Public Welfare*, 1978, *36*, 29–42.

Musgrave, R. A. *The theory of public finance.* New York: McGraw-Hill, 1959.

Sarri, R. S., & Hasenfeld, Y. (Eds.), *The management of human services.* New York: Columbia University Press, 1978.

Stein, H. D. The concept of human service organization: A critique. In H. D. Stein (Ed.), *Organization and the human services: Cross disciplinary reflections.* Philadelphia: Temple University Press, 1981. 24–36.

Thompson, J. D. *Organizations in action.* New York: McGraw-Hill, 1967.

Vinter, R. D. Analysis of treatment organizations. In Y. Hasenfeld & R. A. English (Eds.), *Human service organizations.* Ann Arbor: University of Michigan Press, 1974. 35–50.

Walmsley, G. L., & Zald, M. N. *The political economy of public organizations.* Lexington, Mass.: D. C. Heath, 1973.

Warren, R. L. *The community in America.* Chicago: Rand McNally, 1963.

3
Patterns of Management Activity in Social Welfare Agencies

RINO J. PATTI

The need for additional and augmented master's degree and continuing education programs concerned with preparing students for administrative roles in social welfare is widely acknowledged in social work education. The reason why schools of social work should assume educational leadership in this undertaking has also been persuasively argued,[1] and there are a number of such institutions that have proceeded to develop curricula in this area.[2] However, in the midst of these developments there has been relatively little systematic attention given to the nature of administrative work actually performed in social welfare agencies and the implications of such information for designing educational curricula.[3]

The present study was an attempt to develop an empirically grounded understanding of the tasks and functions that characterize management practice in social welfare that might serve as a partial basis for informing decisions about content to be incorporated in educational programs for administration. More specifically, the study was concerned with deter-

This study was supported by a grant from the Department of Health, Education, and Welfare, Social and Rehabilitation Service, SRS-84-P90261/0-01. The author gratefully acknowledges the contributions of Professor Richard Elmore of the University of Washington, who helped in the design of the study, and graduate research assistants Phillip Osborne, Michelle Hankins, Ronald Rauch, and Elaine Scherba, who assisted in collecting and analyzing the data.

mining what managers did during the course of a typical workweek, the amount of time devoted to these activities, and whether the configuration of management activities varied by administrative level and agency auspice. We were further interested in ascertaining which activities managers considered most significant to the effective performance of their jobs, since it is risky to infer the functional significance of an activity based solely on the amount of time that is given to it.

METHODOLOGY

The survey instrument developed for this study was a semistructured interview schedule adapted from a previous study of management activities conducted by Corson and Paul.[4] The interview schedule consisted of five main sections including identifying data (e.g., agency, job title, education), job history, activity calendar, significant activities, and factors influencing job performance and career mobility.[5] Whenever possible, copies of the questions to be asked were mailed to the respondents before the interview, with the request that they complete a job history and keep a precise account of their activities during the week preceding the interview. The interview itself, usually lasting about 1½ hours, attempted to reconstruct the respondents' work activities in the preceding week in as much detail as the managers' recall, aided by their calendar, would allow. The managers were also asked to select four or five activities from the previous week that they considered most significant to effective job performance and to discuss why these were selected, their purpose, the skills employed, the time spent, and so on.

The sample consisted of ninety managers purposively selected to represent several administrative levels in public, quasi-public, and voluntary agencies in the state of Washington. Since our principal concern was with the management of agencies that provide personal social services to individuals and families, we selected managers who were responsible for programs in which social work services were the principal program elements. Finally, in order to discern if there were substantial differences in patterns of management activity among respondents in agencies serving primarily rural, as opposed to urban, areas, we included a subset of managers in agencies located in a sparsely populated area of the state.

Activity data collected in interviews with the ninety managers in the sample were classified into thirteen functional categories.[6] Ten of the categories represented traditional management functions such as planning, controlling, and supervising. One category, providing direct services, was included to encompass those activities managers engaged in that were directly related to service provision. Another category, information processing, was employed to classify activities devoted to telephoning, paperwork, and correspondence, when it was not possible to determine the management function being performed. Finally, activities devoted to professional development, community service, and the like, where these were not part of a manager's assigned job responsibility, were classified as extracurricular.

ANALYSIS AND INTERPRETATION OF DATA

The following analysis of management activity addresses four major issues. The first concerns the extent to which the sample week for which activity data were obtained was representative of how the respondents ordinarily spent their time. Next, the analysis focuses on how the managers allocated their time across the thirteen functional categories mentioned earlier. Thirdly, the analysis addresses the respondents' judgments regarding those activities that were most significant to the performance of their job. Finally, data are presented that show how patterns of management activity varied by type of agency and management level.

The Sample Week

To what extent were the tasks and activities reported by managers for the week preceding the interview representative of what they do ordinarily? This question is of critical importance, because if the activity data were systematically biased by atypical temporal or situational circumstances, the information would be of little use for curriculum planning. Accordingly, respondents were asked to indicate whether the activities reported for the prior week were typical of those that comprised their job. Of the ninety respondents, sixty-nine (76.7 percent) indicated that the activities reported were typical. The remaining managers who indicated that the prior week was not representative attributed this to requirements imposed by new laws or administrative regulations, seasonal projects, special demands growing out of a legislative session, and assorted idiosyncratic factors. Thus, it is important to note that a substantial majority of the managers were describing activities that were commonly performed by them, though perhaps in varying amounts from week to week. It is also probable that the remaining respondents engaged in some typical activities even though the week was not representative.

A Profile of Managers' Activities

Table 3-1 shows the mean number of hours spent by all ninety respondents in the sample week for each of thirteen activity categories. Perhaps the most significant finding that emerges here is the fact that in the ag-

TABLE 3-1. Mean Hours Spent in Each Activity by Managers

Activity	Mean Hours
Planning	3.9
Information processing	6.2
Controlling	5.4
Coordinating	3.8
Evaluating	1.5
Negotiating	.8
Representing	1.8
Staffing	.9
Supervising	6.7
Supplying	.3
Extracurricular	1.9
Direct practice	4.1
Budgeting	1.0

gregate, managers engaged in a rather wide array of tasks and activities. Respondents devoted at least one hour a week to ten different types of activities, six of which consumed nearly four hours or more. These data suggest the diverse and complex nature of management responsibility although, as we shall see later, the distribution of activities varied substantially by management level and type of agency.

The mean number of hours devoted to various activities compares quite well with conventional knowledge regarding how managers spend their time. As might be expected, substantial portions of the workweek were spent in supervising, information processing, controlling, planning, and coordinating. The large amount of time given to information processing may seem unusual, but it should be recalled that this category encompassed all those activities concerned with reading reports and other job-related materials, making telephone calls, filling out forms, and writing memos and letters (i.e., when such activities were not in the service of some specific purpose or function). Somewhat unexpected was the finding that direct practice occupied an average of over four hours a week. We will later analyze the characteristics of managers who spent significant time in direct practice as compared to those who did not. The other finding that may appear somewhat unusual at first is the relatively small amount of time given to budgeting, since the activities associated with this function appear so ubiquitous in management practice. This datum may be explained by the temporal character of the budgeting process and by the fact that we included in this category only those activities directly related to budget preparation. In addition, it is important to note that a large number of respondents in the sample were in low-level management positions where responsibility for developing budgets per se is not a central element of their job. In the last analysis, however, this finding may reflect the reality that little time is spent in actual budget preparation by most managers. This, of course, does not diminish its importance, nor does it adequately reflect the extensive analytic work that must precede the construction of a sound budget.

Significant Management Activities

In order to obtain some indication of the importance managers attached to the activities in which they were engaged, respondents were asked to choose up to five activities performed in the previous week that they considered significant to the effective performance of their job. In this way we hoped to arrive at some qualitative indication of the tasks and activities that are essential to management and to determine if there was a correspondence between the time spent on a particular kind of work and its importance to management performance.

Table 3–2 shows the number of managers who ranked each activity among the five most significant to the effective performance of their job. Several findings are particularly worth noting. Over two-thirds of the managers in this sample judged activities subsumed under controlling,

TABLE 3–2. Number and Percentage of Managers Who Ranked Activities Among the Five Most Significant to Effective Job Performance

Activity	Number of Times Ranked Significant	Percentage of Managers Who Ranked Activity Significant
Planning	61	67.7
Information processing	24	26.6
Controlling	67	74.4
Coordinating	40	44.4
Evaluating	18	20.0
Negotiating	13	14.4
Representing	25	27.7
Staffing	12	3.4
Supervising	61	67.7
Supplying	2	2.2
Extracurricular	4	4.4
Direct practice	20	22.2
Budgeting	10	11.1

supervising, and planning as the most important ones they had performed during the prior week. Somewhat less than one-half of the respondents ranked coordinating as significant, while one-quarter or less of the managers felt that activities associated with representing, information processing, direct practice, and evaluating were important to effective job performance.

In order to compare the amount of time given to each kind of activity with managers' judgments regarding the significance of these activities, the data were converted to ranks as presented in Table 3–3. An examination of this table reveals that for the most part there is a correspondence between the amount of time given to an activity and the importance attached to it by managers. But there are several interesting exceptions. Information processing and direct practice were not considered as important to effective job performance as the amount of time spent on these activities would suggest. Conversely, planning, representing, and negotiating were generally considered somewhat more significant than the time given to these activities would indicate.

These data suggest that those activities associated with *supervising, controlling, planning,* and *coordinating* are the most important management tasks as judged by both the amount of time they consume in a representative workweek and the significance that managers attach to them. Information processing and direct practice are among the most time-

TABLE 3–3. Ranks of Activities by Time Spent and Significance of Activity to Effective Job Performance

Activity	Time Spent[a]	Significance[b]
Supervising	1	2 (tie)
Information processing	2	6
Controlling	3	1
Direct practice	4	7
Planning	5	2 (tie)
Coordinating	6	4
Extracurricular	7	11
Representing	8	5
Evaluating	9	8
Budgeting	10	10
Staffing	11	12
Negotiating	12	9
Supplying	13	13

[a] 1 = largest amount of time spent.
[b] 1 = most significant.

consuming activities but tend to be viewed as less important to effective managerial performance. While relatively little time was spent on representing and negotiating, a disproportionate number of managers judged these to be among the most significant activities they performed. This suggests that although a relatively small number of managers are engaged in these activities, those who are tend to consider them essential to effective job performance. Managers spent relatively little time in activities related to evaluating, budgeting, staffing, and supplying, and generally did not consider these tasks centrally important to their functioning.

Variations in Management Practice

To this point we have treated all managers in our sample as an undifferentiated group. Such an approach is useful for determining certain commonalities in management practice, but it tends to obscure differences that may be found among those operating in various organizational contexts. In order to explore this question we analyzed patterns of management activity in different kinds of agencies and at five administrative levels. Our purpose in doing so, as we indicated earlier, was to ascertain whether there were significant variations in management practice among the respondents.

Agency auspice. For our purposes, social service agencies were divided into six main types: public-state-urban agencies, public-state-rural agencies, public-local-urban organizations, quasi-public organizations, voluntary-urban agencies, and voluntary-rural agencies.

For the most part, patterns of management activity did not vary substantially among managers in the six types of social service agencies. That is to say, the way managers distributed their time across various activities remained fairly constant regardless of the auspice and/or geographic location of the agency. There were, however, several interesting exceptions to this generalization. For example, the data in Table 3–4 indicate that managers in public and quasi-public agencies spent considerably more time in activities we have characterized as information processing than did their counterparts in voluntary agencies (both urban and rural). While this response pattern may be attributable to chance, it seems more plausible to assume that the functional complexity of public agencies and the extensive overlay of administrative regulations and procedures in these types of organizations may simply require managers to devote more time to formal communication processes. If nothing else, this finding suggests that what is often passed off as "paperwork" is very much a part of the managerial function, especially in public agencies.

Table 3–5 indicates that managers in public agencies spent more

TABLE 3-4. Mean Hours Spent Information Processing by Type of Agency		TABLE 3-5. Mean Hours Spent Coordinating by Type of Agency	
Type of Agency	Mean Hours	Type of Agency	Mean Hours
Public-state-urban	6.9	Public-state-urban	3.4
Public-state-rural	9.0	Public-state-rural	6.0
Public-local-urban	6.1	Public-local-urban	4.8
Quasi-public	6.3	Quasi-public	4.6
Voluntary-urban	4.2	Voluntary-urban	2.4
Voluntary-rural	4.1	Voluntary-rural	1.5
Overall Mean	6.2	Overall Mean	3.8

time coordinating the work of others than did those in voluntary settings. Coordination involved activities devoted to maintaining working relationships between departments and agencies, establishing procedures to ensure work flow and cooperation, and resolving impediments to interunit cooperation. It seems plausible to attribute these differences between managers of public and private agencies to disparities in organizational size (the major exception here would be quasi-public organizations). That is, to the extent that public agencies are structurally and functionally more differentiated, managerial personnel would of necessity have to spend more time establishing linkages, maintaining interunit cooperation, and the like. In addition, public organizations in the sample were generally larger, which means, among other things, that managers in these settings had, on the average, more subordinates. This in itself would explain much of the difference observed, since the greater the number of subordinates, the more attention must normally be devoted to orchestrating tasks.

The data in Table 3-6 indicate that managers in quasi-public and voluntary agencies spent substantially more time in activities aimed at representing their organization than did those in public settings. Respondents in voluntary-urban agencies, for example, devoted an average of three times as many hours to representing than did their counterparts in public-state-urban organizations. However, these findings may be slightly misleading. To the extent that the representing function tends to be lodged primarily in upper-level administrative jobs, the larger number of lower-echelon managers interviewed in public agencies may have had the effect of reducing the overall mean computed for these organizations in this activity category. An alternate explanation might be that voluntary agencies, because of their heavy reliance on multiple funding sources and voluntary input, must give somewhat more emphasis to this function than those organizations supported solely through public sources. Subsequent analysis of these data will be necessary to clarify this information.

The final noteworthy variation in management activities observed for respondents in different types of agencies was found in the area of direct practice. Table 3–7 shows that managers in quasi-public agencies and voluntary agencies spent substantially more time in direct service activities than did those in public organizations. This finding may be attributable to several interdependent factors, among them the fact that voluntary and quasi-public agencies are usually somewhat smaller organizations with more shallow administrative hierarchies. To the extent that this is the case, organizational functions are less likely to be sharply differentiated among hierarchical lines. Under these circumstances, managers are more likely to assume some responsibility for providing direct service. Secondly, observation and experience would suggest that managers in private agencies, especially those at lower and middle levels, keep a hand in practice in order to maintain credibility with subordinates. This is to say that managerial legitimacy in voluntary and quasi-public agencies may in large part be dependent on some evidence of clinical competence. These factors may be operative in some public social service agencies as well, but on the whole, one suspects that private agencies have a more uniformly developed organizational norm that defines clinical expertise as a necessary, if not sufficient basis for managerial competence.

Management levels. Administrative level was the second major variable that we anticipated might influence the nature of management practice. In order to relate the activity data to management level, we assigned

TABLE 3–6. Mean Hours Spent Representing by Type of Agency	
Type of Agency	Mean Hours
Public-state-urban	.9
Public-state-rural	1.2
Public-local-urban	1.5
Quasi-public	2.8
Voluntary-urban	3.3
Voluntary-rural	2.4
Overall Mean	2.4

TABLE 3–7. Mean Hours Spent in Direct Practice by Type of Agency	
Type of Agency	Mean Hours
Public-state-urban	2.1
Public-state-rural	2.8
Public-local-urban	1.3
Quasi-public	4.2
Voluntary-urban	5.8
Voluntary-rural	19.1
Overall Mean	4.1

each of the respondents to one of five job categories that were based principally on the criteria of distance from service delivery. Job descriptions rather than job titles were used as the basis for making these assignments. The five categories were: first-line supervisor, second-line supervisor, department or project head, administrative support staff, and executive or assistant executive director.

As might be expected, the amount of time managers devoted to various activities differed significantly by administrative level. These differences were most obvious in the categories of supervising, direct practice, planning, budgeting, negotiating, and representing.

In general, as Table 3–8 reveals, the more highly placed the manager was in the agency hierarchy, the less time was given to supervisory activities. First-level supervisors devoted an average of almost ten hours a week to these activities, while those in executive positions spent almost one-half this amount of time. Despite these differences, it is important to bear in mind that respondents at all levels engaged in supervision-related activities for a significant portion of each week. At this point it is not possible to determine whether the style and content of supervisory practice varied systematically among levels, but our initial impression is that first- and second-line supervisors were primarily educationally and developmentally oriented in their work with subordinates, while those at higher levels were more likely to be concerned with directing, monitoring, assigning, and the like. Systematic differences in style and content, if any, will have to be confirmed in subsequent analysis.

Data in Table 3–9 suggest a somewhat misleading picture regarding the involvement of managers in direct practice. On the surface it would appear that department heads spent four or five times as many hours in this kind of activity than those in both lower and higher levels. This finding can be explained by the fact that the sample contained a

TABLE 3–8. Mean Hours Spent Supervising by Management Level	
Management Level	Mean Hours
First-line supervisor	9.8
Second-line supervisor	7.2
Department head	6.5
Administrative support staff	6.4
Director or assistant director	5.5
Overall Mean	6.7

TABLE 3–9. Mean Hours Spent in Direct Practice by Management Level	
Management Level	Mean Hours
First-line supervisor	3.6
Second-line supervisor	2.7
Department head	11.2
Administrative support staff	3.2
Director or assistant director	2.0
Overall Mean	4.1

number of persons with departmental level responsibilities (e.g., director of clinical services), who were nevertheless significantly engaged in direct service. A more accurate picture emerges when managers are categorized in terms of the number of subordinates for whom they have responsibility. Table 3–10 indicates that the larger the number of subordinates, the less time was spent in direct practice. Thus it would appear that there were a significant number of respondents, probably in voluntary agencies, who presided over small organizational units. Such persons most likely performed traditional managerial duties but were also heavily involved in working directly with clients.

Table 3–11 reveals some interesting variations in the amount of time spent on planning. Executive level managers and administrative support staff, respectively, devoted 4.8 and 5.4 hours a week to this function. By contrast, first-line supervisors spent an average of only 1.8 hours in the same kind of activity. This finding is not surprising inasmuch as one of the things that is commonly thought to distinguish upper-level from lower-level managers is the emphasis given to analytic and conceptual work. These data seem to confirm this conventional notion.

Although budgeting was a distinct category of activity, it is certainly akin to planning and can even be considered a principal component of the planning process. Thus, it is interesting to note in Table 3–12 that the amount of time given to this kind of activity also increased significantly among managers at higher administrative levels. The major exception was the virtual absence of budgeting activity among those at the administrative support level, which may be explained by the fact that respondents in these jobs had little or no line responsibility for operating programs. Managers in executive level positions, however, devoted an average of more than two hours a week to this budgeting function, as

TABLE 3–10. Mean Hours Spent in Direct Practice by Number of Subordinates

Number of Subordinates	Mean Hours
1–3	9.1
4–19	5.3
20–30	4.7
31–69	2.4
70 or more	.8

TABLE 3–11. Mean Hours Spent on Planning by Management Level

Management Level	Mean Hours
First-line supervisor	1.8
Second-line supervisor	3.1
Department head	3.4
Administrative support staff	5.4
Director or assistant director	4.8
Overall Mean	3.9

TABLE 3–12. Mean Hours Spent on Budgeting by Management Level

Management Level	Mean Hours
First-line supervisor	—
Second-line supervisor	—
Department head	.5
Administrative support staff	.1
Director or assistant director	2.1
Overall Mean	1.0

opposed to the one-half hour or less a week that was spent by those at departmental and supervisory levels. The amount of time given to budgeting probably varies more over the course of the year than other activities, and the discrepancies between top-level managers and others may be even more marked during periods of budget preparation.

Finally, as one might expect, the time spent on activities related to negotiating and representing was greatest among those in the highest administrative level. Tables 3–13 and 3–14 contain these data. This information seems to indicate a bimodal distribution, where respondents at subexecutive levels give little time to these functions, while top managers spend proportionately more. Negotiating in particular appears to be a function that is almost the exclusive domain of executives.

TABLE 3–13. Mean Hours Spent Negotiating by Management Level

Management Level	Mean Hours
First-line supervisor	.2
Second-line supervisor	.4
Department head	.3
Administrative support staff	.4
Director or assistant director	1.4
Overall Mean	.8

TABLE 3–14. Mean Hours Spent Representing by Management Level

Management Level	Mean Hours
First-line supervisor	1.1
Second-line supervisor	1.2
Department head	1.3
Administrative support staff	.9
Director or assistant director	2.5
Overall Mean	1.8

DISCUSSION: IMPLICATIONS FOR MANAGEMENT EDUCATION

If there is a central curriculum idea that emerges from the findings of the survey, it is that education for management must provide a broad base of knowledge and skill for virtually every aspect of social welfare administration. Our data indicate strongly that in a real sense the social welfare manager is a generalist whose job is likely to involve a broad set of responsibilities, requiring both analytic and interactional skills. A configuration of management functions and the emphasis given to them vary somewhat by administrative level and type of agency, but virtually every manager in our sample was expected to perform a wide and varied array of tasks.

A curriculum that seeks to provide students with the skills needed to carry out effectively such a wide array of functions must somehow contend with the dilemma that is inherent in any attempt to train for generalist practice. Put simply, this dilemma involves how to introduce the prospective manager to all the areas of knowledge and skills he/she might conceivably need to draw upon, while at the same time avoiding the dilution and superficiality that would seem to be the inevitable consequence of trying to touch all the bases.

It appears clear that formal degree training programs in management (e.g., master's in social work, master's in business administration, master's in public administration, or some combination thereof) will not be able to provide the in-depth knowledge and skill a student might require to perform the varied functions entailed in any particular job, let alone those that he/she might be called upon to carry out in successive managerial positions during a career. A formal degree program can reasonably be expected to provide the student with a theoretical and conceptual understanding of management processes and entry level skills in certain fundamental areas of administrative practice. Beyond this, it seems essential that continuing education and in-service training programs be available at strategic career transition points to help the manager deepen and extend the basic skills acquired and fine tune them to the demands of a particular job. Thus this survey suggests the need for a fundamental division of labor between degree-related and continuing education programs. The former should focus primarily on the development of basic knowledge and skills that can be adapted to a variety of agency settings and administrative levels. Continuing education, however, would be more usefully directed to in-depth training related to specific skills that are necessary to carry out effectively the responsibilities associated with a particular job. The major exception to this pattern might be those instances in which persons without prior management education are moving into administrative jobs. In this instance the continuing education program might resemble quite closely the master's level curriculum.

In addition to this general guideline for developing management curricula, the findings of this survey also indicate that certain substantive areas should be incorporated in educational programs. While the survey data did not deal with leadership and authority as activity entities per se, the interviews with respondents made it clear that these were, in a sense, the cornerstones of management and a necessary precondition for carrying out those functions that were critical to effective performance, such as supervising and controlling. Managers in this study spent a majority of their time and energy in relations with subordinates where obtaining compliance and cooperation was, at least implicitly, their principal concern. Despite this, many managers with whom we discussed this issue felt that leadership and authority in management practice had been deemphasized in social work education because of the tendency to associate them with bureaucratic dysfunctions such as employee distrust and timidity. Since, with few exceptions, social welfare agencies are formal organizations with well-defined hierarchies, it was felt that the use of authority should be a central theme in the education of mid-level managers.

Supervision was the single most time-consuming and the second most significant activity performed by managers in the survey. Although competencies in using and understanding authority and leadership are an essential foundation for supervision, these data suggest that the development of supervisory skills be given special emphasis in management education. This is particularly important for students who will work in smaller, less differentiated agencies where the middle manager is often responsible for working directly with clinical staff in a relationship that has an educational and professional development dimension as well as a narrowly administrative one.

Skills in communicating also appeared to be an essential competency for social welfare managers. With few exceptions, respondents in our survey spent a large share of their time interacting with others, either verbally or in writing. Virtually every function they performed depended critically upon their ability to receive and disseminate information and ideas in meetings, memos, letters, and on the telephone. The activity category—information processing—accounted for a large portion of the time spent by managers. Perhaps more importantly, communication skills were conceived of as the primary tools used in carrying out such core functions as supervising and coordinating. Representing and negotiating, likewise, depended heavily upon the ability to communicate effectively.

The survey also suggests the importance of competencies in planning and in work organization, delegation, and assessment. The data indicate that managers spend a good deal of their time in planning and organizing the work of their units and departments, delegating and clarifying tasks and responsibilities, and monitoring the quality and quantity of the work performed. Managers are also commonly responsible for translating policy and program goals into operational objectives and concrete work plans and for accounting to superiors when the work is complete.

While the managers in our survey sample spent relatively little time in budget preparation per se, it was generally felt that their own program planning functions depended heavily on an understanding of the budget development and fiscal management processes that served as the context for their efforts.

Finally, the survey findings indicate that competencies in the area of management information systems and program evaluation are essential primarily because of the increasing importance that is being attached to accountability in social welfare agencies. Upper-level managers with whom we had contact attached heavy emphasis to these areas and expressed virtually unanimous agreement that the measurement and quantification of social agency activities and outputs would assume even greater importance in the future. Survey data indicate that middle managers currently give relatively little attention to formal program evaluation, but the amount of time spent on collecting and reviewing information on staff activities was considerable. With few exceptions, both program evaluation and information monitoring were considered areas in need of considerable strengthening.

NOTES

1. Rosemary Sarri, "Effective Social Work Intervention in Administrative and Planning Roles: Implications for Education," *Facing the Challenge* (New York: Council on Social Work Education, 1973); Monica Shapira, "Reflections on the Preparation of Social Workers for Executive Positions," *Journal of Education for Social Work* 7 (1971):55–60.
2. Kenneth Kazmerski and David Macarov, *Administration in Social Work Curriculum* (New York: Council on Social Work Education, 1976).
3. See also Linda Kaiser and Gerald Frey, *Education for Management* (Portland: Portland State University, 1975); Jean M. Kruzich, *Working Paper #4: Analysis of Social Welfare Administration Questionnaire*, Social Welfare Administration Welfare Project (Minneapolis: University of Minnesota, 1976).
4. J. J. Corson and R. S. Paul, *Men Near the Top* (Baltimore: Johns Hopkins Press, 1966).
5. This paper reports data pertaining to the identifying data, activity calendar, and significant activities. Information concerning job history and factors in-

fluencing job performance and career mobility is contained in the report *Educating for Management in Social Welfare* (Seattle: University of Washington, 1976).

6. The thirteen categories included: planning, information processing, controlling, coordinating, evaluating, negotiating, representing, staffing, supplying, supervising, extracurricular, direct service, and budgeting. This scheme was adapted from Corson and Paul, *Men near the Top,* and modified to reflect activities that are unique to social service managers.

4

Who Should Manage a Social Agency?

MORTON I. TEICHER

Who should manage a social agency? This is a question with deep roots and a long lineage. My first exposure to the question came almost four decades ago, when, as a first year social work student assigned to a public welfare agency for field instruction, I learned about the sudden replacement of the distinguished social work leader who was administering the agency by a businessman who was hailed as a person who would bring order and efficiency to the agency. The staff promptly divided into two camps—those who insisted that only a social worker could administer the agency and those who welcomed the "businesslike" approach to management. In all the years since that incident, the descendants of these two camps have continued to vie with each other in answering the question of who should manage the social agency. One camp stubbornly insists that only a professional social worker can manage a social agency. People in this camp have made a slight obeisance to their foes by acknowledging that the social worker should acquire some knowledge of administration in order to function effectively in that role. The other camp—with equal stubbornness and with growing success—insists that administration is a discipline in its own right and that professional managers are required for social agency administration.

My continuing interest in this old battle was recently rekindled by my becoming aware of a similar controversy raging in the museum world. The issue is the same as that in the field of social agencies. Who should manage an art museum? Should it be a professional art historian or should it be a business administrator? The choice of one or the other makes a significant statement. The necessity of making such a choice divides the museum world into two camps, similar to those in the field of social agencies.

A brief examination of the situation in the museum world may be instructive for social agencies.

Those who argue for art historians as art museum administrators hold that the administrator can only make informed decisions about acquisitions, conservation, exhibitions, and publications if the administrator knows art history. By virtue of studying art history, the art historian has demonstrated an intensified appreciation for the art objects in the care of the museum. The art historian has a base in knowledge for furthering the museum's mission of communicating the art of the past and the present. This background is essential if the museum is to serve its primary purpose of educating and providing enjoyment in the visual arts.

Although art museums have become complicated organizations, the traditional requirements for the director remain unchanged. The director must have a thorough knowledge of art history, the director must have keen judgment for spotting and buying great works, and the director must have the tastefulness which is essential for proper display of the museum's possessions.

While the director must be sensitive to issues of museum economics, it is essential that leadership be given in organizing and offering exhibits which serve a useful artistic and educational purpose. The museum is a guardian of art and the director who is an art historian can best help the museum to fulfill this role. The scholar-administrator safeguards the museum's concern for quality.

Since art museums tend to be small organizations, the relationship between the director and the staff is different from such relationships in a large bureaucracy where problems are segmented and authority is delegated. The art historian as director can avoid having to rely heavily on highly specialized experts with narrowly restricted expertise. Background in art history provides the base for the overall view which is necessary for the success of the museum.

Good relationships between the administrator and the staff of the museum are facilitated if the administrator is an art historian. Such an administrator can work with the curators as a co-professional and speak their language. The art historian administrator can provide proper guidance and supervision and can avoid the development of a sense of alienation among the curatorial staff.

An art historian as museum administrator guarantees the primacy and permanence of aesthetic values in the art museum. Only such a person can possess a clear sense of aesthetic standards as the basis for sound artistic judgment. Only such a person can fully understand the purposes of the art museum and maintain its preoccupation with artistic merit. If the museum is to be an arbiter of taste and if it is to influence taste, then it needs an art historian.

The art historian as administrator can shape museum priorities, taking into account what is defensible in scholarly and educational terms. The art historian administrator can help the museum to thrive by making decisions about exhibitions which are in harmony with the basic purposes and long-range goals of the museum rather than on the basis of projected attendance figures.

New acquisitions require careful decisions to allocate the scarce resources which museums have for purchases. Winnowing out what the museum should buy from the thousands of works which are for sale requires the deep knowledge of the art historian. The art historian can separate quality from mediocrity and can discern in the work of the unknown artist the potential for future recognition.

Many museums have to deal with the problem of sifting through works of art which are in their possession but not on display. The art historian director can give leadership to this process, calling on knowledge of art history to rate the works of art, check them for authenticity, correct errors in misnaming and misdating, and determine their physical condition.

All museum planning and all museum decisions are, in the final analysis, artistic decisions. They are ultimately decisions about quality and must be in the service of quality programs.

The development of taste and a sense of quality is painstakingly acquired through study of art history which fosters sensitivity to aesthetic questions. The art historian will not sacrifice knowledge of unchanging standards to the shifting vagaries of popular taste.

The museum director who is an art historian usually achieves the position many years after completing graduate education and usually after a substantial period in curatorial or educational work. By virtue of education and experience, the art historian is ready to give leadership as a scholar and a connoisseur, bringing to the job the kind of professional integrity which is required if the museum is to flourish and fulfill its fundamental purposes.

The rapidly changing nature of the museum world emphasizes the need for creative and innovative adaptations to what has become an open system as contrasted to the stable state of an earlier day. Such adaptations require leadership which is firmly rooted in knowledge of art history. This base for the museum is essential as it confronts an uncertain and turbulent scene.

Administrative leadership of a museum involves a wide range of activities which require a thorough knowledge of art history. Planning, organizing, controlling, and decision making represent the breadth, variety, and interdependence of the museum director's activities. Overall knowledge of the museum's central functions enables the director to engage in these activities productively and effectively.

By contrast, those members of the camp who argue for a business administrator or a professional administrator as museum director believe that the modern museum has become a complicated organization which requires managerial expertise to function successfully. The specific knowledge about art which is needed for decisions can be obtained by the professional administrator from the staff. The professional administrator knows how to exercise leadership so as to make optimal use of talents in the staff to produce a vibrant organization. Appropriate delegation of authority is the basis for a well-managed, smoothly run organization.

Museums require businesslike efficiency. The administrator has to be sensitive to practical matters—to budgets, to board relationships, to fund-raising, to obtaining gifts from important collectors. Since board members and important collectors tend to be wealthy businessmen, a professional business administrator as museum director is more effective. Such an individual can talk the language of the businessman and can understand more readily the psychology of the businessman.

When all social institutions are suffering from financial problems, the museum is no exception. It needs tough-minded decisions about priorities. It needs a director whose head will not be easily turned by an expensive masterpiece or a costly exhibition proposal. Reckless expansion and sloppy management can and indeed has forced some museums to liquidate some of their proud possessions in order to keep the doors open.

A museum should serve the people and, therefore, it is important to attract large attendance. The administrator who is attuned to fiscal matters, to attendance figures, and to membership rosters can best steer the museum into offering exhibitions which are popular, which draw large crowds, and which generate good will and favorable publicity for the museum.

The museum director needs to be familiar with management techniques and management tools. What is required is knowledge about how business decisions are made and about the language and thought processes of the business world. If the administrator is comfortable with budgets and with fiscal projections, then there can be an ease of relationships with the trustees who are concerned with the museum's solvency.

The professional manager can define, categorize, and quantify the work of the museum so as to make it an effective and efficient organization. The professional manager can bring to bear on the museum programs for formalized long-range planning, utilizing sophisticated management information systems which maintain a flow of facts about the operation of the museum in all its aspects. Proper planning, especially in the financial area, will eliminate sublime faith in the unheralded appearance of a wealthy donor who will make up the deficit.

The increasingly complex nature of the museum demands professional management with technical expertise in financial and personnel matters. This expertise is best acquired through study of business administration and through business experience. With such expertise in organizational matters, the professional administrator can plan ahead, formulate goals, make sound decisions, summon the energies of the staff, and generally serve as a successful executive.

The professional administrator has a special capacity for logical organization with clear-cut job descriptions and specific definitions of function. Communication through channels is best sustained through an organization where there are thoroughly understood lines of reporting responsibility and specified delegations of authority. Improvisation, unpredictability, and free-wheeling are avoided when the staff is well-organized and where the pattern of organization can be readily charted. A coherent organization avoids internal ambiguity and inconsistency. It facilitates the development of explicit criteria for performance assessment and measures of accountability.

The professional administrator is concerned with using logic to narrow the scope for decision-making. Problems to be resolved need to be sharply focussed so as to permit maximum concentration and minimum distraction.

What lessons can be learned from this dispute in the museum world which throw light on the question of who should administer the social agency? The arguments advanced by both camps are familiar in the field of the social agency.

The central purpose of the social agency is to provide high quality services to its clientele. All of its activities should contribute to that purpose. Administration is one such activity. It is not an end in itself. Rather, it is an activity the success of which is measured by the degree to which the organization fulfills its purpose. To achieve such success requires a breadth of view, rooted in social work knowledge and values.

The true test of administrative success is not the ability to design and respect organization charts. It is the ability to bring to bear on decision making the knowledge and the information which are essential for wise judgments. Such knowledge and information are painstakingly acquired by education, by experience, and by deep immersion in the work of the social agency.

The notion that the administrator needs sophisticated management information systems implies that running a modern organization requires more data. In fact, what is required is better judgment—judgment based on professional knowledge about the agency's central program activities. Focus on data acquisition and information systems can lead to preoccupation with the minutiae of daily chores and blur the concern for true leadership. A managerial approach which stresses quantitative considerations can override qualitative considerations. Replacing the social work administrator with a professional administrator may represent a corrosion of the concern for quality.

Advocating tough-minded business executives for social agency administration often masks a fundamental hostility to the social programs of the agency. One way of slashing the social program is by utilizing a business administrator rather than a social work administrator. When those with accounting mentalities sit in the driver's seats, they can scoff at the "soft-minded, tender-hearted" social worker who may have difficulty in expressing the value of the social agency in cost-effective numbers. Insistence on gauging effectiveness suggests that one can calibrate the contribution of the social agency to human well-being. This is often an incommensurable activity, no more subject to a numerical count than is the contribution of the artist or the theologian.

The social agency administrator is confronted by innumerable blocks, by countless limits, and by negative attitudes. The ability to perform well and wisely, to steer the social agency constructively for humane purposes, is best acquired by professional social work education and experience, combined with powerful identification with social work values and ethics. The ability to pull it all together is to be sought in the professional social worker rather than in the professional administrator.

PART II

Some Theoretical Perspectives on Social Administration

Editor's Introduction

The literature on social administration is noticeably devoid of material of theoretical interest. A growing list of empirical studies parallels writing devoted to elaborations of practice wisdom. The best that one can find are certain perspectives that help identify the material to be studied and organized.

There are several theoretical streams in the general literature on administration that are potentially useful for the social services. Viewing the social agency as an open system directs attention to the external organizational environment and the host of interorganizational relationships with which it must inevitably interact. In this day of extensive governmental support and regulation, the social agency is increasingly dependent on other organizations for its stability and growth. Few can be self-generating and self-directing.

Furthermore, service-giving organizations are imbedded in a network of constituencies that help define their objectives, policies, and ongoing operations. Each of their universal elements—providers, consumers, and the organization that brings them together—has its essential internal and external constituencies. Practitioners look to unions, staff organizations, and professional societies to help secure their standards and interests. Clients frequently establish parent associations, alumni groups (i.e., ex-offenders), client organizations (i.e., The Welfare Rights Organization). Organizations and their trustees are closely tied to coordinating bodies, funding sources, and, often, accrediting agencies.

Each of the networks in turn, and in common, directs attention to broad, general constituencies that affect public acceptance and legitimacy—the media, legislative bodies, administrative areas of government, and the like. Public relations and social action inevitably become important aspects of administrative action, both individually and collectively. Agencies in special fields band together for the purpose not only of setting standards and advancing levels of adequacy in delivering services, but also to enhance the public awareness of social need and to assure governmental assumption of responsibility where this seems indicated. Thus, open system perspectives help define the broader parameters of administrative behavior, and add important insight to the traditional concern for internal dynamics and management.

Another influential stream of thought comes quite naturally to social administration—human relations theory and reseach. Much that developed since the early Hawthorne research on the effect of social and cultural variables on work organizations parallels similar work on the social and psychological foundations of social work practice. The nature of social system attributes and their effect on social administration provide important clues for administrative practitioners. The significance of value systems, social norms, power constellations, sentiments, reward patterns, goals, and tension management are generally recognized by astute managers as they deal with problems of organizational stability, conflict, and change. Much work remains to be done before the literature of social administration will reflect more of the practice wisdom that grows out of day-to-day experience with organizational encounters.

A recent emphasis in management thought, contingency theory, has hardly begun to influence social administration thinking, yet can potentially provide useful perspectives. Less a theory than a point of view, contingency suggests that few general propositions in administration hold under all circumstances, that it is necessary to specify the unique conditions under which one or another principle is likely to obtain. Such an approach directs attention to the importance of organizational diagnosis, of identifying variables in the organization that condition its ability to achieve its objectives, of highlighting the factors (contingencies) affecting decision making and courses of action that meet the requirements of the organization and the needs and interests of its several constituencies (Morse & Lorsh, 1970).

These perspectives are drawn from the general management literature. It is appropriate to suggest some specific orientations which come from the vantage point of the administration of the social services. One such derives from a view of the often competing interests of the essential elements that contitute the social agency. While client, practitioner, and organization come together to achieve common goals, in practice their requirements and preferences often diverge. Because of their differing interests, internal contradictions abound. Client demands for service availability often conflict with staff convenience. Agency pressures for containing cost run into staff demands for salary increments. Client requirements for comprehensive service compete with agency focus on specialized offerings. Professional dominance, client urgings, and bureaucratic procedures frequently engage with one another in a struggle for control of the service encounter (Freidson, 1970). An essential task of the administrator is to bring these divergent needs, interests, and pressures into some form of balance, moving from one steady state to another in the process of program development.

Where the administrator stands in relation to this force field is crucial with respect to charting administrative strategy. Because of the necessarily interdependent relationships of the several constituencies in the organization, a prime focus on one element directs energy to engender compliance on the part of the others. When agency needs are seen as primary, client and practitioner must conform, often to the ascendancy of organizational maintenance requirements and to the detriment of service adequacy. Such is frequently the circumstance in large bureaucracies. Where practitioner needs are seen as primary, service requirements are often ignored. Thus, medical personnel in hospitals eschew research and treatment of common and widespread illness in favor of "exotic" conditions, such as open-heart surgery.

Finally, when the administrator assumes a client perspective, and client need and service integrity become the primary orientation for administrative action, agency and staff are moved to compliance in furtherance of those objectives. Client service requirements become the constant, and organization and practitioner are encouraged to adapt.

There are two important consequences of such a view. Primacy of orientation to the client and to the integrity of client service leads naturally to a posture of administrative advocacy. While it is true that administrators are formally accountable to their employer—the legal entity that represents the organization—they implicitly assume accountability to the client for the quality of the service. Internal and external constraints on that quality become fundamental targets of administrative action. This may well have the consequence of bringing the administrator into conflict with agency trustees, supporting organizations, and funding sources, as well as members of the staff. The true ethic of professional behavior, however, lies in concern for the clients and their needs. Professional skill is concerned precisely with the ways in which the administrator balances and orchestrates the interests of divergent constituencies, but from a client perspective as an organizing principle.

Finally, the issue of compliance referred to above moves administrators to an interest in organizational change, taking their clue from the shifting environment of social practice and the response of current and prospective clients to the social and psychological pressures that attend such social changes. Organizations rarely remain static, but move from one equilibrium to another, absorbing and adapting to the requirements of both internal and external pressures and circumstances. These processes are akin to Piaget's concepts of assimilation and accommodation (Piaget, 1968), the give and take between the organism and its environment. The process of equilibration, which balances the intrusions of the social and physical environment with the organism's need to conserve its structural systems, describes quite precisely the administrative function. When internal dislocation or external turbulence seem to disturb the existing state of affairs, administrative leadership serves the equilibrating requisites. The ethical guide to this function derives from administrative identification with client service requirements.

The selections in this section deal with a variety of theoretical perspectives for social agency administration. Slavin analyzes the structural life space of the social administrator, identifying in turn the relevant constituencies that perforce engage attention and application of executive skill. Although primary internal relationships between administrator and staff have tended to preoccupy theroretical discussions, the impact of externalities is ever present and often overwhelming. These internal and external networks provide the essential material with which administrators are daily involved. The diversity and contradictory character of the interests that motivate organizational constituencies project an important part of the agenda for executive action. Concepts of administrative advocacy, client accountability, and humanistic ethics flow from this analysis.

Martin presents and analyzes a model of human service organizations that stresses the pressures and influences placed upon social agency administrators by organizations in the external environment. An open systems view reveals the multiple constituencies that affect and direct the professional behavior of administrators and other personnel. Competing interests in obtaining resources and in attracting clients suggest a force field of conflict and accommodation. The prevailing value system of efficiency, productivity, and growth constrains service-providing agencies to stress "business goals" as opposed to service quality or effectiveness. The dilemma this poses to the administrator suggests the need for special training, for feasible models of service delivery, and for a clear focus of the goals of client service.

Mullis reviews several schools of managerial thought and related organizational theory. He elaborates the contingency concepts as they bear on a systems model of organizational behavior. In applying these concepts to public welfare, he analyzes the centralization-decentralization continuum and identifies some of the variables that determine the relative mix of the two strategies.

Glisson elaborates a theoretical model of service organizations that provides a framework for defining and classifying the knowledge and skills necessary for competent management of a service delivery system. The model is based on a contingency view of organization and management that endeavors to incorporate insights from rational-mechanistic, systemic-organic, and human relations theories. In this view, administrative behavior is contingent upon the characteristics of specific organizations and the environment in which they exist. The need is for a "good fit" between the environmental system and the subsystems that comprise the organization. Glisson goes on to detail the attributes of these constructs: goals and values; technology; organizational structure; and the psychosocial aspects of power, human relationships, worker motivation, and job satisfaction. He sees this concatenation of concepts as providing a comprehensive view of the service organization and the requirements for its competent management. Their use as a framework for structuring administrative practice, for knowledge, and for administrative training are suggested.

REFERENCES

Freidson, Eliot. *Professional dominance: The social structure of medical care.* New York: Atherton Press, 1970.

Morse, John J., and Lorsch, Jay W. Beyond theory Y. *Harvard Business Review*, May-June, 1970, 37–44.

Piaget, Jean. *Six psychological studies.* New York: Vintage Books, 1968, 100–114.

5

A Framework for Selecting Content for Teaching About Social Administration

SIMON SLAVIN

In the long line of development of social work, the latter part of the 1970s will be seen as a period that witnessed the coming of age of the conceptual and theoretical underpinnings for the administration of the social services. The growth of programs in schools of social work to train administrators, the recent reports of several studies looking at curriculum issues in administrative teaching, the early development of joint degrees between graduate programs in social work and schools of business administration and public administration, and the appearance of a new journal devoted to the management of the social services all attest to a new interest in an old subject. After all, administration may be the oldest of the practices in social work—the first social agency surely had to be administered.

A paramount interest at the moment is directed to appropriate content for the training of social administrators. What follows is one attempt to develop a framework for selecting such content. The focus here is on the social agency that organizes the delivery of services. This it does in the light of explicit or implicit social policy imperatives. The unit of attention is the administration of specific organizational delivery systems that provide social services to a delineated clientele. (For a comprehensive treatment of these services, see Kammerman & Kahn, 1976.) This is differentiated from other patterns of administration that monitor, de-

---

This paper was presented at the Western Conference on Social Welfare Administration, San Francisco, California, April 28, 1977.

velop, evaluate, and initiate policy prescriptions that bear on actual service delivery. This latter is characteristic of national, state and regional departments of welfare as well as large national welfare agencies and will be discussed in due course.

It is perhaps most convenient to begin with the simplest depiction of a model of the social agency. Essentially it consists of three universal elements and their attributes and relationships: clientele (consumers, users), providers (practitioners), and the organization that brings them together. The administrator has a special relationship to each of these constituent elements, as depicted in Figure 5–1.

These elements constitute the primary constituencies of the administrator whose relationships to client, agency, and practitioner suggest the first approximation of the relevant areas on content that define and enhance administrative skill and understanding. With respect to clients, knowledge concerning populations at risk, client eligibility for service, levels of benefits, focus of service, boundary delineations, and the like constitutes one cornerstone of essential administrative equipment.

The relationship of administrator and staff calls on knowledge and skill in the many aspects of personnel administration. Relevant here are such items as allocating professional roles, providing supervision, developing and training staff, organizing work patterns, establishing professional tasks, providing professional leadership, and managing the personnel process from recruitment and selection of staff through induction, retention, and separation.

Managing the organization's needs, interests, and maintenance requirements directs attention to the development, allocation, and control of physical and financial resources. Budgeting and fund raising are obvious corollary processes. Information and data gathering, processing, and retrieval serve financial planning and research objectives and activities. Central to the organization's existence is the authority structure that provides its sanction and legitimacy and to which the administrator is intimately tied both legally and contractually.

The delineation of these areas of knowledge and skill derives de-

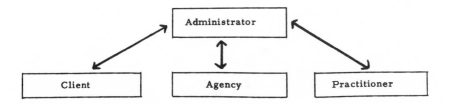

FIGURE 5–1. Model of the social agency, and the relationship of the administrator to each of the elements

ductively from an examination of the key elements of the social agency and their functional technical requirements. The discussion so far has looked at the relationship of the administrator to these organizational building blocks from a linear perspective. As such this constitutes a view of organizational and administrative statics. This line of reasoning has envisioned the organization as a limited and closed system and at its most obvious and simple structure. Clearly the reality of the organizational system is considerably more complicated. It is necessary, then, to look at the organizational elements in their interaction and at the meaning these interrelationships have for the administrator's role behavior. This can perhaps best be seen in the matrix shown in Figure 5–2. Each cell in the ninefold table represents a central relationship in the agency system. Figure 5–2 presents three paired or reciprocal relationships between the organizational elements, and three relationships internal to each element. To comment on the latter first, Cell 1 constitutes patterns of client interactions within the agency. There are at least two classes of such interactions:

1. Those in which clients prepare one another for ways of working the system to their advantage. Thus welfare neighbors orient prospective recipients about ways to approach welfare workers, how to make the case for benefit entitlements most telling, how to dress for interviews, how to deal with hidden resources, and the like. Tenants orient new tenants on how to approach rent control officials and how to extract benefits from landlords. Prospective adoptive parents learn from other clients how to make the best approach to establish acceptability to agency norms.
2. Those in which clients compete with one another, either individually, or in classes, for agency largess. Family service agencies provide settings where selected classes of clients, for example, the poor aged, compete for the organization's resources with fee-paying family clients or with other service demands, such as immigrants. Housing programs deal with competing demands of low-income clients and the economically advantaged.

	Client	Organization	Practitioner
Client	1	2	3
Organization	4	5	6
Practitioner	7	8	9

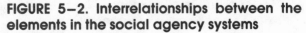

FIGURE 5–2. Interrelationships between the elements in the social agency systems

Cell 9 represents relationships within the practitioner group. This class of constituents is hardly homogeneous. Line workers' needs and interests are often substantially different from those of supervisors, department heads, or practitioners from different disciplines. Conflicts between group workers and recreationists in children's institutions, between social workers, counselors, and psychologists in multifunction agencies, between income maintenance workers and service-providing personnel in the public welfare agency often come to the surface. Much of the administrator's time and attention is devoted to managing these conflicts.

The organization as a legal entity (Cell 5), represented by the Board of Directors or Trustees, similarly tends to incorporate a variety of interests and propensities. Indeed, if a board is properly constituted, it is necessarily composed of members that are representative of different constituencies. The administrator is continually engaged in maintaining consensus on essential organizational objectives on the part of the policy-determining body, and in dealing with internal board differences as they emerge from competing or conflicting motivations for board membership, from differing reference groups interests, or from ideological differences.

The actual service transaction in the agency is reflected in Cells 3 and 7. Practitioners engage clients, and clients engage practitioners, each from distinctive orientations. From the professional's viewpoint, a repertoire of intervention modes and skills furthers the objective of providing a service. A readiness to participate, either voluntarily or under compulsion, on the part of the client makes the service experience possible. The process is reciprocal, and the administrator needs to possess an awareness not only of the professional skills involved but of the ethical and moral basis that lies behind the service delivery. To the extent to which a distinctive methodology and technology is required to provide the agency's service to its clientele, to that extent the administrator requires substantive professional know-how in order to fulfill the professional leadership role so necessary for organizational vitality.

Cells 6 and 8 describe the reciprocal relationship between staff and agency. The agency's policies, purposes, and orientation either attract or repel prospective staff members. Similarly, the physical arrangements, the reward system, the standards of work, the basis of evaluation, and the fringe benefit system all suggest the ways in which organizations are forthcoming in respect to the service providers they engage. Practitioners view the organization as the locus of livelihood and the legitimizer of their professional skill. They approach their self-interest in respect to rewards, working conditions, and security either singly or collectively. Organizational and professional interest frequently diverge, providing an agenda for administrative action that recurs with substantial regularity.

Finally, Cells 2 and 4 depict the ways in which clients view agencies and agencies view clients. There are several classes of issues here, involving such matters as:

- client participation in policy setting;
- availability, accessibility, and sufficiency of services;
- eligibility criteria and fee arrangements; and
- comprehensiveness and continuity of services.

Public welfare agencies are frequently preoccupied with limiting service and establishing eligibility barriers. Troublesome clients may be eschewed, and institutional provision may become oppressive. Social agencies need clients to survive, and clients need agency programs that are responsive to their needs. Keeping this symbiotic relationship in constructive interaction is a significant dimension of administrative competence.

To this point, the social agency system has been viewed as bounded. While dynamic elements of analysis have been introduced, the organizational environment has been ignored. The social agency inevitably exists in a sociopolitical field of related and competing organizations and influences. Resources must be garnered from outside the organization, and increasingly from the public agency. Clients are referred to other services and accepted from them.

The discussion so far has been concerned with the internal, primary constituencies of the administrator. But neither client, nor practitioner, nor Board of Directors exists in isolation. Each is embedded in a network of relationships external to the organization.

What appears at first sight as a simple structure of relationships is complicated by the fact that each of the primary elements involves a complex set of relationships in the form of a multiplicity of constituencies that have a greater or lesser interest in what happens in the process of providing services. From the point of view of the administrator, he is confronted by several tiers of constituencies depending upon their closeness to the actual service provision. It may be convenient to think of primary, secondary, and tertiary constituencies that are the focus of administrative concern. To illustrate, the primary and most intimate concerns of the administrator are the staff group whose roles he allocates and monitors, the clients who are the immediate objects of the service, and the Board of Directors, which represents the legal entity of the social agency. Much of the administrator's energy and time is devoted to managing their activities in the light of the organization's philosophy, objectives, and policies.

None of these relationships, however, develops in an institutional vacuum, for each of the primary constituencies has its own constituencies who are ready to intercede in the ongoing activities of the agency, sometimes implicitly, at other times openly and forcefully. The primary staff group reflects the norms and standards of the profession to which it belongs and to which it refers when questions of professional practice are raised. Similarly, trade union organizations representing the staff constituency actively participate in establishing conditions of work.

In like manner, clients frequently belong to consumer organizations, or parent associations, or tenant groups that reflect client interests and often become part of the process of establishing conditions affecting client service. In some instances, such associations become part of decision-making bodies, thus reflecting formal recognition of this essential interest in the organizations' activities and purposes.

The service-giving agency also has its direct relationship with other bodies in the institutional environment. Of primary interest here are service networks of which they are a part, such as sectarian and nonsectarian local service systems, and city-wide, state-wide or national networks. Funding sources, either voluntary or public, similarly represent immediate organizational relationships that affect the ability of social agencies to provide service. Each of these primary and secondary constituencies is part of the organizational life-space of the social administrator.

There is, finally, a third tier that is part of this organizational reality, one that affects each of the elements in common ways. Located here are the general public, whose sanction is the ultimate source of organizational legitimacy, the media in both press and television, legislative bodies, regulatory agencies, and the like. Each of these has its occasions for making its influence felt on the service-giving function, sometimes to the ultimate detriment of the service, sometimes to its flowering. This hierarchy of constituencies is pictured in Figure 5–3.

This delineation suggests the vast complexity of the administrative enterprise and points to the many forces in the institutional environment with which the administrator must perforce be concerned. (For a somewhat comparable depiction, see "successive environment organization boundaries: [a] organizational environment; [b] task environment; and [c] societal environment," Negandhi, 1975.) Ignoring any one of these elements and their constituencies can only be at the administrator's peril. At different times attention must be focused at specific points in the several networks of relationships. Anticipating when and where this will be is part of the administrative skill and art. Ultimately, the needs and/or interests of these multiple constituencies must be met.

In a nonmarket system of services, client satisfaction leads to organizational stability and continued utilization of the services. Staff satisfaction plays an important part in agency morale and low rates of turnover. Trustee identification with the organization flows from personal satisfaction in the work. With respect to the externalities, parents and con-

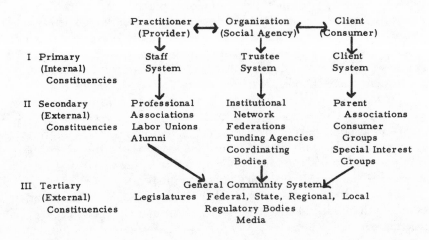

FIGURE 5–3. Organizational life-space of social administration: the constituencies of the social administrator

sumer groups tend to mobilize against shabby or incompetent dealing with clients; professional bodies monitor and often police adequate standards of care; sources of funds attempt to judge the ways in which their resources are expended and provide sanctions where they feel results do not justify continued support. Finally, in a service system network where public funds play an increasingly significant role in supporting service agencies, public policy development and legislative enactments increasingly affect most social services in direct and critical ways.

While the conventional wisdom concerning social agencies suggests the mutuality of interests of organizational participants in achieving organizational objectives, a closer examination of the realities of organizational life reveals a built-in set of contradictions and potential antagonisms. The conflict between professional and bureaucratic orientations has been frequently noted in the literature (Billingsley, 1964; Freidson, 1970, pp. 138–139; Hanlan, 1972, p. 4; Merton, 1957; Rapaport, 1960; Reiff, 1971; Toren, 1969, p. 157). But this is only one aspect of organizational conflict. Others reflect some of the distinctive needs and interests of each of the major organizational elements. Clients come to social agencies out of their need for service; professionals seek income and security, job satisfaction and career development, among other motivations; organizations pursue stability and growth, prestige and status. These needs and the interests they engender are not necessarily syntonic (Epstein, 1973; Schein, 1972, p. 18).

Illustrations of these differences and contradictions abound in actual practice. Practitioner-client divergence of interest is frequently the result of the "abrasive effects of sociocultural differences" (Bolman, 1972). Clients often want and need extended hours for service; practitioners prefer to be available during conventional working hours. The very definition of the client's problem poses a built-in difficulty. Thus, sociologist William Goode (1969) states that "it is the practitioner who decides upon the client's needs, and the occupation will be classified as less professional if the client imposes his own judgment" (p. 278; see also Freidson, 1970, p. 169). Yet, the client's perception of need is an important dynamic in the service transaction.

Practitioners often find themselves at odds with their employing agencies. This is particularly true in public welfare departments where, according to Scott (1969, p. 85), "many of the lay-determined laws and policies . . . constitute a source of strain and tension for the professionals who man the agencies." Organizations tend to eschew programs that are perceived as controversial and unpopular, even though clients and staff might feel they are important. School busing issues and inhospitality to speakers and consultants who express socially deviant viewpoints, for example, tend to be avoided because they might alienate important providers of resources, or affect legislators negatively. Challenges to conventional authority tend to precipitate conflict and hostility between trustees, professionals, and clients (Helfgot, 1974).

Conflicts internal to each of the elements also have their sources. Professional staffs frequently find differences between clinicians and researchers when the latter must deny services to clients in order to prepare tidy experimental conditions. Clinicians of differing theoretical orientations often find themselves in conflict over the preferred behaviors directed to meeting client need. Class and social status differences among trustees often lead to tension surrounding the development of organizational policies. This has been especially prominent in community action-oriented agencies during the 1960s. Finally, client differences get expressed in views about priorities of service, reflecting differences in categories of client need, and in client reference groups.

In summary, the administrator of a social agency always functions in a dynamic field of forces in which conflicting constituency interests contest for attention and response. The varying pressures and demands that result provide powerful constraints on administrative authority. Power and influence tend to be unequally distributed among constituencies and make purely rational behavior by administrators problematical. Organizational maintenance needs necessarily contend with the perceived requirements of clients and practitioners.

An essential task of the administrator lies in the effort to bring these differing needs and interests into some form of balance, of equilibrium—to orchestrate these diverse constituencies. Pusič (1974) refers to the "interest-adjudicating and conflict-handling function of administration in which increasingly interested parties themselves are becoming involved through processes such as representation, bargaining participation, and self-management" (p. 197). This interest-balancing function of administration has frequently been noted (Bach, 1964, p. 191; Vickers, 1965, p. 195; Walton, 1959, p. 32).

I have tried to suggest that the social agency paradigm provides a conceptual scheme for the selection of content relevant for the preparation of social administrators. From the above I derive the following basic dozen areas:

1. Organizational and interorganizational perspectives, including political, sociological, and psychological analysis.
2. Theoretical perspectives, including value assumptions and philosophical propensities.
3. Organization and structure of authority and decision making.
4. Resource allocation, control, and accountability, including budgeting and financing.
5. Policy planning and related program development.
6. Personnel management and labor relations.
7. Organizing and directing service delivery.
8. Evaluation and research.
9. Managerial technology, including information systems, computer use, and selected aspects of operational research.
10. Public relations and information.
11. Training, consultation, and supervision.
12. Organizational conflict and change.

These areas present a formidable repertoire of knowledge, skills, values, and attitudes. Fitting them into a logistical design over a 2-year course of study, given competing demands for curriculum space in schools of social work, is one of the urgent planning tasks for the immediate future.

A cursory examination of these content areas suggests that they include items of central interest to other aspects of the curriculum, and especially to social policy, and in some degree to direct practice. Boundary issues in this connection remain clouded (Gummer, 1975; Spergel, 1977). Schools of social work divide in organizing administration sequences (Kazmerski & Macarov, 1976). Some have an integrated policy-administration set of offerings; others separate the two and differentiate class and field concentrations.

One way to examine these alternative approaches is to look at two central variables: the closeness of the respective practitioners to the actual delivery of services, and the extent to which they deal with intra- or extraorganizational pursuits. Figure 5–4[1] dichotomizes the two.

Cells 1 and 4 represent the polarized alternative patterns of professional behavior. Cell 1 includes the characteristic service-giving social agency. Here, the administrator provides leadership to a staff that includes front-line workers who engage in the service transaction appropriate to the organization's reason for being. Depending upon size, the organization also includes supervisors, subexecutives, and assorted staff positions all concerned with the integrity of the service directed to clients who come to the agency. Where the agency includes offshoots or branches or a network of services, it can be located in Cell 3. A county welfare office would be one illustration.

Cell 4 includes organizations that are concerned with processes that impinge on the service encounter but that themselves are not involved in bringing clients and practitioners together. They deal with a variety of agencies and a multiplicity of clients, and are concerned chiefly with developing policy, planning service development, monitoring programs, stimulating growth (or contraction), financing and evaluating programs they sanction or support. Their contact with actual clients is second- or thirdhand. In a sense, their "clients" include organizations and programs that provide service. Federal, state, and regional welfare offices are prime examples.

Agencies that coordinate specific services in different organizations, for example, halfway houses in a defined area, might be thought to occupy Cell 2. They have an interest in the service experience, and deal with some degree of intimacy with clients, but their tasks have an essentially interorganizational focus.

This sketch is approximate, and is meant to point to some reasonable differences in the tasks that administrators and their staffs perform depending on their structural location in the total social service schema. Depending on the objectives of educational programs, this argues for separating curricula sequences intended to prepare social administrators as opposed to social policy analysts and planners. Yet it remains true that there are demonstrable similarities in much of the work both types of macropractitioners perform. Such work requirements as public rela-

		Intra	Extra
DISTANCE FROM	Close	1	2
SERVICE DELIVERY	Removed	3	4

FIGURE 5–4. Intra-extra organizational focus

tions, budgeting, information storage and retrieval, and the like have as much relevance to one pursuit as to the other. This is true of professional behaviors that go beyond the purely technical. Current experiences in the schools will have to be studied, analyzed, and evaluated in the period ahead before more definitive judgments can be made concerning the two basic curriculum strategies.

I have left for last some comments on the relationship of administration and service delivery. It has frequently been observed that the conventional career line in the social agency moved from direct practice, to supervisory, to subexecutive, and finally executive roles. Administrative learning was essentially on-the-job training. New managerial skills came from modeling on prior institutional practice, flavored with occasional institutes, literature reading, and induction by bookkeepers, accountants, funding auditors, and the like. It is now generally agreed that this experience has been far from satisfactory. It is increasingly recognized that skill in the service encounter is substantially different from managerial skill dimensions, and that the latter requires a professional moulting that is no less profound and demanding. Questions naturally arise concerning the requisite mix between the two for competent administrative leadership. A literature on this issue has begun to appear, particularly in the mental health field (Levenson & Klerman, 1972).

It has generally been assumed that administration as part of macro or indirect practice had intimate conceptual links to planning and policy. I am suggesting that this is no less true of its relationship to direct or service delivery (clinical) practice. Indeed, administration, as discussed above, is essentially concerned with establishing, organizing, and directing direct client service. Otherwise administration would have to be viewed as a technology essentially, though applied to a service system. Other disciplines could then provide the necessary personnel as well as or better than social administration. Indeed, schools of business administration are increasingly becoming schools of management, with the claim of preparing managers for all manner of enterprises, thus opening up an entirely new field for the placement of their graduates. (In part, for this reason I tend to look askance at social work-business school cooperation so eagerly sought originally by the Nixon bureaucracy and pursued by subsequent administrations.)

The historic connection, forged over many decades, between social work, as the core discipline, and the social services, and the intimacy of knowledge and concern of social work practitioners about client need and the purposes of client services, suggests that this profession is better suited to refining social administration roles than are other disciplines. It can do this only by keeping the administrative and service connection at the forefront of attention. This implies that an orientation to the nature and potentials of the service delivery systems, its professional technology, its value base, its ethical prescriptions, are an essential aspect of administrative training. (This also suggests that students preparing for administrative training in the schools might best be recruited from those who have had some minimum of experience with client service.) In a similar and reflexive view, clinicians in social agencies need a familiarity with organizational and institutional factors that enhance or retard clinical objectives for competent professional practice.

There remains a significant dilemma in this general area of discussion: Are middle-management roles essentially related to administrative or clinical (service delivery) orientations? Can middle-management supervisors be better prepared through advanced clinical training with some admixtures of administrative understanding, or the reverse? The dilemma can best be resolved, it seems, through clarifying the specific objectives of the training.

Supervisors, as conventionally perceived, carry essentially clinical teaching responsibilities. To the extent to which their central task is to enhance the capacity of supervisees to perform their professional duties, supervisors need, above all, clinical skills. They perforce need to know more about the service transaction than those they supervise. This comes from advanced training and experience in clinical practice.

While such supervisors fit the mold of middle managers in part, only when they become more distantly removed from monitoring the professional worker-client interaction can they more fully benefit from an administrative managerial focus in training. I would differentiate the service supervisor from the subexecutive in the middle-management realm, and similarly differentiate training protocols. In doing so, it would be necessary to modify the conceptual mix of relevant context.

Little has been said in this paper concerning the philosophical and ethical foundations of the administration function, or its fundamental thrust and conception, Yet this may be the most important aspect of all in preparing social administrators. A clear view of the moral and ethical base on which to build skills can serve to tie together all that has been said above. The executive deals with both empirical-pragmatic and normative propositions, the one descriptive, the other prescriptive. The latter indicates a point of view, an approach to preferences, to the "oughts" of administration. The administrator has a range of choices he can make with respect to fundamental orientation—to organizational maintenance or change, to client advocacy or agency prerogatives. Such choices are not absolute, but reflect preferences, priorities, and primacy of orientation. A complete discussion would involve another paper. For the moment, it may suffice to suggest that no discussion of administration can be complete without reference to social policy and its value orderings, or to conceptions of the functional role and stance of the administrator, as direction and leadership is provided to the many constituencies the organization inevitably involves.

NOTE

1. The author is indebted to Dr. Rosemary Sarri for this line of reasoning.

REFERENCES

Bach, G. L. Universities, business schools, and businesses. In H. Koontz (Ed.), *Toward a unified theory of management.* New York: McGraw-Hill, 1964.

Billingsley, A. Bureaucratic and professional orientation patterns in social casework. *Social Service Review,* December 1964, *38,* 400–407.

Bolman, W. M. Community control of the mental health center. *American Journal of Psychiatry,* August 1972, *129,* 97.

Epstein, L. An autonomous practice possible. *Social Work,* March 1973, *18,* 6.

Freidson, E. *Professional dominance: The social structure of medical care.* New York: Atherton Press, 1970.

Goode, W. F. The theoretical limits of professionalization. In A. Etzioni (Ed.), *The semi-professions and their organization.* New York: Free Press, 1969.

Gummer, B. Social planning and social administration: Implications for curriculum development. *Journal of Education for Social Work,* Winter 1975, *11,* 66–73.

Hanlan, A. Changing functions and structures. In F. W. Kaslow and Associates, *Issues in human services.* San Francisco: Jossey-Bass, 1972.

Helfgot, J. Professional reform organizations and the symbolic representation of the poor. *American Sociological Review,* August 1974, *39.*

Kammerman, S. B., & Kahn, A. J. *Social services in the United States.* Philadelphia: Temple University Press, 1976.

Kazmerski, K. J., & Macarov, D. *Administration in the social work curriculum.* New York: Council on Social Work Education, 1976.

Levenson, D. J., & Klerman, G. L. The clinician-executive. *Administration in Mental Health,* Winter 1972.

Merton, R. K. Bureaucratic structure and personality. In *Social theory and social structure.* Glencoe, Ill.: Free Press, 1957.

Negandhi, A. R. Comparative management and organization theory: A marriage needed. *Academy of Management Journal,* June 1975, *18,* 2.

Pusič, E. The administration of welfare. In F. D. Perlmutter (Ed.), *A design for social work practice.* New York: Columbia University Press, 1974.

Rapaport, L. In defense of social work: An examination of stress in the profession. *Social Service Review,* March 1960, *34,* 71.

Reiff, R. The danger of the techni-pro: Democratizing the human service professions. *Social Policy,* May-June 1971, *2,* 62.

Schein, E. H. *Professional education.* New York: McGraw-Hill, 1972.

Scott, W. R. The professional employees in a bureaucratic structure. In A. Etzioni (Ed.), *The semi-professions and their organization.* New York: Free Press, 1969.

Spergel, I. Social development and social work. *Administration in Social Work,* Fall 1977, *1*(3).

Toren, N. Semi-professionalism and social work: A theoretical perspective. In A. Etzioni (Ed.), *The semi-professions and their organization.* New York: Free Press, 1969.

Vickers G. *The art of judgment.* New York: Basic Books, 1965.

Walton, J. *Administration and policy-making.* Baltimore: Johns Hopkins Press, 1959.

6

Multiple Constituencies, Dominant Societal Values, and the Human Service Administrator: Implications for Service Delivery

PATRICIA YANCEY MARTIN

The aim of the present paper is to analyze the vulnerability of human service administrators and organizations to pressures and influences which are external to the service organization, per se. This is accomplished by identifying the major extra-organizational (i.e., outside the boundary) interest or constituency groups to which the (typical) social service organization must relate. A corollary goal is to explore the consequences of the form which across-the-boundary exchanges take for the delivery of services to clients. In particular, the effects of dominant societal values, locus of control of resources, and external pressures are viewed as fundamental to understanding the priorities which agency administrators emphasize and/or pursue.

Constituency groups external to the organization influence and shape the behavior of human service administrators and other personnel for a variety of reasons. Primary among these is the fact that resources and resource control generally lie outside the boundary of the organization (Walmsley & Zald, 1973). Administrators are required, therefore, to be sensitive and responsive to the activities and goals of important resource controllers. Pressures are great to foresee and forestall anticipated negative effects of changes in public revenues, legislative activities, regulatory requirements, media coverage, and so forth. Resources for the support of social services tend to be limited or scarce, furthermore, with the consequence that different organizations and programs are in competition with each other for their "fair share" of the pie. To remain competitive, human service administrators are under constant pressure not only to justify their programs as providing needed, worthwhile services, but also to demonstrate that they are providing such services in a rational (i.e., pre-planned, logical, well-organized), cost-efficient, and accountable manner (Aldrich, 1978).

Vulnerability to extra-organizational factors suggests that the human service organization (HSO) which survives is the HSO which pays attention to constituents, trends, and developments beyond its immediate boundaries (Scott, 1977). As the subsequent model of organizational constituencies suggests, a sizeable portion of personnel, energy, time, and financial resources are expended by HSOs to influence and/or respond to significant environments (Slavin, 1977). Competition not only for funds but for qualified staff and "valued" clients characterizes the interorganizational arena in which the service organization exists.

A MULTIPLE CONSTITUENCIES MODEL OF SERVICE ORGANIZATIONS

The model in Figure 6–1 identifies for analysis purposes the primary interest groups which have both a stake in and potential influence on the functioning of social service organizations. Five groups are identified as the HSO's internal constituencies, whereas seven are shown as its external constituencies. Although studies of internal organizational structure (Holland, 1973; Martin & Segal, 1976; Glisson, 1978) generally restrict attention to the four (or five, if clients are included) groups inside the heavy lines, the position taken here is that such a "closed system" model of service organizations is deficient. Since the HSO must regularly respond to and/or attempt to influence groups beyond its "accounting unit" boundaries (Evan, 1976), an open systems model is essential for understanding the situational context in which it operates (Walmsley & Zald, 1977; Aldrich & Pfeffer, 1977; Whetten, 1978).

The four groups inside the heavy lines in Figure 6–1 include the following:

1. directors and senior administrators, including their lieutenants and advisory staff;

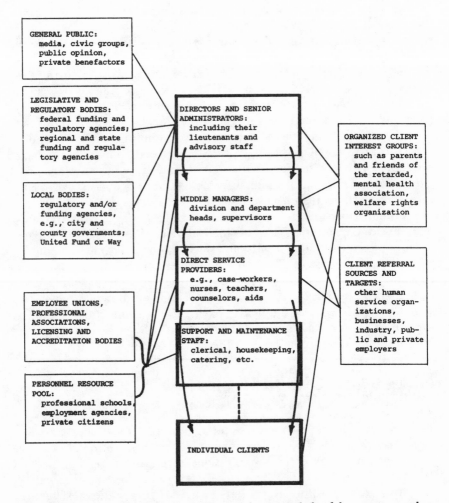

FIGURE 6–1. A multiple-constituencies model of human service organizations

2. middle managers, including department or program heads, supervisors;
3. direct service providers (e.g., caseworkers, counsellors, nurses, teachers); and
4. support staff (e.g., clerical, maintenance, catering, cleaning, etc.).

Beneath this block of groups, and connected to it by a dashed line, are the clients, the group for whose service-provision the HSO is "officially" established.

    Arrows point downward in Figure 6–1 to indicate that power and control inside bureaucratically structured organizations, which most HSOs are, are exercised from the top downward. Senior administrators and their lieutenants establish and enforce policies, rules, goals, and procedures for the middle managers, workers, and clients who fall under their purview (Goldman & Van Houten, 1977). The unequal distribution of power among the organization's internal constituent groups has important implications for considerations of quality of service provision (Whetten, 1977); that is, the goals and the objectives of senior administrators are likely to carry more weight than those of others. An accurate portrayal of the types of goals which administrators are pressured to pursue, particularly by powerful external constituencies, becomes essential for understanding the forces which influence and shape the form of social service delivery systems.

Seven distinctive external constituency groups are shown in Figure 6–1 as having relevance to the human service organization. There are:

1. the general public (including the media, civic groups, private contributors, churches, ordinary citizens, public opinion, etc.;
2. legislative and regulatory bodies (including federal, regional, and state funding and oversight agencies);
3. local funding and regulatory bodies (such as city or county government policies or laws, United Fund standards and grants, etc.;
4. employee unions, professional associations, licensing and accreditation bodies;
5. client referral sources and targets (including other human service organizations, private and public employers, businesses, industries, etc.); and
6. the personnel resource pool (including educational and professional schools, employment agencies, and private citizens seeking employment.
7. The seventh group, clients, are depicted in Figure 6–1 not merely as individuals to be recruited, served, and discharged, but also as collectives (such as parents and friends of the retarded) which organize for purposes of advancing or publicizing various concerns or for lobbying and pressuring HSOs to be more responsive to particular interests and demands.

Connecting lines in Figure 6–1 indicate linkages between groups inside the organization and those on the outside, i.e., across the organization's boundary. As the model shows, relationships or exchanges with important legislative, governmental, and funding/regulatory bodies are primarily the purview of the organization's senior administrators (Katz & Kahn, 1966). High-level administrators not only exercise the most power inside the organization, but they also represent the organization in dealings with powerful groups on the outside as well. As a consequence, senior administrators are generally well acquainted with external resource controllers, thereby being privy to important knowledge and information about which other internal organization members remain ignorant or uninformed.

Close relations between senior administrators and external influentials are fostered not only by frequency and extensiveness of contacts, but also by the processes through which the former are recruited and hired (Aldrich & Pfeffer, 1978). Selection of top administrators is typically influenced, and may be determined, by resource controllers outside the organization, with the consequence that persons chosen for these positions are likely to have qualifications, backgrounds, values, and orientations similar to those of the resource controllers themselves (Offe, 1976; Kanter, 1977). The consequences of this for the types of priorities and goals endorsed by senior administrators versus lower level organization members are of major significance when effectiveness, goal-oriented, or value issues are raised.

Close and continued association between administrators and resource controllers outside the organization poses certain risks both for the administrators and for the social service organization. Unless care is shown, administrators of HSOs are likely to become more responsive to the wishes, aims, and needs of external resource controllers than to those of their own staff and clients (Whetten, 1978). For reasons noted in the next section, persons who control the financial resources of service organizations are likely to be more concerned with "business-related" values and goals—such as growth, productivity, efficiency, and rationality—than with goals reflecting concern for a high quality of service provision or demonstrated service effectiveness. Unless the human service administrator has a clear conception of and strong commitment to a high quality service delivery model, pressures by resource controllers to subscribe to *their* model may be too great to withstand (Whetten, 1978).

An external constituency category whose influence in the social services sector is growing is that of employee unions, professional associations, and licensing/accreditation bodies. As noted by Ayres (1976), "If the present trends continue, more intensive efforts by professionals to unionize seem a certainty." Dissatisfied employees of human service organizations are organizing not only to assure higher pay and better working conditions, but also to combat what they perceive as an increasing tendency by administrators (and/or resource controllers) to stress quantity over quality, efficiency over effectiveness, and system (or "bureaucratic") needs over personal and professional considerations (Fendrich, 1977).

It is accepted knowledge that professional employees of service organizations are unhappy with recent and previous trends toward greater "bureaucratization" of the social services sector (Anderson, 1977). Emphasis by administrators on productivity—i.e., quantity of output—is interpreted by staff as a step in the direction of lowering the level of service quality (Whetten, 1978). Although increases in the levels of centralization and formalization of the workplace have been shown to enhance both productivity and efficiency in a variety of service organizations (Glisson & Martin, 1980), the goals of service quality and of commitment to client well-being may well be contraindicated by such trends.

Recent research by Whiddon (1980) bears on this issue. In a study of the effects of job discretion and participation in organizational decision-making on quality of staff performance and, by extension, quality of service provided to clients, Whiddon finds job discretion to be of primary importance to the direct service provider. Among 200 staff members of a large, statewide social service organization, those who report greater discretion in the execution of their jobs also report themselves and their colleagues as providing services of a higher quality to clients. To the extent that trends toward increasing "rationalization" of the workplace (see below) require a decrease in job discretion for professional employees, Whiddon's results suggest a consequent decline in level of service quality.

Disagreement between professional staff and administrators over definitions of quality and/or effectiveness is an increasingly salient feature of the human services arena (Whetten, 1978). As noted by Salaman (1978), the participation of staff in activities which further the aims or ends of the organization cannot be taken for granted if the organization's ends are seen as contradictory to the goals or well-being of the staff and clients. The success of human service administrators at "balancing" the contradictory pressures which they currently face may well determine the shape of the human service arena in years to come.

Clients are depicted in Figure 6–1 as potentially an internal as well as external group. There is disagreement over whether clients served by an organization are legitimately considered as members of the organization (Bidwell, 1970). Although a welfare agency, general hospital, or public school cannot fulfill its mission without clients, it is also true that clients in comparison to employees typically spend less time "inside" the organization and are less committed to it. Bidwell contends that conceptualization of clients as external constituents served by the organization highlights the problematic and dynamic nature of ongoing client/organization relations and mitigates the tendency to assume that they can be taken for granted.

The omission of linkages among the external groups in Figure 6–1 should not be interpreted as suggesting that they are either absent or irrelevant. Such linkages may constitute essential features of the social and political context within which service organizations operate (Walmsley & Zald, 1977; Aldrich & Pfeffer, 1978). Emphasis here is on ties *between* internal and external groups, however, in order to highlight the diversity of influences and interests which impinge on the HSO and to underscore the extensiveness of the service organization's ties with external suprasystems and environments (Buckley, 1967; Evan, 1976).

DOMINANT SOCIETAL VALUES AND CONTROL OF RESOURCES

Organizations tend to reflect the culture and society in which they are lodged (Fox, 1974; Hickson et al., 1974). Not only their form, but also their values and goals, are reflections of their broader societal and cultural contexts. It is this factor which accounts for the predominantly bureaucratic form of modern social service delivery systems and organizations. In the industrialized west, in particular, the normative organizational form is one which entails a division of labor, a hierarchy of authority, delineation of positions independently of persons, and hiring and advancement on the basis of technical qualifications and/or expertise—i.e., rather than kinship, charisma, etc. (McNeil, 1978).

Recent developments of "collective" organizations (Rothschild-Whitt, 1979), as embodied, for example, in the self-help health and mental health movements, indicate that the acceptance of the bureaucratic model may be less unanimous (and/or ubiquitous) than is generally supposed. Nevertheless, the majority of social and health services provided to clients in the United States are delivered by bureaucratically structured organizations. Because a bureaucracy is premised on certain assumptions and values which also are dominant in the industrialized west, this becomes an important consideration. Bureaucracy rests on the value that relations at work should be highly "rationalized" in order to achieve maximum efficiency and productivity and to minimize waste and inefficiency (Salaman, 1978).

Bureaucracy as the predominant organizational form is buttressed in the United States by the concomitant dominance of a cultural ideology which emphasizes business/capitalist goals as appropriate for formal organizations (Starbuck, 1965). This ideology stresses not only high sales volumes and profits but, more generally, expansion and growth, numbers of units processed (i.e., productivity), and a maximum of outputs for a minimum of inputs or costs (i.e., efficiency) (Glisson & Martin, 1980). It also values rationality in the arrangement of work roles and relations and accountability in the assessment of goal achievement.

Although human service organizations differ from business, manufacturing, and industrial organizations in their absence of profit-making and sales activities, they remain subject to other cultural expectations to demonstrate growth, productivity, efficiency, rationality, and accountability. The dominance of a "business" orientation in the value system of U.S. society pressures directors of human service organizations to pursue "business-type" goals even though their organizations are of a "nonbusiness" nature (Salaman, 1978). Established formally to meet human needs, to "provide services to clients," HSOs are, in fact, pressured to pursue goals which often contradict commitment to high quality service provision.

Although none of this constitutes "news" to the social service arena, it is emphasized here for a number of reasons. External pressures on HSOs consist not only of ideological and/or normative abuse, but also the withdrawal of funds and withholding of needed resources (Imershein et al., 1980). The reputation of many HSOs as "inefficient," poorly rationalized, and non-accountable results in a situation of extreme vulnerability to external pressures and influences (Meyer & Rowan, 1977). Failure to acknowledge and deal with these factors aggressively means that human service administrators often miss the opportunity to circumvent or use them for enhancing service quality and scope (Aldrich & Pfeffer, 1978).

Procurement of resources, and particularly financial resources, is a perennial and pervasive concern among human services administrators (NIMH, 1975). As noted, service organizations generally have less control over their resources than do production-oriented organizations which sell products to customers (Walmsley & Zald, 1973). The role of the customer, in fact, constitutes an important difference between production and service types of organizations. Having a product to sell, the ultimate fate of the profit-making organization depends on whether potential customers actually purchase the organization's product. Concern with "quality" is built into the organization's cybernetic process in that an acceptable (if minimal) level of quality must be maintained or else customers will (presumably) boycott the product (Raymond, 1978). Customer response to the product generates resources which the organization can then use either to create new products or to otherwise alter or expand its services (Aldrich, 1978).

The role of client in the social service arena, as the system presently operates, tends to be much less critical. Unless individually or collectively organized and outspoken, the resource procurement process of human service organizations tends to bypass client responsiveness or concerns (Imershein et al., 1980). As Daniels (1969) notes, the "state" which provides the major source of funds and resources for HSOs tends also to become its major "client"; that is since the state rather than the client generally "pays for the service," concern among administrators tends to focus on the "needs" and requirements of the state itself.

In the case of publicly funded programs, the "state" is embodied in the federal, state, and local elected and appointed officials who pass laws, establish policy, write implementation guidelines, and allocate funds. The types of people who accede to these positions tend, in the main, to personify the values and ideology which are dominant in the society. Running for elective office is costly. Persons who do so are primarily those who have experienced previous financial success in other occupational realms. Coming primarily from legal and/or enterpreneurial backgrounds, political aspirants succeed in political/governmental arenas in part because they have complied with the society's dominant values, goals, and ideologies. Such persons can be expected, therefore, to emphasize the standards by which they have succeeded and from which they have benefited (Offe, 1976).

Elected and appointed officials who have control over the policies and resources which direct and sustain HSOs are likely to stress values, aims, and goals which are consistent with predominant themes in the society at large. Given the general "business bent" of U.S. culture, it is likely that these will be of a business-type or business-like nature as well. Growth, efficiency, rationality, and accountability are likely to be valued over quality or demonstrated effectiveness of services provided. Concern with business-type issues at the level of resource allocation and control pressures administrators of social service programs to be concerned with them as well. In many instances, administrators of human service organizations are selected for their previous records as achievers of productivity, efficiency, and rationality (Imershein et al., 1980). Retention of their jobs, furthermore, may well depend on their ability to achieve these ends in the future.

DISCUSSION AND CONCLUSIONS

A model specifying the multiple and diverse interest groups with which human service administrators continuously interact highlights the dynamic and problematic nature of both daily and long-range operations. Considerations of the dominant values of the culture in which service organizations exist provide insights into the types of goals and aims which administrators of HSOs are pressured by external resource controllers to pursue.

The twin goals of "organizational survival" and "high quality service provision" need not be mutually exclusive although emphasis on one is often viewed as diminishing resources (e.g., money, time, good will, enthusiasm) available for the pursuit of the other (Glisson & Martin, 1980). It appears, therefore, that the human services administrator is faced with a dilemma. Satisfaction of external resource controllers and funding sources may result in a dissatisfied clientele and staff (including employee unions and professional schools and associations), whereas satisfaction of the latter groups may lead to a loss of positions, funds, space, and/or personnel considered necessary to sustain the program. Such contradictions suggest the necessity for considering whether human service administrators are caught hopelessly in a double-bind situation, or whether strategies can be identified which allow for satisfaction of external pressures while simultaneously facilitating provision of high quality services.

The foregoing analysis underscores the necessity for human service administrators to receive training which prepares them for the pervasive and complex dilemmas which are inherent in their jobs (Slavin, 1978). Professional schools and on-the-job training experiences must spell out for administrators those characteristics of the political arena of service organizations, including the conflicting demands of competing constituencies, with which they will be faced. Such preparation entails at least two parallel themes. First, human services administrators must be trained for and skilled in *managing* their external constituents rather than merely *responding* to them (Aldrich & Pfeffer, 1978). They must find out what external resource controllers and opinion shapers want and either give it to them or else convince them that other goals are equally worthy, if not more so, instead. Meyer and Rowan (1977) enumerate the many negative consequences adhering to organizations which openly fail to comply with dominant cultural values and ideology, a category into which many human service organizations presently fall. Human service administrators must be trained in techniques and strategies which will allow them to gain more "control" over powerful external influentials. Such techniques are likely to include innovative ways of actually complying with expectations for greater productivity, efficiency, and/or accountability, while simultaneously "educating" external influentials regarding the requirements and worthiness of high quality service provision programs. An additional approach is to develop and/or court powerful or influential external constituencies which value commitment to a high level of service quality.

Second, the human service administrator must be provided with clear, viable, and feasible models of service delivery systems which foster the provision of high quality services to clients. As noted by Slavin (1977, p. 255), ". . . administration [in the human services] is essentially concerned with establishing, organizing and directing direct client service. . . . *The administrative and service connection must be kept at the forefront of attention*" (emphasis the author's). In this respect, administrators are encouraged to view their own professional staffs as their greatest resource and ally. Professionally educated staff are, in general, both trained for and committed to providing a high quality of client-service. The administrator is advised, therefore, to "charge" the staff with the responsibility for fulfilling this objective. On his/her part, the administrator must likewise protect the staff members' time (e.g., from too much clerical or paper work) and autonomy/discretion so as to maximize opportunities for exercising skill and judgment in the pursuit of their work (Hage, 1974; Whiddon, 1980). As noted by Meyer and Rowan (1977), maximal utilization of professional (or technical) staff requires that they be protected and buffered from external pressures or interference and that they have the leeway to use judgment and innovation in the execution of their work (Meyer, 1975).

It is particularly important, as well, that human service administrators maintain their identification as *professional service providers* (e.g., social workers) while resisting the temptation, though strong and persistent, to identify with powerful (external) resource controllers. Gross and Trask (1976) report that the most effective principals of elementary schools are those who spent many years in classroom teaching prior to becoming principals, and who then retained a strong and primary commitment to curriculum, instruction, and student learning as the school's over-arching mission. If human service administrators identify with external influentials rather than their own profession and professional staff, they are likely to become increasingly concerned with system-level matters and to lose sight of the difficult and problematic but important goal of high quality service provision (Whiddon, 1980).

REFERENCES

Aldrich, H. E. Centralization versus decentralization in the design of human service delivery systems: A response to Gouldner's Lament. In R. C. Sarri & Y. Hasenfeld (Eds.), *The management of human services.* New York: Columbia University Press, 1978.

Aldrich, H. E., & Pfeffer, J. Environments of organizations. *Annual Review of Sociology.* 1977, *3*, 79–105.

Anderson, W. A. *Conflict and congruity between bureaucracy and professionalism: Alienation outcomes among social service workers.* Unpublished doctoral dissertation, Florida State University, Tallahassee, 1977.

Ayres, G. W. An examination of three aspects of the unionization of public employees. *Arete,* 1976, *4*, 81–103.

Bidwell, C. E. Students and schools: Some observations on client trust in client-serving organizations. In W. K. Rosengren & M. Lefton (Eds.), *Organizations and clients: Essays in the sociology of service.* Columbus, OH: Charles E. Merrill, 1970.

Buckley, W. *Sociology and modern systems theory.* Englewood Cliffs, NJ: Prentice-Hall, 1967.

Daniels, A. K. The captive professional: Bureaucratic limitations in the practice of military psychiatry. *Journal of Health and Social Behavior,* 1969, *10*, 255–265.

Evan, W. M. Organization theory and organizational effectiveness: An exploratory analysis. *Organization and Administrative Science*, 1976, *7*, 15–28.

Fendrich, J. Unions help faculty who help themselves: A partisan view of a collective bargaining campaign. *The American Sociologist*, 1977, *12*, 162–175.

Fox, A. *Beyond contract*. London: Faber & Faber, 1974.

Glisson, C. A. Dependence of technological routinization on structural variables in human service organizations. *Administrative Science Quarterly*, 1978, *23*, 383–395.

Glisson, C. A., & Martin, P. Y. Productivity and efficiency as related to size, age, and structure in human service organizations. *Academy of Management Journal*, March 1980, *23*.

Goldman, P., & Van Houten, D. R. Managerial strategies and the worker: A Marxist analysis of bureaucracy. *The Sociological Quarterly*, 1977, *18*, 108–125.

Gross, N., & Trask, A. E. *The sex factor and the management of schools*. New York: Wiley-Interscience, 1976.

Hage, J. *Communication and organizational control: Cybernetics in health and welfare settings*. New York: Wiley, 1974.

Hickson, D. J., Hinings, C. R., McMillan, C. H., & Schwitter, P. P. The culture-free context of organization structure: A tri-national comparison. *Sociology*, 1974, *8*, 59–80.

Holland, T. P. Organizational structure and institutional care. *Journal of Health and Social Behavior*, 1973, *14*, 241–251.

Imershein, A. W., Frumkin, M., Chackerian, R., McDonald, G., Martin, P., Turnbull, A., & Schmidt, W. A critical research framework for assessing services integration in large, human resource agencies: Florida, a case example. *Evaluation*, March 1980, *7*.

Kanter, R. M. *Men and women of the corporation*. New York: Basic Books, 1977.

Katz, D., & Kahn, R. L. *The social psychology of organizations*. New York: John Wiley & Sons, 1966.

Martin, P. Y., & Segal, B. Bureaucracy, size, and staff expectations for client independence in halfway houses. *Journal of Health and Social Behavior*, 1976, *18*, 376–380.

McNeil, K. Understanding organizational power: Building on the Weberian legacy. *Administrative Science Quarterly*, 1978, *23*, 65–90.

Meyer, J. W., & Rowan, B. Institutionalized organizations: Formal structure as myth and ceremony. *American Journal of Sociology*, 1977, *83*, 340–363.

Meyer, M. W. Leadership and organizational structure. *American Journal of Sociology*, 1975, *81*, 514–542.

National Institute of Mental Health. *Halfway houses serving the mentally ill and alcoholics, United States, 1973*, DHEW Publ. No. ADM-76-264. Washington, D.C.: U.S. Government Printing Office, 1975.

Offe, *Industry and inequality*. London: Edward Arnold, 1976.

Raymond, F. B., III. The cybernetic model as a means to accountability: An agency example. *Arete*, 1978, *5*, 23–35.

Rothschild-Whitt, J. The collectivist organization. *American Sociological Review*, 1979, *44*, 509–527.

Salaman, G. Towards a sociology of organizational structure. *Sociological Review*, 1978, *26*, 519–554.

Scott, R. F. Effectiveness of organizational effectiveness studies. In P. S. Good-
man & J. M. Pennings (Eds), *New perspectives on organizational effectiveness.*
San Francisco: Jossey-Bass, 1977.
Slavin, S. A framework for selecting content for teaching about administration.
Administration in Social Work, 1977, *1,* 245–257.
Slavin, S. (Ed.). *Social administration: The management of the social services.* New
York: Council on Social Work Education and The Haworth Press, 1978.
Starbuck, W. Organizational growth and development. In J. G. March (Ed.),
Handbook of organizations. Chicago: Rand-McNally, 1965.
Walmsley, G., & Zald, M. N. *The political economy of public organizations.* New York:
Praeger, 1973.
Whetten, D. A. Coping with incompatible expectations: An integrated view of
role conflict. *Administrative Science Quarterly,* 1978, *23,* 254–271.
Whetten, D. A. Coping with incompatible expectations: Role conflict among di-
rectors of manpower agencies. *Administration in Social Work,* 1977, *1,*
379–393.
Whiddon, B. *The effect of congruence on the relationships between participation/job discretion and staff performance: The case of a social service organization.* Unpublished doctoral dissertation, Florida State University, Tallahassee, 1980.

7

Management Applications to the Welfare System

SCOTT MULLIS

In relating management and organization concepts to welfare programs two clear problems emerge. The first is the degree to which welfare professionals are able to understand principles of management and organization. The second problem, while perhaps more subtle, is the converse of the first. Professional managers have tremendous difficulty understanding welfare.

The purpose of this article is to close some of the differences between management and welfare thinking. It is beyond its scope to resolve most questions, and in particular it is impossible to determine if welfare can, indeed, be managed. Attempted here are two things:

1. an update to management and organizational concepts, and
2. an application of some recent trends in organizational thought to welfare.

In the absence of ongoing education, many middle- and top-level managers today are not generally cognizant of changes in the scope and direction of management and organization theory. Similarly, welfare professionals, often with early training in sociology and political science, are handicapped by their extensive exposure to bureaucracy as *the* form of organization. While we are not about to observe the "death of bureaucracy,"[1] other organizational models are available and an understanding of situations where these contingent forms apply is essential.

An important current trend in management and organization theory is movement away from set, "universal" principles toward a contingency view.[2] This means roughly that the correct organizational structure and management plan is dependent on the situation. Much of the current empirical work in management and organization is directed toward isolating situational variables and developing scenarios where certain principles work consistently. This focus can be exemplified by work in the area of leadership.[3] It was once generally agreed that group participation and concern for subordinates were uniformly good. More recent analysis indicates that in some situations performance requires an autocratic, production-oriented leadership.[4]

So, too, use of the bureaucratic model (and its principles of organization) is increasingly recognized as only one possible form. Longitudinal empirical evidence is scant, but at least three other forms are appearing in organizations. These are project, matrix, and free-form typologies. All of these violate in some way the classical bureaucratic model.[5] They are, however, effective in some situations and for certain kinds of tasks.

The significant generalization seems to be that when an organization is faced with a fairly stable environment, and when tasks are repetitive, a strict bureaucratic structure can work efficiently. However, when goals and objectives are more general, and when the relevant environment can generate great variety, then a more open, less structured, and consequently more responsive organization seems to work well.[6]

MANAGEMENT AND ORGANIZATIONAL THEORY

Management and organizational theory can be traced through four schools of thought: process, behavioral, quantitative, and systems. The currently emerging school described as contingent or situational has potential for uniting these highly divergent approaches.[7]

Process

The process school, as the name implies, sees management as a series of activities. The original thinking in this view goes back to the early twentieth century with Fayol's plan—organize, command, coordinate, and control.[8] Though Fayol's work was published in Europe early in this century, translation into English did not become generally available until the late 1940s. While there has been much elaboration on Fayol's theme, there has been little development in this school beyond the original.

Organizational precepts associated with the process school are bureaucratic. The "universal" prescriptions for efficiency included increasing division of labor or specialization, hierarchy, a set of formal abstract rules, and impersonal relations.

Behavioral

The extreme mechanistic view implicit in the process approach, as well as its failure to provide "universal" answers to organizational problems, led many to seek alternative approaches.

Psychological factors received increasing attention and with the Hawthorne Studies at Western Electric, a behavioral approach was born. The first attempts were primarily a reaction to the mechanics of the bureaucratic model and, in their own way, were severely constrained. Most of the discussion involved looking at psychological factors within the bureaucratic prescription with little attention to other structural forms. The net result was the "happiness equation" of the human relations movement. According to this school, productivity was a function of morale. This simplistic explanation fell rapidly into disrepute as practitioners and students alike increasingly recognized the complexity of the organization-human interaction.

More recently the behavioral approach can be characterized as an assemblage of concepts drawn from all behavioral sciences unified in the conceptual framework of the organization-human interaction as mutually dependent systems. This view is partially the result of influence from the systems approach to management.

Systems

The systems view of management has its roots in developments during and after World War II. The great promise of general systems theory is the idea of tying together many approaches into a unified whole—and therein lies the problem. As a general science of just about everything, it explains just about nothing. As one of its founders points out, there is great difficulty in moving from interesting analogy to a productive model.[9]

This is not to say that general systems theory is without value. As will be developed below, some concepts have great power to assist through "explanation in principle."[10] But the promise is not fulfilled. General systems theory will require years of work and new approaches to mathematics to become the all powerful science of sciences.

Quantitative

The quantitative approach to management, which also developed during and immediately following World War II, is properly viewed as a lineal descendant of scientific management of Frederick W. Taylor (circa 1910). The reason that this merits rating as a major school of management is a function of two factors.

First, in an industrial society there is great impetus to quantify and measure. Often this holds even if it can't be shown that the proper variables are being measured. This emphasis on quantification and measurement is the nemesis of the quantitative school as well as its forte. Too often so much is abstracted from problems in order to force a situation into a given model that any hope of realistic application is lost.

The second factor which brings the quantitative school to the status of a major school of management is the development of the computer. Without the computer many of the techniques and models would never have been developed, much less implemented. As the computer becomes ever faster and more capable in storage and retrieval, quantitative approaches become more viable. The problem of abstraction and consequent oversimplification is ameliorated as the computers become capable of handling models in increasing variety and complexity.

In summary then, students and practitioners of management and organization theory are divided in their approach. This situation has recently changed with the development of a contingency approach. The contingency frame of reference starts with the assumption that universal prescriptions (like universal truths!) are difficult to find.

This approach is not eclipsing the other schools. Contingent analysis has contributed to further development of principles in the four major schools. The behavioralists have for some time now looked to situational contingencies to explain effective leadership. The quantitative approach applies different models to different situations although the methodology remains the same. More important, one of the principles of general sytems theory is that of equifinality.[11] This means that given an open system there is more than one way to accomplish an end. This is the contingency approach in a most abstract form. The following section takes two selected concepts, one drawn from the systems school and the other from the behavioral school, and applies contingent analysis to the welfare system.

CONTINGENCIES IN ORGANIZATION OF THE WELFARE FUNCTION

The Systems Model

The systems school views an organization as having inputs, transformation processes, and outputs which are measured on certain variables. The results of the measurements are then fed back as part of the inputs to the next cycle. Figure 7–1 depicts this conceptual framework.

This framework points directly to three groups of questions ex-

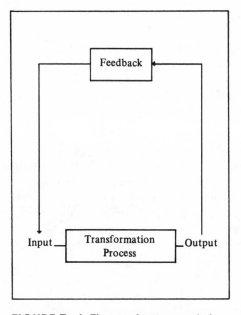

FIGURE 7–1. The systems model

tremely important to organizational analysis. The first set of questions involves the outputs. What is the organization supposed to accomplish? Further, how is this accomplishment to be measured? The second set involves the inputs. What exactly is available to the organization in terms of resources? Also, what is the nature of the environment? What factors beyond the direct control of the organization impinge upon the operations? Finally, the last set of questions looks at the transformation processes. These include: What are the steps that lead to a given end? Can certain steps by bypassed? Can the process be accelerated? Can it be slowed?

These are not surprising questions. An experienced manager would ask these questions and many others if asked to analyze this organization. What this framework does provide is an organized whole—a checklist of areas of possible improvement. Thus, such a framework can at least be used to unify diverse areas of concern.

Beyond such analysis, however, is the possibility of using such a framework to actually structure an organization. It is clear that the kind of analysis alluded to above will not automatically flow from a standard organization chart. Why not use such a systems framework in lieu of the normal bureaucratic organizational chart, thus organizing in terms of process instead of physical entities connected by lines of authority?

Much credit must be given F. H. Allport for his view of structure as a cycle of events.[12]

In looking at a welfare organization such a structure might develop along the following lines:

Output

A welfare department has responsibility for acting on social and economic problems of certain individuals. The desired output then is defined in terms of the proper social and economic variables. The objective in a given case may be a degree of improvement, prevention of a further negative trend, or a deceleration of a negative trend. This definition of output must meet the test of "operationality" to allow measurement. Once the proper output and measurement is determined, the next task is to analyze the inputs to understand the necessary and available transformation tasks.

Inputs

Inputs to the system include physical and human resources, plans, and mandates. The most important input is the people who are to be served. The people that enter the welfare system enter because of some need or set of needs. The input function is charged with defining that set of needs for which the organization can provide. This is done through the eligibility process. Once eligibility is established, the client enters into the transformation process, where transformation includes slowing or stabilizing a regressive situation, as well as improvement.

Transformation Process

In a welfare program the transformation process would be identified as the programs providing aid and services, which generally include income maintenance, and medical and social services. These programs all converge at the individual client level to define a major portion of his life. To artificially separate income maintenance from services at the organizational level as presently mandated really misses the point.

One of the principal reasons for separation of services is to divorce the client-oriented services aspect from the eligibility-oriented income maintenance function.[13] This follows from the idea that the eligibility process is degrading and has highly negative connotations with respect to clients. It should have been apparent that care is required in eligibility determination because a welfare office must be responsible to taxpayers as well as clients (who may also pay taxes). Whenever resources are scarce, and they always are, criteria must be set up. Eligibility is a problem in social services as well as income maintenance.

What follows from this kind of longitudinal analysis of the client as he moves through the system is that the organization could be designed around that flow. Specific recommendations would include the separation of all aspects of the transformation process from the input. Instead of a separation by programs we would implement a separation by flow. When clients entered the system, they would go through the eligibility process once, not twice or more. Out of this screening the client would receive a checklist of all services and other benefits which can be provided by the agency.

Figure 7–2 depicts this kind of systems framework applied to welfare.

CENTRALIZATION-DECENTRALIZATION: A CONTINGENCY APPROACH

The second example of analysis of welfare organization in the context of management and organization theory involves the classic question of whether an organization is more effective when closely controlled at the top through centralization or when lower-level members are given more responsibility and authority for decision making. Most schools of management address this question, and all agree that advantages of decentralization generally outweigh advantages of centralization. The process school sees decentralization as necessary because of the excessive time

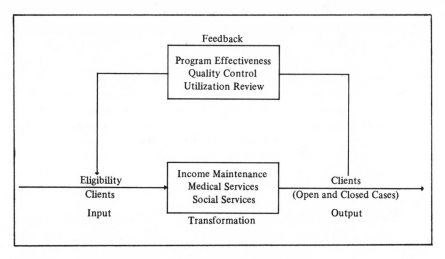

FIGURE 7–2. A systems organization of welfare

lag between a developing situation and remote decision making. The behavioral school points to more satisfaction at lower levels when participants have more input and control on their jobs. The systems school would look not only at increased speed of response but also to the ability of the organization to be more diverse and flexible in its response to nonroutine matters.

Decentralization, for all its popularity, is not uniformly accepted. Many organizations try decentralization but move back to a more centralized form. Decentralization, it is found, is not a universal principle. Rather decentralization is a matter of degree, and the proper degree is dependent on the situation.

This contingency approach to the centralization-decentralization question is generally discussed in terms of the whole organization. The welfare organization indicates centralization of some functions and decentralization of others.[14]

As indicated above, the degree of decentralization involves a trade off of close uniform control against more rapid flexible decision making. The proper degree of decentralization, then, depends on the relative importance of uniformity and flexibility, as well as elements in the specific situation affecting these variables. In the welfare organization, income maintenance and medical and social services each present a different situation; therefore, differing degrees of centralization are appropriate.

Income maintenance involves money, and money is a scarce resource with uniform acceptance by and predictable benefits to the recipient. Equity and uniform treatment of clients dictate a closely controlled centralized operation with minimal variance in policy decisions on an individual basis. The client should know what to expect, and should not be able to "work the system." On the supply side, taxpayers demand accountability and protection from fraud whether perpetrated by client or employee. All of these considerations dictate a highly centralized closely audited payments function.

Client needs, however, are not uniform, nor can they be adequately evaluated in a centralized situation. Provision of social services can, to some extent, pick up the slack. However, it is very likely that local discretionary decisions about money will be required at the local level. Such local discretion should be exercised with a local funds matching scheme and should be centrally monitored for both excessive and insufficient use. The ratio of such discretionary funds to the total aid bill should be low.

Medical, too, should be closely monitored and centralized for services payments. The situation is different from income maintenance, but the result is the same. Medical services are locally provided, but payments for services are centralized.

The problem in medical is to avoid fradulent claims. It is also necessary to assure adequate client care and to avoid experimental treatments. Accomplishing these goals requires a highly integrated utilization-review procedure based on statistical analysis. Centralization of payments provides the opportunity for such close control. The negative aspect of such centralization is turnaround time or the delay of payments. In many states the first requirement is to clean up the medical claims processing; only then can any kind of control become feasible.

Social services provide an interesting variant to the above analysis. Both income maintenance and medical assistance present clear-cut problems when compared with social services. In both cases there are generally accepted, available units of measurement with relatively predictable results in the provision of funds or services. Also, for the most part, in both payments and medical the objective of maintenance is predominant. Social services also involves an implicit mandate to bring about change and prevent deterioration.

Social services do not lend themselves to generally accepted, available units of measurement. This is, of course, because there is little generally accepted operational theory or body of knowledge behind services. This area is emerging as a science and depends to a large degree on an eclectic approach which includes many minor theories, often inconsistent and contradictory, and a smattering of empirical evidence in the form of case histories and poorly controlled experiments and surveys. As a result, there is a great deal of question as to the value of social services in general.

This situation calls for carefully centralized monitoring of services provided, and recording of precedent and subsequent conditions to allow evaluation. But decisions as to which service to provide and the method of provision are most properly made at the local level by truly professional staff. Local decision making provides the variety and the rapid response necessary to cope with the very individual approach required. This is so because the need for service varies significantly between individuals; there is great variety in delivery method as well as availability of service; and finally, local conditions will affect the proper prescription of service. Most services cannot be standardized at this time.

CONCLUSION

This short paper attempts a review of some of the most recent developments in the field of management as applied to the context of public welfare. Application of systems concepts in organizing around client flow and the contingency analysis of relative decentralization of three major functions provide practical examples of how management thinking can contribute to welfare. Purposely avoided are the problems related to federal mandates and matching formulas, which are beyond the scope of this article. It is hoped that some questions have been raised for the practitioner.

NOTES

1. Warren Bennis, "The Death of Bureaucracy," in David C. Cleland and William R. King, eds., *Systems, Organizations, Analysis, Management: A Book of Readings* (New York: McGraw-Hill Book Co., 1969), pp. 11–17.
2. Fred Luthans, "The Contingency Theory of Management," *Business Horizons*, June 1973, pp. 57–72.
3. Fred E. Fiedler, *A Theory of Leadership Effectiveness* (New York: McGraw-Hill Book Co., 1967).
4. Ibid., pp. 142–48.
5. It is beyond the scope of this article to elaborate on these forms. Further development can be found in Fred Luthans, *Organizational Behavior* (New York: McGraw-Hill Book Co., 1973), pp. 168–79.
6. Y. K. Shetty and Howard M. Carlisle, "A Contingency Model of Organizational Design," *California Management Review* 15 (Fall 1972), p. 40.
7. Luthans, "The Contingency Theory of Management," pp. 57–72.
8. Henri Fayol, "Administration Indústrielle et Générale," *Bulletin de la Société de l'Industrie Minérale*, 5th series, vol. 10, pt. 3 (1916), pp. 1–162.
9. Ludwig Von Bertalanffy, *General Systems Theory*, rev. ed. (New York: George Braziller, Inc., 1969), pp. 33–36.
10. Ibid., p. 33.
11. Ibid., p. 46.
12. Floyd H. Allport, "The Structuring of Events: Outline of a General Theory with Application to Psychology," *Psychological Review* 61, no. 5 (September 1954): 281–303; and Floyd H. Allport, "A Structuronomic Conception of Behavior, Individual and Collective. I. Structural Theory and the Master Problem of Social Psychology," *Journal of Abnormal and Social Psychology* 64 (1962), p. 3–30.
13. U.S. Department of Health, Education, and Welfare, Social and Rehabilitative Service, Community Services Administration, *The Separation of Services from Assistance Payments*, HEW pubn. no. (SRS) 73-23015 (Washington, D.C.: Government Printing Office, 1972), pp. 5–8.
14. We are talking now on the state level. The centralization of payments at the federal level in the adult categories was unnecessary and has resulted in untold human misery as a highly efficient centralized bureaucracy, the Social Security Administration, operating in a very stable environment, learned that it is not capable of handling the higher variety and more pressing need of the welfare population. The people and their characteristics did not change by act of Congress. As a result state and county welfare administrators are forced to pick up the slack. The goal of more equitable treatment under federalization should have been accomplished with more leadership from the Department of Health, Education, and Welfare.

8

A Contingency
Model of
Social Welfare
Administration

CHARLES A. GLISSON

The administration of social welfare programs has been identified for
several decades as a practice area in social work. Only recently, however,
have there been efforts to identify the specific knowledge and skills required to successfully meet the demands of managerial roles and functions in service delivery systems. Unfortunately, these efforts have
mainly focused on listing various knowledge and skills with "an absence
of systematic frameworks or models for organizing existing social welfare administrative practice knowledge" (Dumpson, Mullen, & First,
1978, p. 34). The purpose of this paper is to develop a theoretical model
of service organizations and use that model as a framework for defining
and categorizing the knowledge and skills an administrator must possess
to manage adequately a service delivery system.

The framework is based upon the contingency model of organization and management presented by Kast & Rosenzweig (1973). The
model depicts the organization as a social system comprised of interconnected subsystems which exist in a suprasystem, or environment, consisting of other social systems. The administrator's job is to facilitate the
functioning and interrelationships of the organizational subsystems as
well as to insure a relationship with the organization's environment
which contributes to organizational survival. Kast and Rosenzweig argue
that appropriate administrative behavior is contingent upon the characteristics of the specific organization and the environmental situation in
which it exists.

Most contemporary writers would agree that there have been three
major thrusts in the development of organization theory: the rational,

mechanistic models; the systemic, organic models; and the human relations models. The contingency approach integrates these trends, viewing the manager as a decision-maker who must consider the rational, systemic, and human relation dimensions of the organization in choosing alternatives for action.

There are several advantages of applying the contingency model to social welfare administration. First, the model has evolved from over half a century of organizational research and encompasses the major theoretical views of organizations developed during that period by integrating those views into a holistic perspective which avoids the ascription of organizational effectiveness to any single organization variable or subsystem. The contingency approach recognizes that various types of organizations and situations demand different organizational designs and managerial actions. It emphasizes that what spells success for one organization may not spell success for another.

Second, the contingency approach provides a context for the consideration of the unique characteristics of organizational systems which deliver services to human beings. Because the contingency model recognizes the interrelationships among subsystems, the fact that the technological subsystem of a social welfare organization has human beings as its "raw material" (rather than iron ore, real estate, or textiles) suggests that the remaining subsystems should also exhibit characteristics distinguishable from those found in the organizations processing iron ore, selling real estate, or producing textiles.

Third, the contingency model relies heavily on general systems theory in conceptualizing the interrelationships of the organization's subsystems and the relationship between the organization and its environment. General systems theory is familiar ground to social workers and such an approach to understanding organizations is easily integrated into the systemic model of individuals, families, organizations, communities, states, and nations as interconnected elements considered in social work intervention efforts.

Fourth, the proponents of the contingency model define the model in developmental terms. The need is recognized for continued research to establish interrelationships between organizational and environmental variables in order "to understand how organizations operate under varying conditions and in specific circumstances" (Kast & Rosenzweig, 1973, p. 313). While subsystems which comprise organizations have been identified in general, there remains the task of describing the dimensions of those subsystems and their interrelationships for particular types of organizations so that the prescriptive implications of the contingency model can be established (Glisson, 1979). Input from social work can therefore influence the effectiveness criteria upon which the prescriptive implications for social welfare organizations are based.

THE SUBSYSTEMS

A definition of each organizational subsystem presented in the contingency model follows, along with a description of their interrelationships and examples of applications in a social welfare setting. Each subsystem will be described individually. Kast and Rosenzweig's definitions are elaborated upon and applied to social welfare organizations, followed by a description of the interrelationships among the subsystems in those organizations. The knowledge required for social welfare administration is then categorized according to subsystem, and the administrative skills required for the coordination of the subsystems are identified. Social welfare administrative knowledge, then, is presented here as knowledge of organizational subsystems, and social welfare administrative skills are presented here as the skills required to coordinate those subsystems.

It should be clear that each subsystem has been associated in the past with one or more of the previously mentioned theoretical models of organization. In other words, depending on the writer's theoretical orientation, each subsystem has been identified by one writer or another as the most important dimension of a formal organization. The theoretical orientations which correspond to each subsystem will therefore be included in the descriptions. The contingency approach, as stated above, attempts an integration of these theoretical orientations with the assumption that the influence or importance of a given subsystem is dependent upon the characteristics of the individual organization and the existing constraints, both internal and external, under which it must function.

Figure 8–1 provides an overview of the environmental and subsystem components of social welfare organizations based upon the contingency model.

The *psychosocial subsystem* involves the psychological and social relationship factors affecting the behavior of individual workers and, consequently, the performance of the entire organization. Included in the psychosocial subsystem are personality factors and individual characteristics such as motivation, job satisfaction, anxiety, extroversion, etc. In short, this subsystem is comprised of attitudinal, affective, and interpersonal variables which are not a part of the formal organizational charter or structure and are not generally considered explicitly in formal organizational policy and planning.

The human relations model of organizations, which has provided the basis for most of the psychological research into organizational behavior, has identified the psychosocial sybsystem as the crucial subsystem in determining organizational effectiveness, productivity, efficiency, and survival (Argyris, 1957, 1976; Bennis, 1967; Maslòw, 1943; McGregor, 1957, 1960; Likert, 1961, 1967).

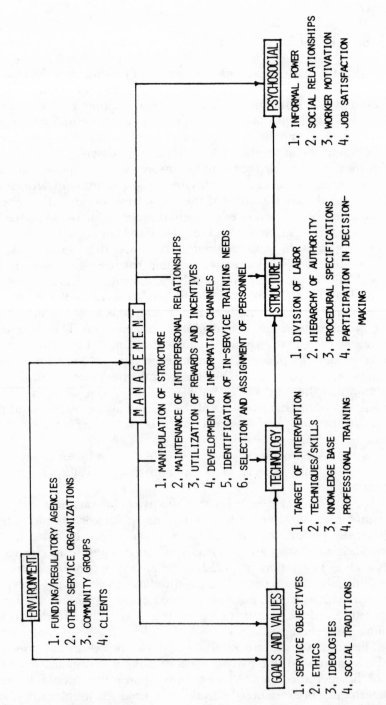

FIGURE 8–1. Environmental and subsystem components of social welfare organizations

While the contingency model relied on here specifies no subsystem as the generally most important, it is recognized that some subsystems may play a more important role in one type of organization than in another. Because the technology of service organizations involves humans attempting to process or change other humans, the psychosocial subsystem consistently plays a primary role in human service organizations. This results from the varied emotional and affective responses to the intense worker-client relationships required in many human service organizations.

In addition to these attitudinal and affective responses, the psychosocial subsystem also includes the informal power structures which evolve through friendships, professional affiliations, shared goals, or the need for a defense against perceived threats from other informal power structures. These informal structures frequently establish hierarchies of authority which are in conflict with those prescribed by the formal structure which is described next. Informal authority within an organization is maintained with the support of an informal structure and is usually expressed in the control of information. Because informal authority has no formal power to actually prescribe procedures, divisions of labor, or decision-making patterns, it is exercised in an organization through the selective sharing of crucial information with other members of a given informal structure.

The *structural subsytem* consists of the formal structure of an organization which can be divided into the broad dimensions of centralization and formalization. The more an organization's structure is centralized and formalized, the more formal control is exercised over work behavior. Centralization and formalization reduce contingencies and increase certainty in the administration of the organization (Thompson, 1967; Glisson & Martin, 1979).

Centralization is defined as the extent to which formal authority and participation in decision-making about planning and policy is confined to a small group. Formalization is defined as the extent to which work procedures are specified in the form of guidelines and the extent to which a division of labor is established which prescribes who is to take responsibility for what duties. The hierarchy of authority, participation in decision-making, procedural specifications, and division of labor can all be determined by management and all, in turn, specify organizational members' interrelationships. The manipulation of centralization and formalization in human service organizations has been shown to directly affect organizational output in terms of productivity and efficiency (Glisson & Martin, 1979).

Rational models of organization such as Weber's (1922) bureaucracy and Taylor's (1916) scientific management traditionally emphasized the structural subsystem as the most potent managerial tool and envisioned the organization as a machine which could be guided and controlled through the proper manipulation of these structural dimensions.

The contingency model, however, includes the structural subsystem in its conceptualization of the organization without overemphasizing its potential for the manager. It is depicted as one of several factors which determine organizational functioning and one which may be effective in some circumstances and ineffective in others.

The *technological subsystem* is an important subsystem within any organization. In social welfare organizations the technology is the knowledge and activities used by workers in processing or changing the recipients of the service. Human service technologies have been characterized as indeterminant because the desired outcomes are intangible and ill-defined, the raw material is variable and unstable, and the knowledge about cause-effect relations in the raw material is incomplete (Hasenfeld & English, 1974, p. 13).

According to the technology model of organization presented by Woodward (1965), Perrow (1967), and others, the technology of an organization defines its structure, so technological indeterminacy would suggest that organizational members who directly work with clients should be given considerable autonomy to handle what is an unprogrammable and unpredictable task.

The dilemma facing the administrator is allowing maximum worker autonomy in solving client problems within the technological subsystem while retaining the degree of control through the structural subsystem that is necessary to coordinate worker activities throughout the organization. Also, the problem of demonstrating the effectiveness of any particular interventive technology increases the administrator's difficulty in selecting the specific repertoire of training and skills desirable in line workers. This problem is sidestepped often by simply emphasizing a specific profession or a specific type of training (i.e., behavioral methods) as the most desirable for a certain position.

The indeterminacy of human service technologies need not prompt the unnecessary routinization of work with clients in satisfying the coordination demands of the organization. While "organizations abhor uncertainty" (Thompson, 1967), the recognition of unpredictable outcomes in working with many target groups enables management to design structures within which line workers may enjoy considerable autonomy. At the same time, the technological indeterminacy emphasizes the fact that management and line workers must also admit the limitations of the incorporated technologies and not assume that increased worker autonomy necessarily leads to increased worker effectiveness. Rather, autonomy must be coupled with evaluative techniques which provide information for documenting and improving the effect of intervention by individual workers or teams. Accountability and autonomy, in other words, can and should coexist in the implementation of an organization's technology (Turem, 1974; Gruber, 1974; Glisson, 1975).

The fourth subsystem consists of the *goals and values* which direct policy, planning, and behavior at all levels of the organization. Although the label "subsystem" seems to be somewhat of a misnomer for goals and values, Simon's (1964) definition of goals as a "set of constraints" within which choices are made helps one to view goals and values as part of a "system." Constraints, or limitations, are placed on the activities of organizations delivering services by professionals, clients, the community, and funders. These constraints vary according to time and place and also vary in the intensity of sanctions elicited when the constraints are not heeded. These constraints may be based on ethics, religion, morals, treatment theories, professional ideologies, tradition, or politics and may be either flexible or impervious to change. They may be supported from within the organization at any level or from the environment. If, then, a set of constraints are described for a specific organization in terms of the origin of support groups, their flexibility, and the intensities of related sanctions, a system is delineated within which the organization must work in defining activities and objectives. This is a boundary system which effectively fences off the territory to which the organization has access. Some of the fences are easily penetrated but others are laid in stone.

The set of constraints limits permissible solutions to individual client problems as well as to organizational planning and policy. An administrator's awareness of these constraints is necessary whether the organization chooses to change them or abide by them, for such systems guide funding legislation, professional training, community support, and the utilization of services by the specific target group. In short, this subsystem, as much as any other, has the potential for determining an organization's survival regardless of a target group's needs and the organization's effectiveness in meeting them.

THE ENVIRONMENTAL SUPRASYSTEM

In addition to the subsystems comprising the organization, the organization is a subsystem of its *environment* which is made up of other social systems. The social systems in the environment having the most impact on the organization are other organizations (Terreberry, 1968), specifically, those which fund and legitimate the organization's activities as well as those with whom services must be coordinated. Other significant elements in the organization's environment include the organization's clients and interested community groups.

The environmental model of organization presents the environment as *the* determinant of an organization's survival (Emery & Trist, 1965; Lawrence & Lorsch, 1969; Meyer 1978). It emphasizes the impact of the availability of resources and legitimation independent of organizational efforts to obtain them. In other words, the organization is depicted as having little effect on the environment although the environment is interpreted as having a major effect on the organization. In contrast, the contingency model presents the relationship between organization and environment as reciprocal, and suggests that an organization may have the potential for determining its own survival as well as for changing its environment. At times the organization is more potent though at other times the environment is more potent, depending on the issue and the characteristics of the particular organization.

INTERRELATIONSHIPS AMONG SUBSYSTEMS AND THE SUPRASYSTEM

Now that four organizational subsystems and the suprasystem in which the organization exists have been described, attention is turned to the interrelationships among the subsystems and the suprasystem and the coordination of those relationships through the administration of the service delivery system. Administrative coordination necessarily overlaps all subsystems as well as the environment and has been labeled the *managerial subsystem* by Kast and Rosenzweig (1973), making a total of five subsystems comprising the organization. The managerial subsystem is used to "co-align" (Thompson, 1967, p. 147) the other four subsystems so that they are mutually complementary and supportive. Co-alignment requires a repertoire of administrative skills which includes the ability to properly manipulate formal structure, the maintenance of positive interpersonal relationships among organizational members, the utilization of rewards and incentives to guide work behavior, the development of organizational channels through which information can be efficiently shared, the identification of in-service training needs to support program objectives, and the appropriate selection and assignment of personnel to assume organizational roles. While this is obviously not a complete list of all skills required of an administrator, these are key skills and will be used to provide examples of administrative co-alignment.

Following Figure 8–1, subsystem and suprasystem interrelationships will be examined along with examples of the application of administrative skills to facilitate organizational survival and effectiveness. Figure 8–1 shows the environment as directly affecting the goals and values and the management subsystems of the organization. It also shows management as directly affecting the other four subsystems, the goals and values as affecting the technology, the technology as affecting the structure, and the structure as affecting the psychosocial subsystem. This particular causal conceptualization of the subsystem interrelationships represents an ideal for organization design and planning, and will provide a format for the discussion of administrative skills.

The importance of the environment in determining organizational effectiveness and survival has been increasingly recognized (Lawrence & Lorsch, 1967; Terreberry, 1968; Meyer, 1978). It directly or indirectly affects all organizational subsystems, but perhaps has the greatest effect on the goals and values of an organization. The funders, clients, and community each place constraints on the organization in terms of goal priorities and permissible approaches to meeting those goals. An administrator must express the goals and values of the organization to its environment in a manner compatible with expectations of funding/regulatory agencies, other related service organizations, and interested community groups, as well as the clients who are to benefit from the service provided by the organization. The administrator must frequently rely on interpersonal and communication skills in effectively expressing the organization's goals. In addition, the selection and channeling of crucial information regarding the organization's activities to various environmental components is an invaluable administrative tool for presenting the organization's goals and values in a positive light.

The goals and values, in turn, have an impact on the other organizational subsystems. Both the target of the intervention and the type of techniques used in the intervention, i.e., dimensions of the technological subsystem, are determined to a major extent by the organization's goals and values. For example, if an organization's goal is to broaden the elderly's use of existing community resources, then skills in urban planning, community organization, and advocacy, in adddition to a knowledge of available community resources for the aging, become crucial to successful intervention. The major administrative skills required for successfully co-aligning the organization's technology with its goals and values are the appropriate selection and assignment of personnel and the ability to identify in-service training needs. That is, an administrator must be able to hire line workers with interventive techniques, the knowledge base, and the professional training that support the service objectives, ethics, treatment ideologies, and social traditions which guide the work of the organization.

Because they attempt to process or change human beings, service organizations face environmental constraints determined more by morals, ethics, and values than those within which their counterparts in business and industry must function. In social welfare services, the demands for productivity, effectiveness, and efficiency may conflict with demands for humane treatment, attention to the individuality of client problems, and the client's right to self-determination. The options for changing or processing people face value constraints not encountered with nonhuman raw material.

The environment exerts influence on social service organizations in another unique way. Clients carry information into and out of the technological subsystem, establishing a link between the technical core of the organization and the environment. It is difficult for line workers in human service organizations to be unaware of environmental variables which affect the delivery of services to clients. While mechanisms can be established which partially buffer line workers by controlling the number and type of clients seen by particular workers or by facilitating referrals to other agencies, social workers are necessarily involved in the maintenance of those mechanisms, usually know how well they are working, and may suggest changes for their improvement.

Technologies which incorporate activities and approaches dependent upon feedback from the raw material itself have been labeled "intensive" by Thompson (1967). He argues that organizations incorporating such technologies must be coordinated through mutual adjustment rather than through standardization. This follows March and Simon's (1958) notion that the method of coordination must be matched with the type of work and that the more unpredictable the technical work is, the more feedback information must be transmitted during the action on the raw material to guide further action. These ideas suggest that characteristics of the technological subsystem should determine characteristics of the structural subsystem if an organization is to function adequately. Perrow's (1967) framework stipulating that nonroutinized technologies require high worker discretion establishes an even more specific relationship between technology and structural design. Based on Perrow's model, organizations delivering social welfare services would be expected to allow considerable line worker discretion through a noncentralized and nonformalized structure. The fact that this does not always exist indicates inadequacies in the administrative designation of divisions of labor, procedural specifications, the hierarchy of authority, and the participation in decision-making.

It has been shown that an inadequate structure may restrict worker discretion and thereby contribute to the routinization of the incorporated human service technology (Glisson, 1978). For example, a social welfare organization which implements a centralized and formalized structure emphasizes control of worker activities, resulting in systematic approaches to working with clients. In other words, the structure actually implemented by management places constraints on the social worker's behavior which affect how the social worker perceives clients and the interventive methodologies utilized. It is crucial, then, that the structural subsystem complements the technological subsystem to insure the optimal utilization of technological knowledge and skill. A less formalized and less centralized structural subsystem is the most appropriate for human service technologies because of the need for worker responsiveness to unexpected client characteristics and because of the absence of consistent client reactions to intervention.

The intervention technologies envisioned by management as appropriate for the goals and values within which the organization must work should therefore determine the structural characteristics of the organization. If the roles of community organizer and direct service worker are to be assumed by the same worker, for example, a less formalized division of labor is crucial to the proper performance of that job. If community organization is identified as an appropriate function for a worker, few required procedural specifications should be developed to guide the worker in that role. If the organization identifies urban planning as an appropriate strategy for workers seeking to affect change in existing public service systems, then line worker participation in organizational decision-making is essential for the organization to be responsive to the ongoing identification of service deficits in the community. And, finally, a decentralized hierarchy of authority is required in an organization which proposes that its social workers become advocates for its clients because a social worker must have the authority to act independently to be effective as an advocate.

The above are examples of how organizational structure reflects the management's view of the appropriate interventive technologies and the goals and values underlying the technologies. Each of the four dimensions of structure—hierarchy of authority, participation in decision-making, procedural specifications, and division of labor—are developed by management to support the technology. The structure of an organization, in short, reveals the organization's philosophy of intervention and the goals and values within which it is attempting to function (Perrow, 1961).

The structure of the organization has an impact on the psychosocial subsystem by encouraging or hindering the development of informal authority structures, by providing opportunities for social relationships, and by influencing the motivation and job satisfaction of individual workers (Vroom & Deci, 1972; Likert, 1967). As explained earlier, the control of information provides the basis for informal power in an organization. To the extent that the organization is centralized, the opportunity for information control exists because *access* is limited. The centralization of authority and decision-making means, in effect, that crucial information is in the hands of a few individuals. The scarcity of the commodity (information) makes it valuable and places power in the hands of those who have access to it. Although the formal structure supposedly dictates who does and who does not have access, information becomes, in effect, contraband, and is illicitly dealt within the organization distributing power in decreasing portion as it passes from person to person. Informal authority and power in an organization can therefore be expected to exist in proportion to the extent to which the organization is centralized.

The formalization of both procedures and divisions of labor within the organization also provides the opportunity for informal power structures to develop. The segregation of worker roles and activities prompts the development of intra-organizational allegiances according to the job performed or procedures followed in the organization. In addition, it has been found that highly formalized structures curtail worker motivation and satisfaction in service roles because of the limitations placed on their activities. Informal structure then becomes a resource for supporting and expanding an individual's influence beyond that specified by the formal structure. It is also important to note, however, that the lack of centralization and formalization of structure results in frustration for workers attempting to accomplish job tasks (Anderson, 1979). Structure, in short, supplies guidelines for worker interaction as well as limitations to worker behavior.

In addition to the appropriate manipulation of formal structure, an administrator may also use rewards and incentives to maintain motivation and satisfaction among organizational members. These may be promotions, titles, office space, secretarial support, commendations, salary increases, or any formal recognition of performance or additional resource allocation to the individual.

The above examples of subsystem interrelationships within a service organization demonstrate the variety and complexity of possible organizational profiles confronting the administrator. This underlines the contingency model's major thesis that the determination of appropriate administrative action is dependent upon the specific organization and its current situation. The environment and each subsystem must be assessed before any action is taken and action must be undertaken with the understanding that the environment and each subsystem may be affected by that action.

While past research has provided information about the nature of subsystem interrelationships among some types of organizations, additional research is especially needed in the social welfare area if valid descriptive models are to be developed which can guide an administrator in improving specific service systems. In other words, prescriptive or normative suggestions must be based upon descriptive models establishing relationships between variables in the various subsystems before profiles of particular organizations can be used to determine effective administration behavior (Glisson, 1979). Just as a family therapist bases the unique intervention plan for a specific family on an understanding of a general model of family dynamics, an administrator must also be able to rely on a valid model of organizational dynamics in determining which skills to use when co-aligning subsystems.

EDUCATIONAL IMPLICATIONS OF THE MODEL

The contingency model presented above provides the basis for organizing social welfare administrative practice knowledge around subsystem and environmental categories. Administrative skills are defined as the components of the managerial subsystem required to coalign the other subsystems. Administrative practice knowledge related to service objectives, ethics, ideologies, and social traditions is categorized under the goals and values subsystem; knowledge of the target population, interventive techniques and skills, theoretical base of the intervention, and professional training is categorized under the technological subsystem; knowledge of the division of labor, hierarchy of authority, procedural specifications guiding worker interrelationships, and decision-making within service organizations is categorized under the structural subsystem; knowledge of informal power, social relationships, worker motivation, and job satisfaction is categorized under the psychosocial subsystem; and knowledge of funding/regulatory agencies, other relevant service organizations, the community as a social system, and the clients as a community subgroup is categorized under the environmental system. The skills of maintaining interpersonal working relationships, developing information channels, identifying in-service training needs, utilizing rewards and incentives, selecting and assigning personnel, and appropriately manipulating formal structure are categorized under the managerial subsystem, which must insure coordination and cooperation among the other subsytems and between the organization and the environment.

The competent administrator must be knowledgeable of subsystem components for a specific organization and must conceptualize their interrelationships and be able to apply the skills required to insure coordination. Competency criteria developed for the administration of a particular type of service system (services delivered to children, for example), would be dependent upon the model's application to that system. The knowledge and skills to be taught in an educational program, therefore, can be developed in sequence as presented in the management model. That is, the program's view of the environment is developed first, followed by the development of criteria in the goals and values, technological, structural, and psychosocial subsystems. The result is a comprehensive description of all components affecting the delivery of services in some practice area such as child welfare. Specific information defined for each component in each subsystem and in the environment comprises the minimum knowledge necessary for competent program administration in that practice area. The managerial skills are more global and can be generalized to a variety of practice areas.

In summary, the application of the contingency model of organization and management to social welfare administration provides a conceptual framework for structuring existing administrative-practice knowledge. The framework can also be used to develop competency criteria to guide training in specialized areas. The paper has outlined the following distinct advantages to using the contingency model as a framework for organizing administrative-practice knowledge. It presents a holistic perspective of organizational theory encompassing the major theoretical models of organization, and it provides a basis for establishing the unique dimensions of organizations which deliver services to human beings. The contingency model has emerged from general systems theory and is therefore easily integrated into other theoretical models of social work practice. Finally, the contingency model is dependent upon research for further development, thus providing a basis for social work input into the refinement of the model and into its application to existing service delivery systems.

REFERENCES

Anderson, W. A. *Conflict and congruity between bureaucracy and professionalism: Alienation outcomes among social service workers.* Unpublished doctoral dissertation, Florida State University, 1977.

Argyris, C. The individual and organization: Some problems of mutual adjustment. *Administrative Science Quarterly,* 1957, *2,* 1–24.

Bennis, W. Organizations of the future. *Personnel Administration,* 1967, *30,* 6–19.

Bennis, W. *Organizational development.* Reading, MA: Addison-Wesley, 1969.

Cyert, R. M., & March, J. G. *A behavioral theory of the firm.* Englewood Cliffs, NJ: Prentice Hall, 1963.

Dumpson, J. R., Mullen, E. J., & First, R. J. *Toward education for effective social welfare administrative practice.* New York: Council on Social Work Education, 1978.

Emery, F. E., & Trist, E. L. The causal texture of organizational environments. *Human Relations,* 1965, *18,* 21–32.

Glisson, C. A., The accountability controversy. *Social Work,* 1975, *20,* 417–419.

Glisson, C. A. Dependence of technological routinization on structural variables in human service organizations. *Administrative Science Quarterly,* 1978, *23,* 383–395.

Glisson, C. A. In defense of determinism. *OMEGA, The International Journal of Management Science,* 1979, *7,* 8–9.

Glisson, C. A., & Martin, P. Y. Productivity and efficiency in human service organizations as related to structure, size and age. *Academy of Management Journal*, 1980, *23*, 21–37.

Gouldner, A. *Patterns of industrial bureaucracy.* New York: The Free Press, 1954.

Gruber, M. Total administration. *Social Work*, 1974, *19*, 625–637.

Hasenfeld, Y., & English, R. A. (Eds.). *Human service organizations.* Ann Arbor: The University of Michigan Press, 1974.

Kast, F. E., & Rosenzweig, J. E. *Contingency views of organization and management.* Chicago: Science Research Associates, 1973.

Katz, D., & Kahn, R. L. *The social psychology of organizations.* New York: John Wiley & Sons, 1966.

Lawrence, P. R., & Lorsch, J. W. *Organization and environment.* Homewood, IL: Richard D. Irwin, 1969.

Likert, R. *New patterns of management.* New York: McGraw-Hill, 1961.

Likert, R. *The human organization.* New York: McGraw-Hill, 1967.

March, J., & Simon, H. *Organizations.* New York: John Wiley & Sons, 1958.

Maslow, A. H. Theory of human motivation. *Psychological Review*, 1943, *50*, 370–396.

McGregor, D. M. The human side of enterprise. In W. E. Natimeyer (Ed.), *Classics of organizational behavior.* Oak Park, IL: Moore Publishing, 1978. Originally published in *Management Review*, November 1957.

McGregor, D. M. *The human side of enterprise.* New York: McGraw-Hill, 1960.

Meyer, M. W. (Ed.). *Environments and organizations.* San Francisco: Jossey-Bass, 1978.

Perrow, C. The analysis of goals in complex organizations. *American Sociological Review*, 1961, *26*, 856–866.

Perrow, C. A framework for the comparative analysis of organizations. *American Sociological Review*, 1967, *32*, 194–208.

Simon, H. A. *Administrative behavior.* New York: The Free Press, 1945.

Simon, H. A. On the concept of organizational goal. *Administrative Science Quarterly*, 1964, *9*, 1–22.

Taylor, F. W. The principles of scientific management. In J. M. Shafritz & P. H. Whitlock (Eds.), *Classics of organization theory.* Oak Park, IL: Moore Publishing, 1978. Originally published in the *Bulletin of the Taylor Society*, December 1916.

Terreberry, S. The evolution of organizational environments. *Administrative Science Quarterly*, 1968, *12*, 590–613.

Thompson, J. D. *Organizations in action.* New York: McGraw-Hill, 1967.

Turem, J. The call for a management stance. *Social Work*, 1974, *19*, 615–628.

Vroom, V. H., & Deci, E. L. *Management and motivation.* Baltimore: Penguin Books, 1970.

Weber, M. *The theory of social and economic organizations* (translated by K. Morris). New York: Harper and Row, 1942. (Original German published in 1922.)

Woodward, J. *Industrial organization: Theory and practice.* London: Oxford University Press, 1965.

PART III

The Structure and Uses of Authority

Editor's Introduction

Social agencies in the United States have evolved a particular and distinctive form of governance. This system of social government establishes organizational authority that is directed to engineering compliance on the part of organizational members and participants, thus assuring organizational stability. Inherent in the working of agencies is a political process in which power relationships and decision-making mechanisms are defined and channeled. The essential bases of sanction and legitimacy of social agencies are several, but always include a legal or legislative source. Voluntary agencies are subject to laws governing membership corporations, their charters specifying rules of organizational conduct. Public agencies providing social services have their origins in legislative enactments or administrative action, and conform to regulations established by public authority.

Although ultimate social agency authority inheres in the board of directors, there is a parallel system of authority that organizes the actual service-giving and that defines the relationship between higher and lower participants in the agency's professional and staff structure. Thus a general system of parallel governance exists, establishing both lay and professional authority. The one consists of board members, officers, committees, the other of executives, associates, and staff. Each is guided by its own distinctive functions and traditions and each is necessarily attached to the other in a symbiotic relationship that makes possible the achievement of organizational objectives.

There is a substantial void in the administrative and research literature on the functioning of boards, on the particular organizational forms that are most conducive to effective work, on the relationship between board leadership and membership, and on the extent to which the traditional views of board prerogatives are operationally verified. Much more has been done with respect to the ways in which professional personnel function in organizations, their styles of work, their motivation, and the supervisory relationships that guide their professional behaviors.

The conventional rhetoric suggests that, in general, boards of directors establish the policies that guide the staff in their service-giving performance—the one establishing direction, the other operationalizing. Practicing administrators know from their experience that the very process in which executives and their staffs provide the essential materials to the board for such determination, in fact, gives them enormous power to skew policy in one direction or another, by the very selection they make of these materials. Experience also suggests that the very act of implementation of policy can enlarge, diminish, or distort the intent of policymakers. Identical policies often yield contradictory outcomes.

There is an appropriate distinction to be made between the relevant actions expected of boards on the one hand and professional staffs on the other. Permeable though they may be, boundaries of authority and responsibility are implicit in the way social agencies go about their business in the context of a democratic, free-enterprise culture. Some of the boundary prescriptions are legally defined, others flow from the tradition and inherent logic of organizational requirements. Thus boards of directors establish the legal entity and legitimacy of the organization; establish and maintain financial integrity, solvency, and accountability; engage and evaluate the chief executive officer; manage financial investments; establish personnel policies; serve as advocates for the organization and its services; serve as communication links between the relevant community and the agency; and establish and monitor the organization's broad policies and goals.

By contrast, executive authority is directed largely to the requirements of service provision, and to the internal and external relationships that impinge on the service. It is preoccupied with engaging personnel; allocation of roles; supervision and evaluation of performance; establishing standards of work; coordinating human and material resources; preparation of budgets and reports; maintenance of records; managing organizational maintenance requirements; managing conflict and tension; and providing professional direction to staff and informed leadership to the board.

The real skill of administrative leadership is seen in the ways in which these inherent functions and responsibilities are discharged by the parallel and coordinate channels of authority, all with respect to fulfilling the organization's purposes and objectives and maintaining the integrity of the service and the organization's response to clients' needs. While the lines of authority are parallel, every relevant level requires explicit attachments one to the other. Thus staff executive and board president inevitably develop a pattern of coordinate work that ultimately provides guidance to their respective constituencies and to the organization as a whole. Presidential authority extends through the lay structure of committees and chairpeople, just as executive authority extends through the professional staff system. These structures are perforce joined by the coordinate activity of committee and staff leadership, each accountable inherently to one another and, explicitly, to their respective structures.

A persistent problem encountered by administrators grows out of the confusion of lay and professional roles, and the resultant conflict that follows upon role invasion. The assumption of authority and behavior inappropriate to one's realm of action inevitably leads to issues of turf and propriety and tends to become organizationally disruptive. Thus, board-executive and board-staff relationships represent important aspects of competent organizational behavior.

A. GOVERNING BOARDS

Selections in this section deal with the place of boards of directors in social agency administration. Mitton describes a particular structure of board committee work—what he calls a matrix type—based on the essential functions of the board and the primary program areas of the agency. He reviews the process pursued by an organization as it sought to make maximal use of the special talents of board members and promote committed involvement. A dual-purpose committee structure was established, according to which each board member belonged to a service or treatment delivery committee as well as to a committee concerned with some functional organizational requirement, such as finance or personnel.

Robins and Blackburn present a study of governing boards of community mental health centers, guided by their postulate that it is necessary to differentiate the effectiveness areas of board members from the effectiveness areas of professional staff. They locate the key to such differentiation in the distinction between program and process objectives, the former concerned with such matters as treatment, disability limitation, rehabilitation; the latter with items such as community responsiveness, availability of services, increasing community support. Whether or not one approves of the specific criteria given, the exercise in differential analysis and the classification of process objectives and variables for measuring citizen boards are most useful.

B. EXECUTIVE AUTHORITY

The selections in this section deal with the exercise of executive authority. They focus largely on internal communication processes, on the engineering of organizational compliance, and on administrative styles. Many administrators find this aspect of their work the most problematic. Authority is clearly lodged in the position of chief executive, but there are constraints that circumscribe the free play of authority. Executives quickly learn that they can rarely rule by fiat, but need to engender consent on the part of organization participants. How administrative behavior is shaped in response to organizational demands, managerial judgment, and decisional challenges shape an executive's administrative style. The debate as to whether there is one preferred approach (Blake & Mouton, 1982) or whether style is situationally defined (Reddin, 1970) has been vigorously engaged. Issues underlying this discussion are pursued in the following selections.

Berg explores the various leadership styles in social agencies, and suggests that pressures both internal to the organization and in the organizational environment make their impact on individual predilections. Administrators fashion their approaches in a field of forces that are frequently turbulent. Personal needs and motivations of executives may or may not make a "good fit" with particular organizational needs, whether for stability and consolidation or for change, growth, and development. Berg locates four styles of leadership utilizing two major constructs—orientation (proactive or reactive) and professional identification. The appropriateness of style in any particular situation can then be readily determined.

Russell et al. report the results of an empirically based research study that explored various administrative styles of social work supervisors. The research tools used were based on the managerial grid developed by Blake and Mouton. Concern for production and concern for people define alternative and interacting approaches to fashioning administrative styles. The polar opposites, laissez-faire (1,1) and cooperative team management (9,9) have their counterparts in styles of supervision. Suggestions to move from the least desirable (1,1) to the most desirable (9,9) patterns flow from the analysis, and deal with team management, personnel policies, training, communication, and evaluation.

Kotin and Sharaf use an analysis of bureaucratic succession in a mental health agency to highlight the concept of administrative style. This is defined as the executive's professional behavior in structuring his or her role and in influencing the roles and functioning of others in the organization. In exploring *how* the executive does this, they pose two polar types, "loose" and "tight," and review the virtues and shortcomings of each in the context of a particular experience in leadership change, where issues of authority, consensus, conflict, and change inevitably intruded. They conclude that executive effectiveness depends upon an appropriate fit between an incumbent's administrative style and the needs of the organization at a given time. In a 1974 postscript to their original 1967 article, the authors ponder the effect of decentralization on their early formulations, and suggest areas for future study of succession, style, and organizational structure.

C. BOARD-EXECUTIVE RELATIONSHIPS

The ways in which the two systems of authority intersect and interact is addressed by the selections in this section. Stein looks at some realities that surround this relationship, in the course of which he examines the motivation of trustees, responsibilities of board and executive in relation to establishing agency policies, issues in the evaluation of the executive by the board, the informal structure of power of boards, board-staff relationships, and the important issue of the responsibility of voluntary and public agency boards to respond to social welfare issues, particularly those which contain elements of controversy.

Levin discusses the current "crisis" in board-executive relationships, and reviews in historic context the patterns of conflict that have evolved over the decades. Although perceptions of overlapping functions frequently engender differences and antagonisms, questions of relative power and control of agency activities serve covert interests. Recent developments in the social and political environment affect funding sources and create new constituencies for board participation. In some ways it has become more difficult to locate meaningful activity for trustees. Executives are cautioned to view this arena of activity with care. Strong boards make for strong agencies and strong executives.

D. MINORITY AND FEMALE EXECUTIVES

Much attention has been paid during the past decade to the special problems faced by minority and female administrators in the human services. Similar developments have been noted in the general field of management. Not only has the literature, particularly about the female executive, been fairly extensive, but many more members of these groups have moved into managerial responsibility, albeit frequently into middle-management roles. It seems apparent that the social movements of the sixties and the seventies with their legal, economic, and political concomitants have created a new personnel resource for administrative skill.

Although Herbert discusses the administrative processes of government, his argument and observations are as relevant to the voluntary social service system. After reviewing the data on federal minority employment rates and the modest extent to which minority members are located in administrative posts (even in social programs, where they tend to do best), Herbert examines the multiple role demands and dilemmas confronting minority administrators. He suggests that two basic and difficult questions inevitably call for response: responsibility to minority group people and responsibility to the needs of all the people. In negotiating this hazardous terrain, Herbert rejects value neutrality in implementing policy decisions and makes the case for the necessity to research, develop, and articulate minority group perspectives on public policy questions.

Chernesky discusses the difficulty women have encountered in entering the managerial ranks and reviews the evidence concerning sex differences in group and organizational behavior. Women who are the sole representative of their sex in a male-dominated hierarchy face severe challenges, and are often constrained to adapt to an unsympathetic organizational culture. Fashioning a leadership style that makes for a good fit between organizational demands and patterns of female socialization represents a major challenge. Dealing constructively with these strains remains an important arena for further study and experience.

The dilemmas faced by women and minority executives come together in the instance of the Latina social service administrator. Here a three-way confluence of forces is at play. The Latina struggles as a member of a minority group, as a woman in a male-dominated American culture, and as a Hispanic subject to traditional views of women in that culture. Rincon and Keys discuss the barriers to socializing a Latina into traditional male-dominated managerial roles. They review the developmental tasks necessary to accomplish this transformation, as well as several recurrent themes that underlie this effort.

E. PARTICIPATION IN EXECUTIVE MANAGEMENT

One key to successful management lies in the ways in which executive authority and decision making is shared with organization participants. Such sharing can involve staff members at all points in the hierarchy—direct practitioners, supervisors, department heads—as well as client and ex-client groups. Participatory management is increasingly extolled in business and industry, stimulated by successful experiences in Japan, with its quality circles and theory Z philosophy. Although a participatory orientation is hardly foreign to social work practice, practical problems attend many efforts in this direction. It is generally recognized that participation must be relevant to the tasks at hand and involve people with a significant stake in the consequences of decisions made and activities taken. Productive participation also depends on the possession of relevant knowledge and skill.

Issues bearing on these matters are addressed by the selections in this section. Fallon reviews the experience of two social agencies that were introduced to a new participatory management pattern of democratic decision making. Some characteristics of this process and the essential constraints and limitations that invariably follow are detailed. A study of perceptions and attitudes toward management orientation in one agency is reported. A strong desire by the staff for participatory management as opposed to exploitive-authoritarian, benevolent-authoritarian, or consultative patterns was indicated.

Client participation in the delivery of mental health services is the subject of Kopolow's article. He sees the potential value of establishing self-help programs in the day-to-day operations of community mental health centers. Among the benefits of well-conceived client involvement are enhanced motivation, reduced resistance to treatment, increased self-esteem, and recovery optimism. Diminished cost, improved outreach, and significant advocacy action are also potential gains. A variety of ex-patient operations, both independently and collaboratively organized, are reviewed. Some are concerned with human and legal rights of patients, others deal with mutual support and aftercare, but all suggest that the client group can become an important community resource.

Weatherley analyzes the experience of a state public welfare agency in developing a series of changes in the delivery of social services using participatory techniques that involved frontline staff. Staff were generally eager to have a voice in shaping policies and procedures that governed their work; however, a number of constraints inherent in the public bureaucracy limited the potentialities for effective participation. Suggestions to overcome these difficulties are offered by the author.

REFERENCES

Blake, Robert R. and Mouton, Jane S. A comparative analysis of situationalism and 9,9 management by principle, *Organizational Dynamics*, Spring, 1982.
Reddin, William J. *Managerial effectiveness*. New York: McGraw-Hill, 1970.

9

Utilizing the Board of Trustees: A Unique Structural Design

DARYL G. MITTON

The board of trustees is charged with the general stewardship of the agency. The specific professional expertise and directorship of the administrator must be combined with the diversified talents of the board. A balanced and objective board and a capable director have to interact with each other.

But how can board members become acquainted with agency operations and staff? How do they tune in on current attitudes or catch the spirit of the agency? How do they sense the psychological, sociological and physiological impact of the total program and the impact of the aura of the physical facility itself?

Further, how can one design a system that will elicit board members' talent in a manner consistent with their usual talent delivery, so as to utilize their skills effectively and foster greater enthusiasm and commitment to service?

These are questions all private agencies ask themselves over and over again. The agency of which I am a board member, the San Diego Children's Home Association, like many other agencies, has sought answers.

The agency conscientiously screens its board nominees for applicable talent and for representation and commitment. The nominees are familiarized with the general service performed and with the agency itself through selected literature and reports—the history of the agency, its bylaws, long-range plans, budget, programs, newsletters, current board membership, sample case histories and periodicals or articles relevant to agency approach. In addition, they are requested to spend 4 hours on 2 separate days in agency indoctrination—observing staff meetings, lunching with staff and children, observing ongoing programs, getting acquainted with intake procedures and meeting staff personnel.

THE USUAL TRAP

In the past, the agency has been extremely sensitive to its continually changing programs and new developments. Accordingly, much board meeting time was devoted to staff reports and demonstrations of ongoing projects—so much so that the board found itself spending all its meeting time validating administrative actions and just trying to keep abreast of agency changes. But regardless of staff diligence in keeping the board informed, the information always seemed peripheral and noninvolving.

The committees of the board operated in somewhat the same way. They were only sporadically active, with major initiation and input coming from staff. Substantive board input was largely limited to individual board member performance in contributing to specific problems—fiscal interpretation, endowment investment advice, obtaining financial support, etc. It is not without significance that all the examples cited are in the fiscal area. Traditionally, if board members have any clout, it's here. But this leaves areas of agency concern (improved client care, needed community service, agency administration effectiveness, etc.) untouched by board talent.

A BREAKTHROUGH IN APPROACH

Several years ago, a particular circumstance involving minority representation brought realization to the board that its abilities could be tapped in a more creative way. The administration and staff, anticipating community and governmental pressure for affirmative action, initiated the formulation by the board of an affirmative action statement and policy. The board recognized the worth of the suggestion and set itself to the task.

The nominating committee did not have to wait for the setting of specific policy to recommend talented minority nominees to fill recurrent board vacancies. Population parity in board representation was reached quickly. All the members were concerned about the problem, understood its ramifications and worked on it with skill and zeal. The

Personnel and Service Committee roughed out the initial draft. It was received and adjusted by the Executive Committee and forwarded to an ad hoc Minority Committee comprising both board and staff. Again the draft was reviewed by the Executive Committee and sent to an ad hoc Legal Committee, then back to a joint committee review and to the board for final review and adoption. Not only was an excellent document produced, but the involvement of board and staff was outstanding. Policy formulation and policy implementation within the agency were achieved simultaneously. Board, administration and staff worked together for a significant accomplishment.

ANOTHER BREAK

More recently the board found itself in another interesting circumstance. Consultants from the Human Interaction Research Institute, operating on a grant from the Office of Child Development of the Bureau of Social Rehabilitation Services of the Department of Health, Education and Welfare, were making a pilot study using the agency. They hoped to develop, demonstrate and make available strategies, intervention models and tools to improve the operational effectiveness of child development agencies.

The agency board invited the consultants to observe it in action, and out of this grew a program of self-examination and realignment. The board examined its interpretation of board objectives, and the individual members' interpretation of board worth and potential use to the agency. The self-analysis revealed the usual frustration resulting from a desire to serve and the helplessness of being underutilized in a ritualistic, validating manner.

An ad hoc committee was set up to study board structure and function, and eventually developed a structural design that serves both as a system of information gathering and education and as a system of emitting functional information and action.

INFORMATION-GATHERING COMMITTEES

The global overview of the agency and the board members' role revealed an urgent need for a more specific understanding of the many services the agency was performing. Gradual change and adjustment had made the agency a full-fledged, multiservice organization. But the ramifications of this change had not been acted upon, and questions went unanswered. For example: What were the overt and subtle differences in the treatment programs? What really determined these differences—client need, financial necessity or agency talent and inclination? What treatment mix best suits community needs? What treatment deserves what agency priority? What unique problems do the treatment units have?

Accordingly the board determined to set up committees related to each service or treatment unit in the agency: Residential (24 hours, 7 days a week therapy); Day (8 hours, 5 days a week special education and treatment); Satellite (24 hours, 7 days a week community treatment units); and Outreach (day care, consortium and cooperative efforts with other community, public and private agencies, pilot programs). The board felt that this type of committee setup would allow it to address directly the complex of changes in treatment patterns continually evolving within the agency. Experience has proved this to be the case. This committee structure allows for information gathering with a problem orientation. It involves the members and provides specific and utilitarian input to the board. The approach is worth consideration by any multiservice agency.

FUNCTION-EMITTING COMMITTEES

Up to this point, the board had been operating with traditional functional committees. It was decided the board needed policy-formulating, action-oriented committees, but with an emphasis on function and a makeup somewhat different than before. The obvious question was asked: What needs doing?

Pursuit of the obvious provided significant results. Functional committees matched to basic functional agency needs were set up—a structure applicable to most agencies in public service. The committees are: Finance (for getting, allocating, monitoring the utilization and management of funds); Service Appraisal (for determining community needs, reviewing programs and determining service effectiveness—the degree to which the agency is treating or merely warehousing children); Personnel (for establishing and monitoring personnel policies and practices); Management Audit (for reviewing agency operation and performance, appraising administrative structure and procedure, and monitoring resource utilization); Policy Review (for providing legal expertise and interpretation and legislative guidance, and updating bylaws).

There is also an Executive Committee, which functions in the absence of the board and addresses itself to long-range strategy and planning and public relations. In addition, there are a Nominating Committee, for recruiting and screening potential members and preparing slates of future officers, and an Affirmative Action Committee, made up of both board and staff members, to monitor minority-population parity throughout the agency.

A MATRIX ORGANIZATION

With this enlarged and dual-purpose committee structure, the board looked for some way to combine and tap effectively the information-gathering and function-emitting services. What was evolved is essentially a matrix-type organization structure applied to the board itself. Each board member is automatically a member of at least two committees—one oriented toward service or treatment delivery, the other toward a functional requirement. The concept of the matrix plan was to set up a system by which board members could achieve immediate involvement and learn about the agency while playing an active role, rather than learning about the agency and then trying to do something.

The board structure is depicted in Table 9–1. Each square in the grid represents a member. The vertical dimension determines the member's service or treatment committee designation. The horizontal dimension determines his functional committee.

In the assignments for the various committees, all board members were asked to indicate their first, second and third choice of combina-

TABLE 9–1. The Board's Matrix Organization

Service Function	Residential	Day	Satellite	Outreach
Finance	Member A[a]	Member F[b]	Member K[b]	Member P[c]
Service appraisal	Member B[d]	Member G[a]	Member L[c]	Member Q[b]
Personnel	Member C[b]	Member H[c]	Member M[d]	Member R[a]
Management audit	Member D[c]	Member I (V.P.)	Member N[b]	Member S[d]
Policy review	Member E[b]	Member J[d]	Member O[a]	Member T[e]

[a] Chairman, Service Committee
[b] Vice Chairman, Function Committee
[c] Vice Chairman, Service Committee
[d] Chairman, Function Committee
[e] Group Coordinator, Service Committees
(Note: Chairmanship slots vary from year to year, depending upon talents and interests. All 21 board members are in some form of leadership capacity.)

Executive Committee: President, Vice President and all chairmen of Function Committees ([d]) and the service Group Coordinator ([e])

Nominating Committee: Vice Chairmen of Function Committees ([b])

tions of committees to serve on. There was a variety of interests wide enough so that in all but about three instances (on a 21-member board) it was possible to comply with first requests.

After the member assignments were made, a chairman and a vice chairman for each of the treatment service committees and for each of the functional committees were designated. Under the setup, each member of the board acts in some leadership capacity. As shown in Table 9–1, Member A is chairman of the Residential Committee and a member of the Finance Committee; member M is a member of the Satellite Committee and chairman of the Personnel Committee, etc.

Each service committee chairman has a liaison staff contact. The service chairmen are coordinated by a "group coordinator" (Member T, Table 9–1), who is also a member of the Executive Committee. The chairmen of the functional committees are also members of the Executive Committee. The president and vice president complete the Executive Committee roster (in the old arrangements the Executive Committee consisted of the officers). The vice chairmen of the functional committees make up the Nominating Committee.

The matrix concept provides a mixed representation on all committees, for a balanced input and output of information and activity. This structure not only achieves a balance, but provides a mechanism for ongoing involvement. Each member becomes a contributing participant rather than a passive, validating observer. The majority of activity takes place outside the board meeting. Direct interaction of board members and of board and staff evolves as a work pattern in place of everything from major problems to trivia having to come before the administrator and board president for approval or coordination.

THE BOARD IN ACTION

Taking a specific problem area as an example, here is how the model works. The Finance Committee, in monitoring the budget, notices a continuing rise in the cost of care in the community treatment units. Administration is questioned and two apparent causes are uncovered:

1. relatively high staffing costs due to the special nature of the programs, and
2. limitations on occupancy in the units in the agency.

The Satellite Committee undertakes the task of physical facility adjustment—exploring the possibility of remodeling to increase occupancy or selling existing homes and buying residences more suitable to needs and more consistent with city, county and state code requirements. The Policy Review Committee assists in legal interpretations and recommends legislative advocacy. The Service Appraisal Committee, its members familiar with all phases of treatment and sensitive to community needs, seeks alternatives to the high-cost community treatment concept or ways of increasing treatment cost effectiveness. The Finance Committee explores the availability of funds for any kind of physical plant or treatment adjustment to alleviate the problem.

When the issue comes before the Executive Committee, the input is real, the problem is understood and a rational solution can be attained. Neither Executive Committee nor board feels it is merely validating an administration-sponsored program.

The former procedure would have been for administrative staff to explain away the cost rise—or take an arbitrary action to solve the problem; ask for board approval; pick someone on the board cognizant of real estate dealings to help switch properties or someone on the board cognizant of building or architecture to facilitate remodeling.

THE ULTIMATE GOAL

The use of a board as outlined here is no panacea. It is, however, food for thought for any multiservice agency. It does offer a possibility for tapping the talents of board members in ways they are used to. It provides a setting to utilize fully the time the board member gives, without usurping the administrator's authority. It demands a kind of board-member performance that makes the nonperformer uncomfortable, and therefore transient.

If a board member gives good service he will be rewarded with the recognition that he is constructively utilized. At very least, he should be able to realize that he is working with other equally committed persons and that he has a real opportunity to make the agency a little better through his service.

10

Governing Boards in Mental Health: Roles and Training Needs

ARTHUR J. ROBINS
CHERYL BLACKBURN

INTRODUCTION

A concept which has guided the development of community mental health centers (CMHCs) is the importance of the participation of members of the local community in the development and operation of center programs. Chu and Trotter (1972) contend that the stress on community participation was an afterthought on the part of the NIMH policymakers. Nevertheless, many centers from their inception have recognized the need to establish the semblance, if not the substance, of community participation. Although the relevant Federal guidelines are loosely drawn, it is mandatory that a center demonstrate the requisite responsiveness to community needs by including some form of citizen participation in program planning and implementation. The individual States, exercising the discretionary powers delegated to them by the 1967 amendment to the Community Mental Health Centers Act of 1963, may specify the form that participation takes.

Traditionally, administrative volunteers have been the means for expressing the role of the local community in the development and implementation of health, education, and welfare services, under either public or voluntary auspices. Most CMHCs have some kind of board, in conformity either with State provisions or with convention.

At the same time that State-imposed constraints bring about homogeneity, even boards within the same State may vary considerably in their stated goals and authority and the nature and extent of actual power that they wield. The authority of the boards may be directive, advisory, administrative, or some combination of these. The areas for which they have authority may be circumscribed or may extend to every aspect of agency operation. Despite the formal provisions of the constitution and bylaws, they may serve primarily as a facade (Stanton, 1970). Some boards serve an organization of which the center may be a minor component. For example, the university-affiliated center may have the same board that serves the entire university; the hospital- affiliated center, the same board that serves the entire medical complex.

Performance Criteria vs. Structural Criteria

The Federal injunction that CMHC boards be broadly representative of the community may lead to State requirements concerning the groups to be "represented"; still, there is no way to assure more than the achievement of token representation of various strata in the center's catchment area population. In any event, the effectiveness of boards is not ensured by provisions regarding composition and constitutional authority; rather, effectiveness is probably a function of the clarity of objectives assigned to a board, the competence of a board to achieve the explicit objectives, the formulation of objective criteria to measure achievement, and the tying of tenure of board members to achievement. The board and staff should apply the same management-by-objective approach to their respective efforts (Robins, 1974). This is not to say that efforts at representativeness be abandoned; however, it may be a disappointing instrument for attaining the desired responsiveness to community needs. It would be better to achieve consensus on the specific task of the board and to select people who have characteristics believed to be relevant to successful task performance.

Program and Process Objectives

We believe that it is important to differentiate the effectiveness areas of board members from the effectiveness areas of professional staff. Good management practices should eliminate duplication and unnecessary overlap of the objectives of various components of an organization and should define clearly the output toward which the effort of any work unit is addressed. We see the professional staff as composing one general work unit; the board another. Failure to differentiate their functions may lead to conflict between the professional staff and the board, or it may lead to one or the other abdicating its responsibilities in its proper areas of effectiveness. If it is not possible to differentiate functions, then obviously one group or the other is superfluous. Indeed, the professional staff not infrequently sees its board as an unnecessary burden. This is a deplorable outcome, because we believe that organizational effectiveness depends upon a joint effort.

We see the professional staff as responsible for achieving what might be called program objectives; the board, for achieving process objectives. The former have been discussed in a paper by one of the authors (Robins, 1972). Using a public health frame of reference, he classified the program goals as health promotion, specific protection, early recognition and treatment, disability limitation, or rehabilitation. The direct outcome of successful professional service is the reduction or elimination of a mental health problem of an individual, group, or community.

Process objectives have been explicated by Spaner and Windle (1971), who identify five desirable characteristics of center programs: responsiveness to community needs; availability of services to community members; continuity of services; shift of locus of care to community; increasing community support. The common theme of these objectives is their community orientation: the priority of services, the effectiveness and efficiency of the service delivery systems, and the adequacy of logistical support. The difference between program and process objectives becomes clear as one contemplates the possibility that a professional service can achieve program objectives, yet be ineffective with respect to process objectives. For example, it is conceivable that an inpatient service may be very effective in achieving its program objectives with respect to the patients who receive treatment; nonetheless, the program may not be directed toward the category of patients whose problems should receive the highest priority, according to the community's assessment of its needs. "A responsive program in one community may be quite inadequate in another" (Ozarin, Feldman, and Spaner, 1971).

"Felt" Needs or "Real" Needs

Many professionals would hold that laymen do not have the competence to determine needs. (This belief probably accounts for many of the situations where the board, selected for its docility, is at best dormant.) The criticism by professionals is not easily dismissed. The concept of "felt" needs has long been a fetish of many workers in the human services. It need not lead to passivity by professionals, who should attempt to influence the selection of social goals. Professionals should educate and should undertake research that suggests policy and program directions. But the decisionmaking rights belong as much to the community as they belong to the patient.

Citizen participation in the planning of research may be crucial to utilization of findings. Limitations of objective studies need to be recognized. For example, epidemiological studies, even when the center possesses professional staff competent to execute them, cannot provide the final professional answer to program development. Our experience with the effect of social forces on human behavior must be considered in the light of human values. Value judgments must enter the process of selecting questions to which professional effort and other resources are to be committed. Professionals do not have exclusive possession of the competence to render value judgments. They can and should point out the consequences of alternative courses of action, but the values to be assigned to the outcomes are the responsibility of those who "own" the center.

The Committee on Community Mental Health, National Association of Social Workers, has flatly stated that the community must make decisions about "program priorities, deployment of resources, the interaction between staff and board, and, above all, how the community has come to grips with the social problems which contribute to social dysfunction in its citizens" (NASW, 1968). The committee warned against center professional personnel's becoming an "isolated professional elite who regard themselves as the proprietors of a highly specialized establishment."

THE STUDY

An a priori assumption of our study, and not tested by it, was that the equity of a community in its CMHC should be expressed through a citizen board, the members of which have the power and authority to implement their responsibility for achieving specified objectives. The board's objectives are distinct from the objectives of the professional staff, although some overlap is inevitable. The study was undertaken with the idea of ascertaining goals for the training of board members that would enhance their competence to achieve those distinct objectives. It should be clear, then, that the study was not designed to derive a definition of task objectives for board members. Beginning with a preconception of what the output of a board should be, we expected to assess the extent to which these objectives were achieved and the factors that might be predictive of effectiveness, and to describe the role that board members presently play in achieving the goals of a center.

Major Questions

A study by Meyers et al. (1972) on measuring citizen board accomplishments was reviewed in order to obtain items that would be helpful in rating the achievement of process objectives. Although not explicitly addressed to the process objectives, that study derived a set of effectiveness areas which overlap the process objectives. The effectiveness areas factored out were:

1. service creation (we see this as roughly equivalent to responsiveness to community needs);
2. mobilization of outside resources dealing with the board's role in obtaining funds, but including Federal funds as well as the local sources;
3. local autonomy (roughly equivalent to a combination of the development of local funding sources and responsiveness to local needs;
4. coordination (roughly equivalent to continuity of service).

The items used by Meyers to measure effectiveness areas were used in the present study, when equivalence could be assumed, to measure achievement of process objectives. A list of the process objectives and their defining variables appear in Table 10–1.[1]

At the time of our study, there were eight comprehensive CMHCs in the state and all were invited to participate. One center elected not to participate in the study; two of the centers were excluded when it was ascertained that the boards had only a token relationship to the center. The state in which these centers are located has no requirements concerning boards, their structure, or function.

After initial contact with the center directors concerning the nature of the study, the directors provided lists of board members and a copy of the constitution and bylaws. A random sample of board members of the participating five centers was selected for contact. The board president was always included, being considered best qualified to answer detailed questions about board structure and function. The total sample was 23 (the second author interviewed 20 of the 23 board members), all interviewed individually in their communities. The center directors provided data relevant to effectiveness measures.

Separate schedules were constructed for board presidents, board members, and center directors. In addition, the Community Mental Health Ideology Scale (Baker & Schulberg, 1967) was administered to each board member and center director for purpose described in the findings section below. The interview schedules comprised items related to the following questions:

1. What are the characteristics of the members?
2. What are the practices relative to selection and orientation of members?
3. What does a member perceive to be his authority and responsibility?
4. How effective is the board as perceived by the member and as rated by investigators?

TABLE 10–1. Process Objectives and Variables for Measuring Citizen Boards*

Responsiveness to community need (Service creation)

1. The total number of services the board was involved in creating or improving (weighted for degree of importance and stage).
2. The average degree of involvement of the board in service-oriented activities weighted for importance.

Availability of services to community members

1. The length of time center has been comprehensive.
2. The number (by position) of staff members.
3. The size of the inpatient service.
4. The size of the outpatient service.
5. The size of the partial hospitalization service.
6. The total number of other services offered.
7. The size of the total budget.

Continuity of services (Coordination)

1. The total number of contacts by the board with service institutions weighted for kind of contact (informal to regular meetings).
2. The coordination of services with schools, clinics and hospitals, and law enforcement agencies.

Increasing community support (Mobilization of outside resources and local autonomy)

1. The amount of money obtained by the board from the State Government.
2. The amount of money obtained by the board from the Federal Government.
3. The amount of money raised by the board from within its area.
4. Attempts to gain support from the Governor, legislature, and Commissioner of Mental Health.
5. Frequency of contact by the board with the Governor's Office of Finance or the Bureau of the Budget.
6. Attempts to write, call, and meet with State and Federal legislators.
7. The input of the board on the annual plan of the center (the greater the input the higher the score).
8. Is the board privately incorporated?
9. The board's use of mass media within its area.
10. Is there an active mental health association within the area?
11. The amount of gifts and bequests the board has obtained.
12. The amount of funds the board administers in trust.

Shift of locus of care to the communities

1. The number of new admissions to State hospitals from the area (in terms of the population percentage).

---

*In parentheses are the counterpart factors used in the Meyers study. The items in those categories are suggested by that study. The second and last categories were created for the present study.

FINDINGS

Characteristics of Board Members

The typical board member in the study was a 47.5 year-old, married, white, Protestant male employed as a professional or as a business executive. He had a college education and had completed some graduate work. A long time (24 years) resident of the community, he had a fairly high degree of participation in formal social organizations. Prior to joining the board, he was as likely to have had no previous interest in the field of mental health as to have had such an interest. In any case, he had not sought to serve on the board.

The Community Mental Health Ideology Scale (Baker & Schulberg, 1967) was used to measure the degree to which the board members subscribed to a community mental health orientation. The major aspects of this orientation emphasize a feeling of responsibility for a total population instead of only the individual who comes for treatment, the importance of primary prevention, treatment directed toward social adjustment goals rather than basic personality change, continuity of care within an integrated network of services, and viewing the mental health specialist as only one member of a community team dealing with the mentally ill. The typical board member's score indicated a low degree of orientation to community mental health ideology, his score being similar to those obtained by criterion groups known to lack commitment to community mental health.

Recruitment and Orientation

The major criterion used to nominate him was the fact that he was deemed to be representative of the "people," or some portion of the total community, such as an organization, a profession. Other criteria were his demonstrated interests in mental health, leadership qualities, and civic mindedness. There had been no problem in finding candidates who met those broad criteria. The staff had played no role in his selection, the nominating committee having requested his services. The typical board member would be willing to serve indefinitely; in fact, he usually accepted additional terms on the board in accordance with the constitutional authorization to do so.

He was unlikely to have received any formal orientation to his role on the board. Demands on his time could be considered minimal; he attended all of the meetings per year (median number of meetings: six). The example of time devoted to fund raising gives an indication of the time required beyond attendance at regular meetings. Those who had this responsibility by reason of membership on the finance committee found that it took a nominal amount of time annually, perhaps only the time required to accompany a group on a visit to the official who held the purse strings in one county of the catchment area. A member rarely was a volunteer in service programs operated by the center.

Authority and Responsibility of Board Members

The constitution and bylaws of the centers gave comprehensive responsibility and authority to each board, and clearly indicated that ownership resided in the board. The global statements in those documents called for the board to plan, implement, and evaluate mental health services for the population of the catchment area. The usual board organization to implement this authority included an executive committee composed of chairmen of other committees, a personnel committee, a finance committee, a nominating committee and sometimes a public relations committee. This structure is consistent with the report of the members that the specific matters on which they spent the most time concerned personel needs and overseeing the center's use of funds. Although most of the board members believed that they had administrative authority rather than advisory, almost half of the respondents thought that their actual power to influence the administration of the center was quite limited.

In response to the probing, more than half the members believed that they exercised no responsibility for program development. Most of the respondents reported that the board had nothing to do with organizational structure of the center; however, most were involved in personnel actions such as selection and evaluation of upper echelon staff. They reported responsibility for overseeing the leadership of the center and assessing its effectiveness. The data for this assessment was "feedback" from the "community." However, they tended to fulfill their liaison role with the community rather than vice versa. This is consistent with findings of the recent study of community involvement (Bloomfield, 1972). Essentially, members of the board felt accountable only to each other, except for fiscal accountability to the governmental funding sources. With respect to obtaining funds, the board members played primarily a supportive role. Most of the funds came from Federal and State sources and were obtained largely through staff effort. On the other hand, the amount of money obtained from local sources, such as county and municipal governments and United Fund organizations, was believed to be a function of the persuasiveness of the board members.

Effectiveness

Most of the members believed that their center was effective in meeting the needs of the community. The response, however, to probes specific to the five process objectives elicited the fact that about two-thirds of the members felt that the center had a record of achievement in these areas. However, the same proportion did not believe that the board had contributed significantly to effectiveness in those five areas.

The work of Meyers et al. was used, when relevant, to generate effectiveness scores for each objective, and a composite score developed for each board. None of the characteristics descriptive of members was significantly related to the effectiveness of achievement of process objectives. Operational definitions of responsiveness to need, availability of service, and continuity of care were slippery and enabled us to rank the centers with respect to each other but not to assess absolute effectiveness. Measuring shift of locus of patient care from State hospitals to the community was difficult because the period since the centers had become comprehensive was too brief to expect any significant impact upon state hospital admission rates; however, each had offered most of the essential services, except for in-patient care, that could have been expected to have had some effect on those rates over the years.

The increase in local community support was assessed both in terms of annual changes in the proportion of the total budget collected from local sources and in terms of annual changes in the absolute amount. The proportion of the total budget coming from local sources showed little fluctuation prior to the centers' becoming comprehensive, but dramatically decreased after achievement of that status. Despite that proportional decrease, most of the centers achieved a substantial percentage increase in the amount of local support at about the time that they became comprehensive.

Analysis and Interpretation

The findings regarding board member characteristics are consistent with other assessments (New, Holton, & Hessler, 1972) of the elitist nature of boards. Despite their apparent high status in the community, most members recognized the limitations to their power over the activities of the center with which they were affiliated. They appeared to "reign but not rule." They were not highly oriented toward the goals of a CMHC. This is not surprising, adherence to a community mental health

orientation not having been a criterion for selection for board membership.

Almost none of the members had any experience as program volunteers at the center, and usually gave only a minimal amount of time to
their duties as administrative volunteers. While they tended to view
themselves as representatives of the community, activities directed toward the identification of community needs were meager and unsystematic.

The rhetoric of the constitution was inconsistent with the spotty activities of the board. Members did not have any well-defined set of objectives to which their activities were systematically related. One wondered
whether the most important activity of the board had not been that directed toward the establishment of the center and the construction of
the physical plant.

Although the members rated the center as effective in serving the
community, they did not display the same unanimity in assessing the
achievement of each process objective. We assume that this discrepancy
was the outcome of more focused consideration of progress toward specific objectives not considered in their earlier evaluation. They were
frank in assessing their lack of contribution toward the degree of effectiveness that had been achieved. Even the increase in local support may
have been stimulated by the huge increase in funds from the State and
Federal sources, dependence upon which had not been reduced.

The lack of relationship between factors that had been believed to
be potentially related and the effectiveness of achieving process objectives may be explained in the following ways:

1. The characteristics, in fact, had no significant association with effectiveness.
2. The scores fell within a narrow range on the effectiveness scale. In
   other words, the centers were a homogeneous group with respect to
   effectiveness; they were all equally effective or not effective.
3. The operational definitions of the process objectives were inadequate.

Reliable and valid performance criteria are needed not only for research purposes but for center operations. Evaluation must become an
integral component of the administrative process. Board members
should make inputs into the process of establishing performance criteria
for the achieving of their objectives.

Implications for Training

The difficulty of measuring effectiveness in achieving process objectives
means that the selection of training objectives is dependent upon self-
reported performance discrepancies and observations concerning the

lack of clarity of goal definition and the unsystematic nature of programs directed to goals. We believe that the study demonstrated a need for a training program which would help the board members understand and develop values that are implicit in the community mental health movement and the goals that are appropriate to that value system. The training should be directed toward helping the board members define their unique goals as explicitly as possible. They should become familiar with the effort of the NIMH staff to utilize a center's annual inventory report as a source of data for measuring the achievement of board objectives (Bass, 1971; Windle, 1973). Training would help the members develop performance programs designed to achieve their goals, accept responsibility for evaluating their progress, and revise their efforts in accordance with an analysis of the outcomes.

The high motivation of board members for acquiring the relevant competence was clearly evident in the interviews. The provision of training opportunities for citizen participants is essential to fulfillment of the potential of the community mental health movement. It is gratifying to note that the Department of Mental Health of the State in which this study was done has contracted with the senior author's organization to provide training addressed to the objectives indicated above. The program will be offered to executive committee members. Participation in training may be burdensome but there is no place for the honorific board in the community mental health field. The head of the NIMH Citizen Participation Branch has unequivocally summed up the task: "The live dynamic board makes demands on its members for persistence, ingenuity, and dedication" (Rooney, 1968).

NOTE

1. Too late for use in our study, we learned of the work (Bass, 1971) being done in the Office of Program Planning and Evaluation, NIMH, on the development of measures specific to the process objectives. This effort has since progressed rapidly. Wherever possible the Annual Inventory is being utilized as a source of items related to each process objective (Windle, 1973).

REFERENCES

Baker, F., & Schulberg, H. C. The development of a community mental health ideology scale. *Community Mental Health Journal*, 3(3):216–225, 1967.

Bass, R. D. *A method for measuring continuity of care in a community mental health center*. Department of Health, Education, and Welfare Publication No. (HSM) 72–910. Washington, D.C.: Superintendent of Documents, U.S. Government Printing Office, 1971.

Bloomfield, C. *Evaluation of community involvement in community mental health centers.* New York: Health Policy Advisory Center, Inc., 1972.

Chu, F., & Trotter, S. *The mental health complex, part I: The community mental health centers.* Washington, D.C.: Center for Study of Responsive Law, 1972.

Meyers, W. R., et al. Methods of measuring citizen board accomplishment in mental health and retardation. *Community Mental Health Journal,* 8(4):311–310, 1972.

National Association of Social Workers. Position statement on community mental health (Mimeo.), 1968.

New, P. K., Holton, W. E., and Hessler, R. M. *Citizen participation and inter-agency relations: Issues and program implications for community mental health centers.* Boston: Department of Community Health and Social Medicine, Tufts University School of Medicine, 1972.

Ozarin, L. D., Feldman, S., and Spaner, F. G. Experience with mental health centers. *American Journal of Psychiatry,* 127(7):912–916, 1971.

Robins, A. J. Administrative process model for community mental health centers. *Community Mental Health Journal,* 8(3):208–219, 1972.

Robins, A. J. Management-by-objectives for community mental health programs. *Hospital and Community Psychiatry,* 25(4):April, 1974.

Rooney, H. L. Roles and functions of the advisory board. *North Carolina Journal of Mental Health,* 3(1):33–43, 1968.

Spaner, F., & Windle, C. The perspective of national program development and administration: Program needs and evaluation activities. Paper at 79th Annual Meeting of American Psychological Association, Washington, D.C., 1971.

Stanton, E. *Clients come last: Volunteers and welfare organizations.* Beverly Hills: Sage Publications Inc., 1970.

Windle, C. "The Community Mental Health Program—1971: Performance Indicators Derived From the CMHC Inventory." (Discussion draft) 1973.

11

Evolution of Leadership Style in Social Agencies: A Theoretical Analysis

William E. Berg

In recent years, social agencies have been forced to invest an increasing proportion of their time and energies in activities associated with administration and management. To some extent, this trend reflects a growing awareness among human service professionals of the role that effective management plays in the development of integrated social service delivery systems. In a much larger sense, however, this development represents a response to an environment that has become increasingly complex and diverse in the demands that it makes upon such agencies.

Agencies have, wittingly or unwittingly, been forced to recognize the role of management as a result of the growing demand for program evaluation and accountability, the related concern that is evident at all levels of government with cost effectiveness, and the need to regulate the expenditure of public funds. Confronted by an environment that has become increasingly aggressive in its demands, the agency system has responded in a manner that is designed, at least temporarily, to guarantee their survival. Thus, agencies have moved toward increasingly sophisticated information storage and retrieval systems; they have placed considerable emphasis upon those internal processes designed to provide the data necessary for administrative decision making; they have developed some expertise in monitoring the external environment and in working within interagency networks; and they have rewarded those skills and capacities that are normally associated with administrative or managerial functions.[1] Although these developments have had a number of positive implications for agency operations, including perhaps a relative increase in operating efficiency, they have also produced a growing centralization of power and authority within the agency system.

One of the questions that this emphasis upon management raises concerns the relative quality of an emerging leadership group. This chapter represents an attempt to analyze, within a theoretical framework, some of the dimensions of administrative leadership within human service agencies. Dimensions that are of particular concern here are those of leadership style and the relationship between variations in leadership styles and the relative quality of organizational life found within these agencies.

LEADERSHIP BEHAVIOR AND LEADERSHIP STYLE

Administrative leadership may be defined as relatively distinctive patterns of behavior that are associated with the position of leader, behavior designed to influence or direct individuals or groups along a predetermined path toward a set of specified goals and objectives.[2] Within most formal organizations, therefore, leadership may be viewed as the enactment of a formal role.[3] Leadership is, in this sense, subject to the normative values, beliefs, and expectations of the organizational system.

These expectations associated with the role of the leader provide a structure that lends a measure of stability and predictability to the leader's behavior. As in any other role, however, the leader's actual performance of the role is influenced by those unique skills, attributes, and capacities he or she brings to this role.[4] Thus, we may assume that leadership includes both those common traits or characteristics that are inherent in the role itself, and those unique social and psychological factors that lead to variations in interpretation and performance.[5]

The commonalities that exist as a part of the leadership role have been examined in an unusually rich and extensive literature.[6] As Stogdill has suggested, this literature tends to approach leadership from four distinct perspectives: it may be associated with the personality characteristics of the individual leader; it may be viewed as an instrumental function for the attainment of organizational goals and objectives; it has been analyzed as the locus of power and influence within the organization; or it may be viewed as a group process that involves certain rituals or routines.[7]

The approach that the leader adopts to his or her role has also been analyzed in relationship to the functional needs and requirements of the group or organization. In general, these analyses have attempted to delineate between two characteristic modes of leadership behavior: behavior directed toward the maintenance of the group or organization, and behavior concerned with the achievement of its goals and objectives.[8] Perhaps the most widely known example of this analysis is found in Bales and Slater's distinction between the task-oriented and the socioemotive dimensions of leadership behavior.[9] As Bowers and Seashore have indicated, this approach can also be extended within a four-dimensional framework, which includes behavior designed to enhance the individual's sense of self-worth or value, behavior that encourages the development of positive working relationships, behavior involved in the attainment of organizational goals and objectives, and work-facilitative behavior involved in organizational planning and coordination.[10]

Although these approaches to the study of leadership have provided a useful basis for analyzing leadership and leadership behavior, it is apparent that they do not exhaust those variations that may be observed in the practice of leadership. A "good" leader is clearly one who adapts his or her behavior to the demands of a given situation, one who is task-oriented or socioemotive as the circumstances dictate. The author's view of such a leader tends, however, to incorporate those rather subtle differences in behavior that are a part of the concept of leadership style.

Leadership style may be tentatively defined as the distinctive and dynamic patterns of behavior that are exhibited by a leader, patterns that make the leader's behavior unique, and patterns that provide some measure of consistency and predictability to his or her behavior. The concept of leadership style involves, therefore, those social and psychological attributes of the leader that determine how he or she will act as a task-oriented or socioemotive leader. This suggests, of course, that leadership style may require a distinct and a more descriptive mode of analysis.

LEADERSHIP AND LEADERSHIP STYLE IN SOCIAL AGENCIES

One of the problems encountered when one attempts to analyze leadership in social agencies is that the functions associated with leadership in these agencies are different from those found in most industrial or business firms. Most industries and businesses operate with a defined set of

organizational goals and objectives, with a technology that is clearly defined in relation to its products, and with a degree of commitment to
and consensus about its system of values and beliefs. As Cohen and
March have suggested in their analysis of educational leadership, however, most service-oriented organizations may be characterized by a
loose collection of changing ideas rather than a defined set of goals and
objectives, tend to operate on a trial-and-error basis rather than through
clearly defined technologies, and possess a limited and fluid commitment to organizational values.[11]

These differences are important to an understanding of leadership
within the social agency because they imply, following Cohen and
March, that the standard theories of management and administrative
leadership that have been developed in terms of business or industrial
firms may not be applicable to the realities of the social agency.[12] What
this suggests, in part, is that it may be necessary to develop a framework
of analysis that reflects some of the unique circumstances and conditions
involved in administrative leadership within these agencies.

The existing literature on administrative leadership within the social agencies suggests some of the dimensions that may be involved in
this role. Hawkes has, for example, analyzed those forces or factors that
constitute the role of psychiatric administrator.[13] He indicates that
these include those legal and political bases of support for the agency, its
technical and professional support systems, and the client population
served through agency programs. The professional and moral value systems that are frequently associated with these agencies have, as Street,
Vinter, and Perrow have noted, an impact on the power of the administrator and on the delegation of responsibilities within the agency structure.[14] Finally, Zald's analysis of the interaction between the agency executive and the board of directors underlines the often important role
that they play in determining agency structures and processes.[15]

These three forces or factors influence the leader's interpretation of
his or her role. The relative weight that any single factor achieves in this
process is a function of the perceived needs of the agency and of the relative intensity of the leader's interaction with these various groups.[16] In
cases, therefore, where operating budgets are imperiled, or where they
are maintained on an insecure and tentative basis, one would normally
expect to find that the administrator would take his or her behavioral
cues from those groups or organizations involved in the funding process, and that they would be less inclined to respond to the expectations
of the agency staff or the client population. In other circumstances or situations, however, these priorities might be reversed, and the leader's behavior would reflect the influence of other members of the role set.

This suggests that leadership style in social agencies represents a
complex and interactive process. It goes beyond the personal prefer-

ences of those occupying the role of leader and involves a set of constraints inherent in the operations and in the organizational environment of the agency.

A MODEL OF LEADERSHIP STYLE

In order to analyze leadership style in these settings, it is necessary to develop a theoretical framework broad enough to incorporate those constraints found in the role and specific enough to provide a meaningful basis of analysis. Most attempts to develop such an analysis have relied upon a dichotomous approach to a leadership style.

Anyone who is familiar with social work education is aware of the importance that is placed upon the distinction between the "inside" versus the "outside" dean or director. The behavior of certain deans or directors may, according to this distinction, be defined in terms of the emphasis placed upon internal concerns and processes on the one hand, and the external environment of the university setting, the professional community, or various governmental agencies and bureaus on the other.

Proactive vs. Reactive Patterns

A much more meaningful distinction between leadership styles can be found when they are viewed in terms of the proactive versus reactive executive.[17] The proactive executive is "guided by the motivation to actively influence and shape the external environment of the organization as well as its internal structure in order to fulfill the organization's mission."[18] The reactive executive is devoted primarily to maintaining the status quo and to avoid risk-taking situations or circumstances.

Both of these distinctions imply certain qualitative differences in the behavior of the leader; differences that involve a mixture of personal motivations and organizational requirements. The internal dean or director is, in other words, not simply a psychological type who chooses to define a role in terms of the internal structure and processes of the school because of some unique personal attributes or capacities. He or she may also be responding to the priorities dictated by the perceived needs of the school. Whatever the source of such needs, the style of administration that results represents the product of the interaction between personal and situational factors.

Leaders may, of course, choose those agencies or organizations that are most compatible with their own personal needs and motivations. Those qualities of leadership that Hasenfeld and English associate with the proactive leader—qualities of innovation, change, and risk taking[19]—may be appropriate to certain agencies and inappropriate in others. In the best of all possible worlds, these two dimensions will be identical; reactive leaders will be found in those agencies that require stability and gradual evolutionary change and proactive leaders will be associated with agencies that demand rapid growth and development.

One of the difficulties involved in the analysis of leadership style in these settings is that the concept of style includes something more than the distinction between internal versus external, or proactive versus reactive patterns. If these were the only dimensions of leadership in the social agency then one might, with some adjustments, apply a similar analysis to any bureaucracy and to many private firms. The element that makes leadership in such agencies unique is the relationship of the agency to a profession or a group of related professions.

Levels of Identification

The level of identification with professional values and beliefs represents a critical element in determining the leader's interpretation of the role. It is critical because it influences the leader's perception of the agency and of its processes. In this respect, the level of identification may be viewed as an internalized motivational system that is responsive to external groups. Leaders who are highly identified with their profession will be more responsive to professional interests and concerns, and will be more likely to place a higher priority on those dimensions of agency practice that reflect these concerns.

Four Styles of Administrative Leadership

The orientation or the motivation of the leader and his or her level of identification with the profession interact to create four distinct styles of administrative leadership within the social agency. Although these styles reflect qualitative differences in these dimensions of leadership, they imply quantitative differences in the actual performance of the role. Thus, "professional managers" are different from the "community influentials," not just in terms of those forces that determine their approach to the roles, but in the way they organize their time, the groups with which they relate, the value they place upon different aspects of agency operations, or the way they present themselves to others.

These styles represent the organizing frameworks within which the leader perceives, interprets, and enacts his or her role. In this sense, the styles reflect those permutations that exist in both the value systems and the personal motivations of the leader. As Figure 11–1 suggests, moreover, there are two pairs of opposing styles evident in the interaction between these dimensions (that is, the "local" versus the "cosmopolitan"

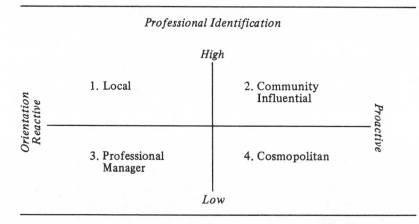

FIGURE 11–1. Dimensions of leadership and leadership style

style, and the "professional manager" versus the "community influential"); all of the remaining pairs share either a common orientation toward the role or a common level of identification with the profession. In order to examine some of the possible behavioral implications of the model, it may be useful to compare some of the characteristic differences between these pairs (see Table 11–1).

One of the important elements in determining these characteristic modes of behavior can be found in the relative perspective that the leader adopts toward the role. Although the "local" and the "community influential" styles are both committed to the prevailing professional values and beliefs, they differ in their behavior because they associate these commitments with different fields of practice. Thus, the "local" leader defines his or her field in terms of the professional practices of the agency; the "community influential" maintains a field that includes both local and national professional groups or organizations.[20] Similarly, the "professional manager" differs in his or her perspectives from the "cosmopolitan" leader in the focus upon the internal processes and operations of the agency, rather than on the relationships between the agency and external organizations or agencies.

SOME EVOLUTIONARY TRENDS IN LEADERSHIP STYLE

The style of administrative leadership found in most social agencies tends to change over time in relationship to the quality and the texture of the organizational environment.[21] The present environment of most social agencies includes two forces or developments that have combined to influence leadership styles.

TABLE 11–1. Leadership Styles and Behavioral Modes

1. Local

(a) Socioemotive leader.
(b) Spends major proportion of time in agency.
(c) Focuses on internal dynamics and operations of agency.
(d) Highly committed to primary and secondary agency norms.
(e) Identifies with agency reference group
(f) Promoted from within
(g) Concerned with professional aspects of agency practice.

2. Cosmopolitan

(a) Task-oriented leader.
(b) Spends major proportion of time outside agency.
(c) Focuses on external relationships of agency.
(d) Minimally committed to primary and secondary agency norms.
(e) Identifies with external reference group(s).
(f) Recruited from outside.
(g) Concerned with goal attainment.

3. Professional Manager

(a) Task-oriented leader.
(b) Spends major proportion of time in agency.
(c) Focuses on internal processes and operations.
(d) Minimally committed to agency norms.
(e) Identifies with professional manager reference group.
(f) Recruited from outside.
(g) Concerned with goal attainment and operating efficiency.

4. Community Influential

(a) Socioemotive leader.
(b) Spends major proportion of time outside agency.
(c) Focuses on relationships with local/national professional groups.
(d) Committed to primary agency norms, minimally committed to secondary norms.
(e) Identifies with a professional leadership reference group.
(f) Recruited from outside.
(g) Concerned with goal attainment.

An Unstable Environment

The first of these has been alluded to earlier and includes the increase in the regulatory authority of various governmental and private funding sources, the emergence of sophisticated accountability and evaluation processes, and the proliferation in those policies and programs that relate, at one level or another, to the operations of the social agency. All of these have combined to produce an environment that is increasingly unstable in its demands upon the agency; an environment in which the demand for agency products tends to fluctuate over time and the resources necessary for agency operations are subject to competitive pressures.[22]

An unstable environment is one in which growth and development tend to move in rapid and frequently unpredictable paths, one which requires organizational structures and processes that are "dynamic," as Hage and Aiken have suggested,[23] in order to provide that flexibility necessary to an efficient and effective organizational response.[24]

In stable environments, on the other hand, both the demand for agency products and the availability of resources remain constant or grow in a predictable manner. Such environments place fewer adaptive pressures upon the agency and, as a result, it is able to operate effectively with "static" organizational structures and processes.[25]

Deprofessionalization

The second force present in the agency environment involves a relative deemphasis upon the role and the functions of the professions. That special status that the professional has historically occupied in American society has, in recent years, been subject to a critical reassessment and reevaluation.[26] This represents, in part, a reaction to some of the excesses of the professions themselves (for example, the role of lawyers in Watergate or the actions of health care professionals in the abuse of public and private medical insurance programs) and must, in part, be viewed as one of the products of a larger process of social change and development.

In either case, the move toward deprofessionalization has a number of important implications for the future growth and development of the social agency—implications that have already had an influence on the shape of administrative leadership.

The pressures exerted by these developments within the agency environment have produced an emphasis upon those leadership styles that are capable of dealing with the problems of rapid and unpredictable change. Agencies have, as a result, tended to emphasize managerial skills and capacities in the recruitment of leadership personnel, rather than the more traditional reliance upon professional experience and expertise.[27] At the same time, agencies have also moved toward more complex administrative structures and processes,[28] a move that reflects the need for greater flexibility in the organization and enables the agency to include more than one leadership style within the administration.

Thus, it is possible, following Patti and Rausch, to have a "local" leadership orientation at the supervisory levels, while moving toward the "professional manager" style in the middle-management positions.[29] For the foreseeable future, however, it would appear that the characteristic leadership style that is required by the agency as a whole includes those qualities associated with the "cosmopolitan" leader; that is, qualities that involve a deemphasis upon professional values and the capacity to monitor the environment.

SUMMARY

The future of the professional within American society is, according to Yarmolinsky, contingent upon his or her ability to develop a role that includes both the commitment to professional skills and capacities, and some recognition of the larger contexts of professional practice.[30] Although this dual role makes certain demands upon the professional, demands with which he or she may be unaccustomed to dealing, the alternative may be that professionals will find that their power and authority has been taken over by the professional manager.[31]

The analysis presented here suggests that this trend is evident in the social agency, where the pressures exerted by the agency environment have placed a premium on those leadership skills associated with deprofessionalized leadership styles. The danger this presents to the social agency is that it will lose, in its structures and processes, that sensitivity to the needs of each client that is characteristic of a professional role.

In order to deal with these dangers, in order to circumvent the bureaucratic constraints inherent in the present environment, it will be necessary for social work professionals to possess broader administrative skills. In order to achieve this goal, however, professionals must, in their training and in practice, acquire more skills in management and administration and become more sensitive to the role that effective management plays in social work practice.

NOTES

1. See Jerald Hage and Michael Aiken, *Social Change and Complex Organizations* (New York: Random House, 1970).
2. Jeffrey Barrow, "The Variables of Leadership," *The Academy of Management Review* 2 (April 1977): 51–63.
3. Eric Hollander, "Style, Structure, and Setting in Organizational Leadership," *Administrative Science Quarterly* 16 (March 1971): 153–65.
4. Cecil A. Gibb, "Leadership," in *Handbook of Social Psychology*, vol. 2, ed. Gardner Lindzey (Reading, Mass.: Addison-Wesley, 1954).
5. Robert L. Peabody, *Organizational Authority* (New York: Atherton, 1964).
6. Barrow, "Variables of Leadership," pp. 52–53.
7. Ralph Stodgill, *Leadership: A Survey of the Literature* (New York: Creative Research Corporation, 1968).

8. Dorwin Cartwright and Alvin Zander, *Group Dynamics: Theory and Research* (Evanston, Ill.: Row, Peterson, 1968).

9. Robert Bales and Phillip Slater, "Role Differentiation in Small Decision-Making Groups," in *Family, Socialization, and Interaction Process,* ed. Talcott Parsons and Robert Bales (Glencoe, Ill.: Free Press, 1955).

10. Donald Bowers and Stanley Seashore, "Predicting Organizational Effectiveness with a Four-Factor Theory of Leadership," *Administrative Science Quarterly* 16 (March 1971): 166–79.

11. Michael D. Cohen and James G. March, *Leadership and Ambiguity* (New York: McGraw-Hill, 1974).

12. Ibid., p. 4.

13. Robert W. Hawkes, "The Role of the Psychiatric Administrator," *Administrative Science Quarterly* 6 (June 1961): 89–106.

14. David Street, Robert D. Vinter, and Charles Perrow, *Organizations for Treatment* (New York: Free Press, 1966).

15. Mayer A. Zald, "The Power and Functions of Boards of Directors: A Theoretical Synthesis," *American Journal of Sociology* 75 (July 1969): 97–111.

16. Robert Merton, "Reference Groups and Social Structure," in *Social Theory and Social Structure,* ed. Robert Merton (Glencoe, Ill.: Free Press, 1957).

17. Yeheskel Hasenfeld and Richard A. English, eds., *Human Service Organizations* (Ann Arbor: University of Michigan Press, 1974): p. 155.

18. Ibid., p. 155.

19. Ibid., p. 154.

20. Alvin W. Gouldner, "Cosmopolitans and Locals," in *Organizational Careers,* ed. Barney G. Glazer (Chicago: Aldine, 1968).

21. Shirley Terreberry, "The Evolution of Organizational Environments," *Administrative Science Quarterly* 12 (April 1968): 590–613.

22. James Thompson, *Organizations in Action* (New York: McGraw- Hill, 1967).

23. Hage and Aiken, *Social Change,* pp. 68–72.

24. Richard M. Cyert and James G. March, *A Behavioral Theory of the Firm* (Englewood Cliffs, N.J.: Prentice-Hall, 1965).

25. Hage and Aiken, *Social Change,* pp. 74–75.

26. See, for example, Burton J. Bledstein, *The Culture of Professionalism* (New York: W. W. Norton, 1976); Paul Starr, "Medicine and the Waning of Professional Sovereignty," *Daedalus* 107 (Winter 1978): 175–94; and Adam Yarmolinsky, "What Future for the Professional in American Society?" *Daedalus* 107 (Winter 1978): 159–74.

27. Rino Patti and Ronald Rausch, "Social Work Administration Graduates in the Job Market: An Analysis of Managers' Hiring Preferences," *Social Service Review* 52 (December 1978): 567–83.

28. Terreberry, "Evolution of Organizational Environments," pp. 611–12.

29. Patti and Rausch, "Social Work Graduates," pp. 580–82.

30. Yarmolinsky, "What Future for the Professional?", p. 173.

31. Ibid., pp. 164–67.

12

Administrative Styles of Social Work Supervisors in a Human Service Agency

PAMELA A. RUSSELL
MICHAEL W. LANKFORD
RICHARD M. GRINNELL, JR.

The various patterns of administrative approaches that supervisors bring to their jobs are said to be their supervisory styles (Hersey & Blanchard, 1972). The supervisors' unique personality characteristics and value systems, as well as skill, are integral parts of these supervisory styles (Sheriff, 1968). Included in this definition as well are the subjective and objective methods that a supervisor employs in assuring that activities of others, especially supervisees, are geared toward meeting the broader organizational goals (Jaco & Vroom, 1977).

The majority of supervisor/supervisee style studies have been executed in business or industry settings, with human service agencies being largely ignored. This is true even though there is presently increased public awareness of the relationship of supervisory styles to productivity—seen here as a cost to the taxpayer as well as inclusive of quality services (York, 1977). Similar to some of the business and industry studies, the social work profession has largely viewed styles of leadership from a model of consideration versus structure or a minimal amount of control versus rigid authority. Viewed similarly as a path-goal theory, social work research has generally suggested that the "people" orientation is more important than the "organization" orientation (Hammer & Dachler, 1975).

The majority of studies that have been executed in social work settings relate supervisory styles only to "given" situations. Additionally, few empirical studies have been executed on the various supervisory styles utilized in social work settings. This article presents the results of an empirically based research study that explores the various supervisory styles of social work supervisors employed in a large human service agency.

METHOD

Setting and Population

The study was conducted in one of the twelve state regions in the Texas Department of Human Resources (DHR), one of the largest DHRs in the Southwest region of the United States, with about 13,000 employees. The Region is comprised of 23 northeast Texas counties having about 750,000 total population. Over half the Region's population is in five urban counties, while the remaining counties are rural.

The DHR, by legislative mandate, provides medical, financial and social services to children, adults and low income families of the state. The eight major social programs provided by the DHR are: Food Stamp; Aid to Families with Dependent Children; Child Support; Medicaid Eligibility; Early and Periodic Screening, Diagnosis and Treatment; Alternate Care for Aged, Blind and Disabled; Family Services; and Protective Services. Expenditures under these programs exceed $1,000,000 annually.

The Region is under the direction of a regional administrator (and an assistant) who has the overall responsibility for coordination of the programs administered by the DHR for community relations and planning. Five regional directors have the responsibility for the development and implementation of the programs providing direct delivery of services to clients. Program directors are responsible for the supervisors who direct the specialized areas of service delivered by individual units. Direct social services are delivered by the workers in these units. The Region has 142 employees in Support Units which include: Personnel; Business Management; Data Transmissions; Continuing Education and Budget and Planning; Regional Attorneys; Civil Rights Officers; and Volunteer Coordinators.

The eight major social programs have several supervisors who in turn supervise several supervisees. Each of the eight social programs and the specific number of supervisors (a) and supervisees (b) in each program are: Food Stamp, $a = 9$, $b = 118$; Aid to Families with Dependent Children, $a = 7$, $b = 103$; Child Support, $a = 2$, $b = $

28; Medicaid Eligibility, $a = 4$, $b = 42$; Early and Periodic Screening, Diagnosis and Treatment, $a = 2$, $b = 23$; Alternative Care for Aged, Blind and Disabled, $a = 6$, $b = 70$; Family Services, $a = 3$, $b = 23$; Protective Services, $a = 11$, $b = 103$. Thus, the population for this study is the 44 supervisors and their 510 supervisees in addition to the 142 employees who are employed within the Support Units mentioned in the previous paragraph (totaling 696 people).

Operationalization of Supervisory Styles

This study utilized the *Management Appraisal Survey* (Hall, Harvey, & Williams, 1973) and the *Styles of Management Inventory* (Hall, Harvey, & Williams, 1980) as the operational definition of the various known supervisory styles. These two instruments are based on a grid concept developed by Blake and Mouton (1978). In order to understand the supervisory styles of the social work supervisors within the DHR it is necessary to have an understanding of the Managerial Grid Model utilized in the two instruments. A brief overview of the model is presented below.

The Managerial Grid Model. The model represents a two-dimensional analysis of supervisors' behaviors. The two most basic concerns supervisors have serve as the two dimensions:

1. a concern for production, and
2. a concern for people.

Supervisors have personal values about how these two concerns should be related to one another, and depending upon the particular values they hold, supervisors will adopt particular sets of behaviors in satisfying their concerns; these behaviors may be considered to constitute "supervisory style." The five supervisory styles depicted by the model are presented in summary form in Figure 12–1.

As the model indicates, a grid notation is used in identifying specific supervisory styles. With the value 9 denoting a maximum concern and the value 1 denoting a minimal concern, supervisory styles can be interpreted in terms of the degree of concern for production vis-à-vis the employees which the supervisors experience. Thus, the 9,1 style reflects a maximal concern for production coupled with a minimum concern for supervisees; the 1,9 style reflects a minimal concern for production coupled with a maximal concern for subordinates; the 1,1 style reflects minimal concern for both dimensions; and the 5,5 style reflects a moderate concern for each. The 9,9 style suggests a maximal concern for produc-

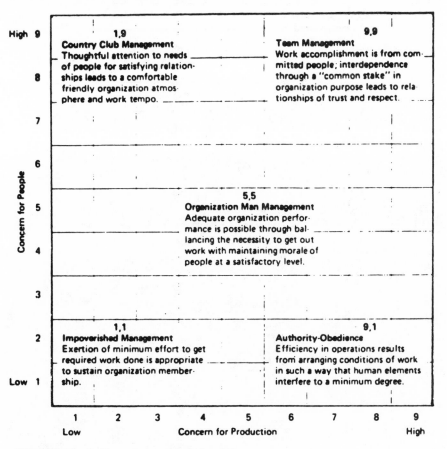

FIGURE 12–1. The managerial grid
Source: Blake & Mouton, 1978. Used by permission.

tion and supervisees. Obviously, different behaviors are used by supervisors adhering to the pressure of such different combinations of concerns; it is these behaviors—and the overall style which results—that the two instruments were designed to measure. The four specific components measured by the grid are:

1. philosophy of management,
2. planning and goal-setting,
3. implementation activities, and
4. evaluation practices.

Each of these components is defined in terms of the style orientations toward each and displayed graphically in Table 12–1.

TABLE 12–1. An Overview of Managers by Management Component and Supervisory Style

Component	Supervisory Style	
	9/9	5/5
Philosophy of Management	The 9/9 manager sees people as basically productive and creative. He attempts to maximize employees' involvement in the planning and doing of meaningful work since he feels this promotes productivity and job satisfaction. Rejecting the philosophy that the needs of people and work are in conflict, he feels there can and should be an "integration" of production goals and human potentials. He may err in granting people more autonomy than they are ready to accept. To avoid such an abuse of the 9/9 style, he should be sensitive to the cultural backdrop which has conditioned people's expectations and practices.	Somewhat an extension of the philosophy that people and production concerns are in conflict, the 5/5 manager attempts to take a compromise approach in dealing with conflicting employee needs and organizational needs. Assuming that people can only be moderately productive and have moderate job satisfaction, he further assumes their need for pragmatic leadership and "flexible" management. Despite denial and defensiveness if confronted, he likely feels people are gullible and can be manipulated. He is quick to rationalize his actions due to his ability to compartmentalize his thinking.
Planning and Goal-setting	An attempt is made by the 9/9 manager to involve all employees who are to be affected by decisions in the planning and setting of goals. People who are to be directly affected by decisions are included in discussions about those decisions. Through participation, the manager feels he increases the possibility of commitment. Creativity, he feels, is an outgrowth of increasing the number of resources which can best be achieved by the increased participation of the employees involved.	The 5/5 manager favors a "tell and sell" and/or consultative approach to influencing decision-making, goal-setting and planning activities. He feels if he can get employees to see the logic of the steps he outlines for them, then they will go along. An attempt is made to find a delicate balance between exercising major control over the situation while taking into account the opinions of the majority of his employees. He prefers that employees "feel like the ideas are theirs", but he supplies the ideas first, and works on the feelings secondly.
Implementation	In implementation, the 9/9 manager tries to develop a team from the work group in which he functions as a member of the team. Because of the advantages of special resources he may have as a manager, he readily makes these available to the team. Encouragement is given to other members of the work team to contribute whatever special resources they may possess. Under such an ongoing team effort approach, implementation becomes but a logical extension of the planning phase and, indeed, may have re-planning built into it.	The 5/5 manager prides himself in maintaining an "open door" policy during implementation activities. In this stance, he considers himself to be "on call" when problems occur or when plans need reviewing or revising. Although the manager may feel he is making himself available, this approach is essentially one of minimum participation, when possible, or fire-fighting when necessary. Such practices serve to reinforce the manager's view of himself as extremely flexible.
Evaluation Practices	The 9/9 manager views evaluation, in which his and his employee's performance is candidly appraised, as a learning experience. Usually these sessions are conducted on some kind of regular and ongoing basis and are viewed as being an integral part of implementation activities. Sessions may take a one-to-one or team format; the guiding rule-of-thumb is: treat the problem within the context in which it exists.	With an effort at focusing on both mistakes and successes, the 5/5 manager underplays evaluation. The whole process of evaluation is likely to be rather informal and may not be recognizable as evaluative in substance to an observer. It is not uncommon for the 5/5 manager to be so uncomfortable with dealing with the failures of employees that he rather routinely rewards successes in a group setting while attending to failures in private one-to-one sessions. Sessions tend to be indirect, cliche-ridden, and "pep talk" oriented.

TABLE 12–1. An Overview of Managers by Management Component and Supervisory Style

Supervisory Style		
9/1	1/9	1/1
Assuming that people and production concerns are mutually exclusive, the 9/1 manager's philosophy is therefore reflected in his feelings that people do not like to work and that to get them to produce requires that he exert strong authority. For work to be accomplished, he tends to feel people have to be directed, coerced, and controlled. His pessimistic beliefs about people's responsibility and competency are so all-inclusive that there are no exceptions. Such an unvarying philosophy becomes the best defense for his practices since he must compensate for the perceived inadequacies of his personnel.	With a basic underlying philosophy which is very similar to the 9/1's, the 1/9 expresses his philosophy with a different set of behaviors. He feels people are not very competent, that they do not like to work, and that they are not very responsible. As a manager, he feels that his employees require shelter and protection which he feels they are not capable of providing for themselves. Obviously underlying this philosophy is the notion that production and people concerns are in conflict; but this is often denied by the 1/9 manager. Because of his own need for acceptance, he avoids negative commentary about others.	Perhaps in reflection of his own self-image, the 1/1 manager sees employees as not liking to work, not competent, hesitant to assume responsibility, and trapped. People and production concerns are felt to be in conflict; so, rather than choosing one or the other, the manager feels his best option is one of withdrawal from employees and isolation from organizational issues. The 1/1's philosophy is often manifested in a cynicism which is likely borne of frustration traceable to his powerlessness to have any meaningful impact on his organization.
Using their authority and power as a base, 9/1 managers reserve the "right" to keep planning activities, decision-making, and goal-setting to themselves. Most decisions are made on the basis of personal subjective criteria. To yield to others by including them in decision-making would be viewed as an admission of weakness and inadequacy as a manager. Decisions are made "for" employees, not "by" them under this approach.	Managers with a 1/9 approach to planning and goal-setting permissively abdicate decision-making and planning responsibilities so that the employee group has total control. In the extreme, the manager will withhold his own views from the employees. So strong is his need for acceptance that he feels employees will not "like" him if he imposes decisions that affect them.	In an effort to avoid personal risks, the 1/1 manager tends to rely on precedents that have been set by past decisions or on authorizations from his superiors. He is quick to quote from the "manual" in making decisions and developing plans. Such an approach is likely designed to free him from personal involvement and responsibility since he can always say, "I can't do otherwise; my hands are tied."
With a firm insistence upon close and constant step-by-step supervision of implementation activities, the 9/1 manager may often give the appearance of doing the work himself. Such actions, of course, reflect a basic distrust of people and their ability to assume responsibility. During implementation activities, the 9/1 manager's power and authority are likely to be most in evidence. The manager expects strict and speedy compliance which, in turn, may be his major mechanism for protecting himself from managerial failure.	The 1/9 manager provides little direction for his employees. He tends to function as a support person or administrator who occupies himself with providing satisfaction for the morale and technological needs of his employees rather than providing any direction. Encouragement checks as to what is needed or how people are feeling are his major implementation activities.	During implementation activities, the 1/1 manager tends to specify his directions as clearly as possible. After having taken this step, he avoids any contact or involvement with the work except when things do not go according to plan. If things are not going according to plan, he is likely to resort to policy or rely on the decisions he can solicit from superiors. A "management by exception" climate prevails, with the 1/1 manager serving primarily as a behind-the-lines tactician.
The focus of attention for the 9/1 manager in evaluation sessions is on the mistakes and failures of individuals in one-to-one sessions. He shuns group meetings for this purpose. Essentially negative and somewhat punitive, he is concerned with fixing the blame and deciding on the penalties he sees as necessary so that the same mistakes will not happen again. It is not uncommon for him to "sacrifice" an employee as an example to bring others into line. The evaluative session will be dominated by his thoughts and feelings to the extent that the employee who is "called on the carpet" will always be on the defensive.	With a "don't say anything if you can't say something nice" approach, the 1/9 manager focuses his attention on the maintenance of high morale among his employees. He tends to avoid any discussion of employee mistakes or failures. Such an approach may have as its basis the underlying distrust of people in that he likely feels they are too fragile to be confronted with their shortcomings and therefore must be protected from such unpleasantries. He would prefer to play the role of confidant, rather than that of censurer.	The 1/1 manager customarily conducts evaluation sessions only if they are required by existing policy. When he does evaluate, he will attempt to find a method which limits his personal involvement and is fairly "safe" and impersonal. Such a method is often found through the use of a formal checklist with which the employee is familiar. He tends to avoid extreme ratings of either favorable or unfavorable, lest he be called on to defend them. Yet, he is rigidly influenced by other's ratings in making personnel decisions.

155

Philosophy of management. The supervisor's philosophy of supervision often reflects the basic set of attitudes and assumptions one has about one's supervisees, their competence, and how best to accomplish work through them. The model is based on three different philosophies about the relative importance of the employees versus production issues. The first philosophy assumes that the employees and the production concerns are in conflict and are mutually exclusive. This position reflects the notion that employees do not like to work and are generally not very competent. Therefore, one's supervisory style under this philosophy is typically an attempt to compensate for the shortcomings of the supervisees as they pertain to the major concern of their supervisors. The 9,1, 1,9, and 1,1 styles fall under this philosophic orientation. The second philosophy calls for moderation and compromise, and it may be thought of as an extension of the conflict theory since the production and the supervisees concerns are still considered incompatible. The 5,5 style is characterized by such an orientation and is aimed at working out compromises between the needs of the organization and the needs of its employees. A manipulative approach results, and this is founded on the assumed gullibility of employees. The third philosophy lends the philosophic basis for the 9,9 style and is based on the assumption that the employees are most satisfied and produce most when they have the opportunity for doing meaningful work. Thus, such an integration approach is aimed at concerns through the creation of meaningful work conditions by the supervisors. The philosophic orientation of the supervisors are thought to predispose them to use specific behaviors during the remaining phases of the supervisory process.

Planning and goal-setting. The supervisors' approach to planning activities are typically colored by their philosophies. This phase of supervision concerns the making of supervisory decisions, planning of work flows, identification of evaluative criteria, and the like. As such, it is the first action step in supervision. Given the philosophic orientations described above, the handling of this phase by the various styled supervisors is generally as follows: 9,1 supervisors keep the planning process to themselves and use subjective criteria in making decisions; 1,9 supervisors permissively abdicate decision-making and planning responsibilities—even to the point of suppressing their own desires in order that the employees have total control; the 1,1 supervisors avoid personal involvement and rely instead upon precedent and/or "the manual" in making decisions and working out plans, especially when they are unable to get the opinions of their superiors; the 5,5 supervisors try to exercise major control while taking into account the opinions of a majority of their employees, and they favor a "tell and sell" approach to influencing decision-making and planning activities; the 9,9 supervisors involve all those affected by decision-making and planning in the activities in an attempt to gain commitment via participation and creativity by way of an increase in the number of resources.

Implementation activities. This component phase concerns the actual translation of plans into action and the accomplishment of the task. Again, the behaviors of supervisors differ according to their preferred styles. The 9,1 supervisors, being basically distrustful of people, insist upon close and constant step-by-step supervision of the work to such an extent that they might well seem to be doing the work themselves. The 1,9 supervisors function as support people and occupy themselves with providing satisfaction for the morale and technological needs of their employees rather than direction. The 1,1 supervisors approach implementation on the basis of the "management by exception" principle and, having specified their directions as clearly as possible, avoid any contact or involvement with the work except when things do not go according to plan. The 5,5 supervisors employ an "open door" policy during implementation and consider themselves to be on call when problems occur or plans need reviewing or revising. The 9,9 supervisors function as members of the implementation team and contribute their special resources where most appropriate while encouraging their supervisees to do the same.

Evaluation practices. Following the accomplishment of work, it is necessary to review how the work was performed in an attempt to learn from both successes and failures. Similarly, the individuals involved must have feedback on their own roles during the implementation phase. Providing this type review is the central task of the evaluation component. The 9,1 supervisors focus all their attention on mistakes and the failures of the employees in one-to-one meetings, and are primarily concerned with fixing the blame and affixing penalties so that mistakes are not likely to be repeated. The 1,9 supervisors focus their attention upon the maintenance of morale and tend to avoid discussions of mistakes in a "don't say anything if you can't say something nice" manner. The 1,1 supervisors do not usually conduct evaluation sessions unless they are required by existing policy; when they do evaluate, it is typically according to a formal checklist with which the supervisees are familiar and upon where they are rated impersonally. The 5,5 supervisors try to focus on both mistakes and successes in rather informal underplayed evaluation sessions; they are likely to reward successes in a group setting, while dealing with attending failures in private one-to-one sessions. The 9,9 supervisors approach evaluation as an ongoing process and intersperse evaluation sessions with implementation activities; they stress the utility of evaluation sessions as a learning opportunity and conduct regular review sessions with all the employees in which everyone's performance—their own included—is candidly appraised.

Administration of the
Management Appraisal Survey

The *Management Appraisal Survey* was group administered between October 7 through October 31, 1980 to 636 of the 696 supervisees (60 supervisees refused to participate) in 36 DHR offices in the 23 county region. A minimum of one session and a maximum of nine sessions were held in each county. Supervisors and their supervisees attended joint explanation sessions which included a brief (approximately 15 minutes) oral presentation focusing mainly on how the *Management Appraisal Survey* and *Styles of Management Inventory* instruments would be used in the study. Questions were answered regarding the study prior to distribution of the instruments.

The average age of the supervisees was 36.9 years old (S.D. = 11.2); 556 were white, 67 were black, and 13 were of other ethnic origins. Their highest educational level attained was: high school diploma, 82; some college, 263; Bachelor's degree, 145; some graduate courses, 83; graduate degree, 56; and missing data, 7. Five-hundred eighteen were female and their average length of employment in the DHR was 6.6 years (S.D. = 5.8). The average length of employment within their present program areas was 4.0 years (S.D. = 3.5).

The *Management Appraisal Survey* is an eight-page self-administered inventory that measures supervisees' perceptions of their supervisors' supervisory styles through the use of vignettes. It takes about 75 minutes to complete the instrument. All of the supervisees' *Management Appraisal Survey* scores (over 200 variables for each supervisee) were calculated (by standard procedures outlined in the accompanying scoring manual) if they were supervised by one supervisor. For example, if one supervisor supervised 13 subordinates, then his/her subordinates' scores were constructed to form an "average perception" of his/her supervisory style.

Administration of the
Styles of Management Inventory

The *Styles of Management Inventory* was group administered to forty-three of the forty-four supervisors (one supervisor refused to participate). The average age of the supervisors was 40.3 years (S.D. = 11.6); 38 were Anglo and five were black. Twenty-five were female and their average length of employment in the DHR was 11.3 years (S.D. =

6.4). The average length of employment within their present program area was 6.9 years (S.D. = 2.5). Ten supervisors had completed some college; 18 had a Bachelor's degree; eight had completed some graduate courses; and eight had received a graduate degree.

The *Styles of Management Inventory* also is an eight page self-administered inventory that measures a supervisor's perceptions of his/her own supervisory style through the use of vignettes. Like its counterpart, the *Management Appraisal Survey*, it also takes approximately 75 minutes to complete. There are over 200 variables in the instrument where they are eventually scored, coded and manipulated to form an individual style of supervision score for each supervisor.

FINDINGS AND DISCUSSION

Table 12–2 presents the perceptions of the supervisors (left side) and their supervisees (right side) as to how the supervisors supervised their subordinates broken down by the five supervisory styles and program area. As can easily be seen from Table 12–2, 24 (55.9%) of the supervisors perceived themselves as possessing the 1,1 supervisory style whereas 21 (48%) of the supervisees rated their supervisors as the same. When viewing the totals in Table 12–2, and ignoring program area, it can easily be determined that on a general level, the 43 supervisors and the 636 supervisees mutually agreed to the supervisory styles that were being utilized by their supervisors. However, it must be pointed out that a majority of the supervisory styles perceived by the supervisors and their supervisees were 1,1.

To break Table 12–2 into raw scores, Table 12–3 displays the means, standard deviations and difference scores of the five supervisory styles broken down by the perceptions of the supervisors and their supervisees. To determine if there were any statistically significant differences between the perceptions of the supervisors and their supervisees for all five supervisory styles, five *t*-tests were calculated and found to be statistically insignificant at the .05 level (two-tailed test).

The average score of the 24 1,1 supervisors identified in this study represents two standard deviations above the mean score of the norm group identified by Teleometrics International. The mean is based on data from business, industry, government and service organizations representing 4,819 supervisors. Based on the norm group, it would be expected that only 2-1/2% of the supervisors in this study would fall above two standard deviations from the mean. However, 50% (and over) of the supervisors in this study were above 2 standard deviations above the mean. This unusually high proportion of 1,1 supervisors ranked the

TABLE 12–2. Supervisory Styles of Supervisors as Perceived by the Supervisors and their Supervisees Broken Down by Program

Program	Perspective											
	Supervisors (N = 43)						Supervisees (N = 44, n = 636)					
	9,9	9,1	5,5	1,9	1,1	Total	9,9	9,1	5,5	1,9	1,1	Total
Food Stamp	2	2	1		4	9	2		1	1	5	9
Aid to Families with Dependent Children		1		1	5	7		1		1	5	7
Child support					2	2					2	2
Medicaid eligibility				3	1	4		1	1	1	1	4
Early and periodic screening, diagnosis, and treatment		1		1		2				2		2
Alternate care for aged, blind, and disabled			1	1	4	6		1		1	4	6
Family services			1		1	2ª		1		1	1	3
Protective services	2			2	7	11	1	1	1	5	3	11
Total	4	4	3	8	24	43	3	5	3	12	21	44

ª One supervisor refused to complete the inventory.

DHR supervisors in one percentile of organizations that have such a high percentage of 1,1 supervisors.

The remaining four supervisory styles (i.e., 9,9; 9,1; 5,5; and 1,9) fell below the mean: The average score for the group of 9,9 supervisors was 2.4 standard deviations below the mean; the 5,5 supervisors were two standard deviations below the mean; the 9,1 supervisors were one standard deviation below the mean; and the 1,9 supervisors were .7 standard deviations below the mean. Figure 12–2 displays graphically the results of the supervisor/supervisee total styles of supervision component T-scores comparing the supervisors' and supervisees' perceptions of supervisory styles.

TABLE 12–3. Distribution of Total Supervisory Style Scores as Perceived by the Supervisors and their Supervisees (from Table 12–2)

Supervisory Styles	Perspective						
	Supervisors			Supervisees			
	N	Mean	S.D.	N	Mean	S.D.	Difference[a]
9,9	4	39.9	7.5	3	38.6	3.1	1.3
9,1	4	40.5	6.5	5	39.4	2.7	1.1
5,5	3	37.6	6.7	3	38.5	2.3	−.9
1,9	8	42.3	7.5	12	40.8	3.7	1.5
1,1	24	45.1	7.6	21	42.7	2.6	2.4
Total	43[b]			44[c]			

[a]Not statistically significant at the .05 level (two-tailed test).
[b]From the totals of the supervisors' perceptions in Table 12–2.
[c]From the totals of the supervisee's perceptions in Table 12–2.

Not only did the supervisors and supervisees agree to what their supervisors' total styles of supervisory patterns were (Table 12–2), but they also agreed as to what their supervisors' four component supervision styles were (Table 12–3). As mentioned in the Methods section, each supervisor's supervisory style score can be broken down into four subcomponents: philosophy, planning, implementation, and evaluation. Through data manipulation, Figure 12–2 represents the four component T-scores derived from Table 12– 3.

Components of supervisory T-scores have a S.D. of 2. A theoretical target band representing 2 points (1 on either side of an "ideal" line) on the component graphs separates the "stronger than desirable" from the "weaker than desirable" practices. A deviation of 4 or more points from the band on either side of any of the styles is a significant departure and worthy of consideration. In interpreting these, special attention should be given to the diagonal gray band for this constitutes a *theoretical target plot*; that is, it represents the plot that would have resulted if one had scored *ideally* on each component. Therefore, obtained scores can be compared with this ideal target as a means of identifying significant departures from ideal practices. Any score plot which falls above the target line is indicative of more than theoretically desirable usage of the plotted style and should suggest a search for other style alternatives which will result in a decreased use of the currently overused style. Similarly, any style plot which falls below the target line may be interpreted as reflecting less usage than is theoretically desirable of the plotted style. Ways of

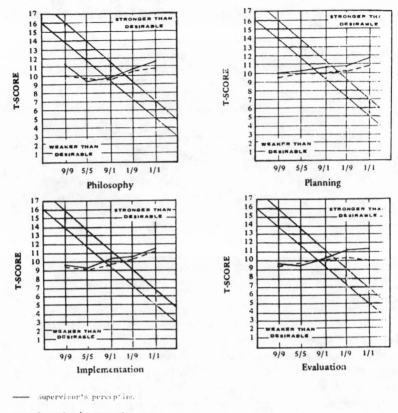

—— Supervisor's perception

---- Supervisee's perception

FIGURE 12–2. Comparison of supervisee/supervisor total styles of management component T-scores comparing supervisor and supervisee perceptions

strengthening such styles in one's practice should be ascertained. Thus, on a general level, the four plots in Figure 12–2 can be interpreted to reflect a significant over-reliance on 1,1 behaviors coupled with too few 9,9 behaviors. The plots reveal an appropriate amount of 9,1 behaviors.

The most important finding of this study was the extremely high number of supervisors who utilized the 1,1 supervisory style, the most undesirable style of supervision of all. Not only did the supervisors and supervisees agree as to what their supervisors' total styles of supervisory patterns were, but they also agreed as to what their supervisors' four component supervision scores were.

Only four supervisors utilized the 9,9 style of supervision as perceived by themselves and three as perceived by the supervisees. Thus, less than 10% of the supervisors utilized the most desirable form of supervision regardless of perception.

Research described in *The New Managerial Grid* indicates that the 9,9 "team builder" supervision style is most positively associated with productivity and corporate profitability, career success, and satisfaction, along with physical and mental health. However, this is not true in the present study.

The most unexpected finding of this study was the high number of supervisors who utilized the 1,1 supervision style. It was not anticipated that the prevalence of the 1,1 style would be two standard deviations above the norm as found in this study. Findings of this study indicate an organizational culture exists which supports 1,1 supervision styles.

The 1,1 style of supervision is usually not considered as a dominant style but as back-up style to which supervisors retreat when the environment is tense or stressful. They may also retreat to this style when they feel frustrated, threatened, or when they are meeting resistance from others.

One possible explanation for the large number of 1,1 supervisors in the Region is that the prior administration can easily be characterized by the old line, authority-obedience philosophy. This style is closely related to a paternalistic 9,1 style of supervision. Decisions were made in the central office and approved by the administrator. This type of organizational climate breeds dependency and apathy and supports the development of a 1,1 culture. The recent change in supervision philosophy may not yet be clearly perceived as a change in supervision behavior. This type of change may be slow and made more difficult by the resistance to change of a 1,1 style at lower levels of supervision.

Secondly, the historical definition was that the line-level supervisors' functions were technically oriented to the tasks of the subordinate's job. It has only been in recent years that a supervisor's job included responsibilities for developing unit goals and objectives, planning activities, implementing action plans, and evaluating results. This new role requires human relations and conceptual skills not previously recognized as valuable. This type of change is often slow.

A third possible cause could be related to the rules, regulations, and strict lines of communication which are inherent in large bureaucratic organizations. When work is over-regulated by manuals, policies, and procedures, a situation develops where individual autonomy, creativity, and innovation are not encouraged, but discouraged. Supervisors thus become frustrated at their inability to have any meaningful impact on the organization and may withdraw into a 1,1 supervision style.

A fourth reason may relate to the funding base of the agency. Tax supported organizations are made exceedingly turbulent by "soft money" funding and incessant changes in the general objectives and missions of agencies, as well as in the very life of specific programs. This results in frequent periods of job insecurity which, in turn, breeds inactivity and an effort to maintain the status quo.

A fifth barrier may be that obtaining genuine involvement, participation and commitment is often perceived as very time consuming and is viewed as being too great a task to attempt.

A sixth factor may be the resistance to quantify outputs or the lack of an accurate way to measure the unit's activities in relation to the goals and objectives of the program. This absence of accountability can lead to a 1,1 culture and allow it to continue.

Yet, the final and greatest difficulty may be that the knowledge, skills and abilities needed for supervising work in a 9,9 manner are scarce. This involves supervision practices which increase individual involvement and requires commitment to sound problem solving and increased production. Supervisors must have the ability to develop within each employee positive mental attitudes, interpersonal openness, and candid communication which, in turn, insures effective decision making. Also needed is the willingness to evaluate organizational traditions and precedents which stifle productive effort and creative thinking, replacing them with standards and values which promote efforts toward excellence and innovation.

Past practices that have long ordered, regulated, and stabilized many public organizations are under serious attack. Resources are shrinking and increased funding is not forthcoming. Client needs are changing. Agencies are struggling with how human energies and physical resources can be harnessed to provide better service to clients.

The 1,1 culture identified here can present serious problems to an organization when the times call for dynamic change rather than order and regularity. This culture looks to traditions and past practices for guidance in decision making, even though the past may be outmoded. It persists because what is widely known and recognized is produced for non-1,1 supervisors to conform to the culture. This creates a drag on the organization's capacity for change and slows down progress. There is no communication, problems are ignored, decisions and risks are avoided, and innovation is not encouraged; thus, good employees leave or become stagnant.

RECOMMENDATIONS FROM FINDINGS

Due to the large number of 1,1 supervisors as identified in this study, a Regional Management Team was formed and met on January 6 and 7, 1981, to review the project findings and implications. It was the concensus of the Team that a systematic and deliberate plan must be developed in order to operationalize a participatory management (9,9 supervision style) concept throughout all levels of supervisory staff. The Team agreed that this effort must begin with the Team and then be expanded in a planned manner.

The Team recognized that reality was reflected in how individual staff perceived their supervisors as well as how they received the overall organization. The Team also recognized that change is continually occurring—the challenge is recognizing the quality of change and managing it. The Team also recognized the inherent value of each employee's input because the quality of the agency is the aggregate of the qualities of the employees. Goals were formulated as a result of this realization and as a basis for moving toward a 9,9 style of supervision.

Six goals were established in trying to improve the overall supervision within the DHR in the areas of: team management; personnel policies and procedures; training; communication; commitment to future research and experimentation; and evaluation. The objectives of the goals are as follows.

1. Team Management

- to become knowledgeable of team management concepts and develop participatory management skills;
- to develop a team approach to meeting agency objectives;
- to set team goals and objectives which reflect a consistent regional philosophy of management;
- to clarify areas of Team decisions versus areas of program decisions;
- to practice concensus planning across program lines;
- to integrate all individual program perspectives into one regional identity;
- to increase Team visibility and role model Team supervisory behaviors; and
- to individually assume responsibilities for continual self-evaluation as a team member.

2. Personnel Policies and Procedures

- to utilize the existing personnel policies and procedures in a manner which reflects a fundamental dedication by regional supervision to the selection of high potential, team-oriented supervisors;
- to develop performance plans for supervisors based on a balance of exhibited concern for production and for staff; and
- to develop a reward system which will promote team supervision behavior.

3. Training

- to develop a time-framed, formalized training plan for the Team that is congruent with team management concepts;
- to develop a training plan for middle level, line-level, and potential supervisors to promote participatory supervision; and
- to promote skills sharing among supervisors.

4. Communication

- of attitudes which promote standards of excellence; cooperation and support among the various programs;
- of a belief that each individual is free to grow, develop, and use to full potential, his/her capabilities and resources;
- of information to improve the credibility between supervisors and other staff; and
- of confidence in employee's inherent desire to perform well.

5. Commitment to Future Research and Experimentation

- to foster the development of an attitude within the region receptive to a quest for knowledge through experimentation and research.

6. Evaluation

- to continually assess the progress of the Region toward meeting these goals.

The Team realized the importance of the development of action plans to accomplish the above goals. Action plans were developed through task forces. A task force was formed for each of the above goals. Each task force was the responsibility of a Team member and included staff from all program areas and at various levels.

REFERENCES

Blake, R.R., & Mouton, J.S. *The new managerial grid.* Houston, TX Gulf Publishing Company, 1978.

Hall, J., Harvey, J.B., & Williams, M.S. *Management appraisal survey.* Woodlands, TX: Teleometrics International, 1973.

Hall, J., Harvey, J.B., & Williams, M.S. *Styles of management inventory.* Woodlands, TX: Teleometrics International, 1980.

Hammer, T.H., & Dachler, H.P. A test of some assumptions underlying the path goal model of supervision: Some suggested conceptual modifications. *Organizational Behavior and Human Performance*, 1975, *14*, 60–75.

Hersey, P., & Blanchard, K.H. *Management of organizational behavior: Utilizing human resources.* Englewood Cliffs, NJ: Prentice-Hall, Inc., 1972.

Jaco, A.G., & Vroom, H.V. Hierarchical level and leadership style. *Organizational Behavior and Human Performance*, 1977, *18*, 131–145.

Sheriff, D.R. Leadership skills and executive development: Leadership mythology vs. six learnable skills. *Training and Development Journal*, 1968, *22*, 29–36.

York, R.O. Can change be effectively managed? *Administration in Social Work*, 1977, *1*, 187–197.

13

Management Succession and Administrative Style

JOEL KOTIN
MYRON R. SHARAF

This study of management succession is the second of two articles dealing with the events that occured at a state mental hospital following a change of superintendents. In the first article we explored the ideological elements of the accompanying intrastaff controversy.[1] In the present study we are concerned with the interaction of social structure and executive personality in determining the successor's role. This is in contrast to most previous studies of management succession, which have been focused primarily on sociological factors. Conceptually, this study is part of a recent trend toward the inclusion of personality in studies of occupational roles and organizational processes.[2] We shall consider one aspect of an executive's personality, namely, his administrative style. We shall introduce the concept of tight and loose administrative styles in order to understand more fully the successor's behavior and subsequent events in the life of the institution.

PREVIOUS STUDIES

Perhaps the most significant treatment of succession in the theoretical literature is Gouldner's study of the succession of a new manager in a gypsum plant.[3] Here the successor was faced with problems of commu-

Editor's Note: "Management Succession and Administrative Style," by Joel Kotin and Myron R. Sharaf was originally published in *Psychiatry: Journal for the Study of Interpersonal Processes* in August 1967. We have now asked the authors to examine their article in the light of developments in the field since that time and share their reactions with our readers. With permission of the publisher, the original article is reprinted below. "Management Succession Revisited" follows.

nication and control. His information and authority via the existing formal system were inadequate, and he had no access to the existing informal system, especially the corps of "old lieutenants" who owed their loyalties to the former leader. These old lieutenants were under the spell of what Gouldner called the Rebecca Myth, namely the idealization of a departed chief to whom loyalty belongs and a corresponding derogation and suspicion of the new chief.[4]

In countering this opposition, the new manager utilized two important techniques. First, he replaced some of the "old lieutenants"—some of the middle-management supervisory personnel. The replacements were loyal to the new manager and faithfully supported his policies. Gouldner calls this technique "strategic replacement." Second, he enhanced communication and control by what Gouldner calls "increased bureaucratization." As Gouldner points out,

> Barred from effective use of the informal system of controls, the successor was compelled to rely more heavily upon the formal system. . . . There is a close connection between succession and a surge of bureaucratic development, particularly in the direction of formal rules.[5]

At the gypsum plant this increased bureaucratization took the form of the institution of new rules and stricter enforcement of existing ones; the introduction of required daily and weekly reports that provided the new manager with a more careful check on production results and on accidents and breakdowns; and the introduction of formal "warning notices" to be sent to delinquent workers.

Guest's study of the succession of a new manager in an automobile plant focused on how the new leader improved the plant's performance, rather than on sociological elements of the succession, but certain points can be inferred from his well-documented presentation.[6] Although the new manager did make some strategic replacements, mostly by promotion from within the organization, there was no surge of bureaucratic development; indeed, Guest describes the plant's organization as considerably looser following the succession.

Another aspect of Guest's study that contrasts sharply with Gouldner's is the description of the mythology that evolved concerning the new and departed leaders. At the automobile plant the retired manager was disliked, while the new man was immensely popular. Hodgson, Levinson, and Zaleznik suggest that these two types of response represent alternative attempts by members of the organization to deal with the loss of the departing figure and the difficulties of adjustment to a new administration. Furthermore, they add, ". . . it would appear that both types can coexist, with cyclical variations in the predominance of one over the other."[7] Thus the concept of the Rebecca Myth must be expanded to include the reverse reaction; the polarization of affect may be in either direction.

RESEARCH SETTING AND METHODS

Since the research setting has been described in detail previously,[8] we will present only a brief summary of it here. Eastern State Hospital[9] is the largest mental institution in its state, with a capacity of 2200 beds and an annual admission rate of 2000. The staff includes more than 1100 persons. Complete medical and administrative responsibility for the hospital is invested in the superintendent, under whom are an assistant superintendent and various divisions, such as medicine, nursing, and finance.

In April, 1963, Dr. Smith, eminent in psychiatry, president of various prestigious professional associations, and highly esteemed within the hospital, resigned after 17 years of service. A new superintendent, Dr. Lattimore, also of considerable renown in psychiatry, took office.

In July, 1963, the second author began recording informal observations; the research was formally begun in the spring of 1964. Between May, 1964, and August, 1965, over 100 interviews were conducted by the first author. Those interviewed included the entire senior medical staff, the heads of all major departments within the hospital, plus many others. Also interviewed were Dr. Smith and those psychiatrists and department heads who left the hospital after Dr. Lattimore's succession. However, no systematic attempt was made to interview persons in the lower levels of the organization—residents, nurses, aides, and patients. Most of the senior medical staff and many department heads were interviewed twice, with about a year intervening between the first and second interview. In addition to interviewing, the authors regularly attended numerous meetings and conferences throughout the hospital.

INITIAL PROBLEMS CONFRONTING THE SUCCESSOR

Although Dr. Smith had been concerned with developing a many-sided treatment program for the hospital, it was during his administration that the battle for psychoanalytically oriented psychotherapy had been fought and won in the state hospital. At the end of his term of office the major theoretical orientation of the hospital was psychodynamic. Psychoanalytically oriented psychotherapy was the "prestige" treatment and the core of the residency training program, even though the hospital had pioneered in an impressive number of developments in community psychiatry, including day and night hospitals, a patient employee program, and a Home Visit Unit.

Dr. Lattimore came to the hospital with a well-known interest in social psychiatry and research. Although social psychiatry and research programs had aroused little opposition during Dr. Smith's regime—in part because they never challenged the central emphasis on psychodynamics in the training program—Dr. Lattimore's increased emphasis on and more rapid implementation of these programs led to resentment in many analytically oriented staff members, who felt that individual psychotherapy was being downgraded. A good deal of controversy accompanied many of the programs, whether they were entirely new to the hospital and paid for by outside agencies or extensive modifications of existing hospital programs.[10]

There were several other complicating factors. After the arrival of Dr. Lattimore, a number of changes among the hospital's top-level personnel occurred, many of which were unrelated to the succession or the new programs. In the two-year period following Dr. Lattimore's succession, new personnel included the assistant superintendent, two successive clinical directors, the director of nurses, the head dietitian, and the head occupational therapist. Thus, the new superintendent was confronted with the loss of some key persons soon after his arrival, at a time when he was just beginning to find his way in a new social world.

In addition to the specific problems of resistance to new programs and staff turnover, Dr. Lattimore, like all successors, was faced with the general problems of communication and control. Lacking informal contacts, he could not easily find out what was going on in the system. Lacking fullhearted cooperation from some "old lieutenants," and confronted with the inertial properties of a large government institution, he found it difficult to implement change.

Finally, the prevalence of a Rebecca Myth was both a reflection of and a factor contributing to the difficulties encountered by the new superintendent. Many staff members, especially psychiatrists, were quick to note what they perceived to be flaws in Dr. Lattimore's psychiatric emphasis or his administrative methods or both. They tended to remember Dr. Smith nostalgically as the "good" superintendent and to look upon Dr. Lattimore as the "bad" one. The polarization described by Gouldner was very much in evidence.

However, the situation was not completely bleak. The "myth" did not affect all personnel. Some persons were indifferent, and others supported Dr. Lattimore and hoped that he would make needed changes. This feeling was especially strong in persons more in ideological sympathy with Dr. Lattimore than with Dr. Smith, and in persons—often the same ones—who felt that they had not received sufficient support under the old regime. Nevertheless, the dominant initial feeling was nostalgia for Dr. Smith and resentment toward Dr. Lattimore.

Like Gouldner's new manager, Dr. Lattimore approached his problems of communication and control by making numerous strategic replacements. This was facilitated by the departure of some key personnel. Dr. Lattimore was also able to use State and Federal funds to create several new positions at the middle management level, so that he could recruit new personnel without having to replace anyone. However, in some instances, the choice of a new man was heavily influenced by pressure from the old lieutenants, which tended to make the replacement less useful to Dr. Lattimore in furthering *his* plans for the hospital. As James points out, high-status professionals within an organization frequently influence the administrative decision-making process in this manner.[11]

In addition to bringing in strategic replacements from outside the hospital (assistant superintendent and clinical director), Dr. Lattimore varied the technique by making many promotions from within the hospital (several senior psychiatrists). In some instances the promoted persons were sympathetic to his aims and methods, and their promotions enhanced their enthusiasm and loyalty to the new management. When established in their new positions, they were model strategic replacements. In other instances Dr. Lattimore promoted persons who were not particularly sympathetic to his aims, but who were regarded as "entitled" to the promotion by most of the staff. Conceivably, one intent of these promotions was to win over the recalcitrant lieutenant. Very often, however, these staff members simply felt that they had received their due, and there was no increase in enthusiasm or cooperation.[12]

Strategic replacements, whatever their form, take time. As Gouldner states:

> If the new manager is at all sensitive to what is going on, he does not wish to be accused of failing to give the old lieutenants a "chance" nor of seeking to install his favorites with indecent haste. He has to spend some time looking for possible allies and lining up replacements. In the meanwhile, the breakdown of upward communication to the new manager grows more acute. It is, in part, as an outgrowth of this crisis that the successor elaborates the system of "paper reports," the better to keep his finger on things and to check up on the "old lieutenants."[13]

Striking in the succession of Dr. Lattimore was the fact that he did not rely on increased "rules" or "reports." There was no "bureaucratic surge" following his succession. In order to understand this more fully, we must turn to a new concept, that of "administrative style."

TIGHT VS. LOOSE STYLES OF ADMINISTRATION

With the exception of Hodgson, Levinson, and Zaleznik,[14] studies of succession have emphasized sociological factors. For example, Gouldner emphasizes "the kinds of pressures and problems" which confront the successor because of his role.[15] He discusses the advantages and disadvantages of the various strategies a successor can employ. He also analyzes the particular strategies the successor of his study did in fact employ, but his analysis does not relate the successor's choice of strategies to his personality.

It is our thesis that the process of succession can be understood more fully if one examines more closely the influence of the successor's personality on his role performance and the role performances of others. We argue that the choices the successor makes reflect the influence of *both* institutional exigencies and the successor's personality. Of the many different facets of personality that might be studied, we have selected one in particular—the successor's administrative style.

Administrative style refers to an executive's professional behavior, the characteristic way in which he functions as an executive, how he structures his role, and how he influences the roles and functioning of others in the organization. It is, for the most part, unrelated to policy: it is not *what* he does, but *how* he does it. We are especially concerned here with two contrasting types, the "tight" and the "loose" administrative styles.

A tight administrative style relates to the military model, sharing with it an emphasis on hierarchical authority and communication. A tight style implies:

1. clear-cut delegation of authority and responsibility,
2. an orderly and hierarchical chain of command through which communication flows upward and downward, without skipping levels,
3. a reliance on formal communications—for example, regular meetings, reports, printed forms,
4. formal expression of power—for example, hearings, written notification of promotions and dismissals,
5. reliance on explicit, written rules, or, in their absence, on tradition.

A loose administrative style is characterized by flexibility, with fluid lines of authority and communication. A loose style implies:

1. absence, in many areas, of clearly designated authority and responsibility,
2. considerable tolerance of role ambiguity and role diffusion,

3. frequent bypassing of the chain of command, both in communication and authority,
4. informal communications,
5. informal exercise of power,
6. relatively little reliance on rules and tradition.

Using Presidents Eisenhower and Kennedy as examples, Arthur Schlesinger, Jr., illustrates some of the differences between a tight and loose administrative style:

> The President [Kennedy] was in this respect very much like Roosevelt or Churchill. If he was interested in a problem like the Congo and wanted to control what was going on, he would not follow the chain of command as President Eisenhower, I gather, did. In other words, say, tell something to the Secretary of State, who would tell it to the Under Secretary of State for Political Affairs, who would tell it to the Assistant Secretary of State for Africa, who would tell it to the Congo Desk Officer, and similarly the Congo Desk Officer would reply through the same chain of command. This would often dilute the message, both ways, divesting it of any pungency of character. President Kennedy's instinct would be to call the man and ask him, and this had the effect of not only giving the President much fresher information and sharper opinion, but it also would imbue the machinery of government itself with the sense of his own purposes.[16]

Schlesinger goes on to emphasize that Kennedy used his White House staff in a very flexible way. He disliked the notion of staff assistants with fixed assignments and sharp demarcations of authority. Moreover, the boundaries between the White House staff and other governmental agencies became blurred. The Presidential assistants took an active role in defending the interest of the President and were often aggressive in invading what a particular bureaucracy regarded as its own domain. In this way the President, through his staff, could seek out those people in the government machinery who were capable of innovation and could support such persons in their own internal conflicts. It is not surprising that these efforts by the White House staff were often labeled as "meddling" and resented by officials who were wedded to the status quo.

Schlesinger emphasizes the advantages of a loose-style—for example, it gives the leader fresher information and permits him to strengthen the influence of innovative and creative persons throughout the organization. However, when Hans Morgenthau describes Kennedy's administrative style, it is difficult to realize that one is reading about the same style that Schlesinger cites so positively. Morgenthau criticizes Kennedy for the "disorderliness" of his administration:

He [Kennedy] would receive information from, and give orders to, second-level officials without informing their chiefs, and it happened that when an issue was later discussed in the formal councils of government, he had forgotten that he had already given an order contrary to his present position. From Schlesinger's discussion of Kennedy's Vietnam policy emerges a melancholy tale of ignorance, miscalculations, confusion, and absent-mindedness. The initial decision to withdraw support from Diem derived from a Presidential misunderstanding of the actual position of the different executive departments concerned. The result was confusion.[17]

Commentators tend either, like Schlesinger, totally to approve the loose style, or, like Morgenthau, totally to condemn it. The critics are more numerous than the supporters. Cumming and Cumming, in discussing administration in the mental hospital, write:

... The authority holder should always be alert for skipping and should try to divert communication back through the correct channels. ... Persistent skipping always demoralizes the person skipped—first, because it cuts him out of the communication stream and, second, because it gives presumptive equality to those under him who, by other criteria such as salary and training, are not his equal.[18]

One of the few supporters of a loose style is Zaleznik, although he labels it differently. Zaleznik speaks of "bureaucratic" and "circumventive" styles of management. He writes that "bureaucracy" fosters "orderliness, equality, and proportionality," whereas "circumvention" fosters "ambiguity, competitiveness, and shifting rewards."[19] Eisenhower is his example of an executive functioning in the "bureaucratic" mode, and Franklin Roosevelt is the prototype of the "circumventive" style. Zalezink's own sympathies are clearly with the latter, since his special concern is the fostering of innovation and initiative within an organization rather than the maintenance of order and harmony.

ADMINISTRATIVE STYLE AT ESH

At ESH one of the outstanding characteristics of the succession was the change from a tight to a loose style of administration. Dr. Smith was widely known as an excellent administrator, and under his administration the hospital was a model of tight organization. The following excerpts from Dr. Smith's writings on administration illustrate his views:

The efficiency of bureaucratic administration depends upon the reliability of its responses and its adherence to regulations.

He [the administrator] must delegate responsibilities to others. . . . the formal channels for authority will let everyone know who is responsible for what.

The good leader supports those to whom he delegates authority by avoiding *over-ruling, undercutting,* or *bypassing.*

To the best of the authors' knowledge, the hospital bureaucracy functioned as it should, with a maximum of efficiency and a minimum of nonproductive red tape. Dr. Smith delegated medical authority to his clinical director and concerned himself largely with the administrative aspects of the hospital. His personal manner was characterized by one psychiatrist as follows:

Typically Dr. Smith would get up and say, "This is our twelfth administrative meeting of the year, and I have the following to report." When changes were made, all of the appropriate people were consulted—the various levels of staff conferences, separately and together. Then there would be a barrage of memos. Then, at 12:01 A.M. on January 1, you would do it the new way.

Dr. Lattimore unquestionably had a looser administrative style. He frequently cited the remarks of a former superior:

All rules of procedure are to be neglected to a large extent. Personnel are to be taught that they are to use intuition, imagination, initiative, judgment, rather than to be constrained by rules or procedure. For example, let the nurses decide whether or not they are to wear uniforms, and the best way to get along with patients. If they want a type of ward organization, they do not need special permission, unless it unavoidably collides with something else.

We want continuing change, not by ukase but by discussion and argument, perhaps continuing for months, with respect for the opinions of all. Issues can be decided by logical debate rather than direct orders. The "High Moguls" should be willing to justify themselves to the "Low Moguls." . . . Look for capacities additional to those imparted by training or required by the role. Especially important are those qualities which are submerged, seeking outlet, but inhibited by rigidities in our system and in our thinking. . . . These concepts are not new, only the doing is new.

Dr. Lattimore's administration was characterized by flexibility and fluid lines of authority and communication. Several comments from staff members illustrate the difference in the styles:

A *psychiatrist*: The old way was to do things through regular channels; the new way is not.

A *clinical director*: With Dr. Smith there was a clear-cut assignment
of roles. He was very much involved with administrative problems.
With Dr. Lattimore this is not so.

A *senior psychiatrist*: I think Dr. Lattimore is much more flexible
than Dr. Smith. He's younger and more flexible. He's less apt to say:
"No, that's impossible," and more inclined to say: "Let's see how that
works out—why not go ahead and do it?" That's the main difference.

Dr. Lattimore's personal manner was folksy and equalitarian. He
would sometimes begin a meeting saying, "Does anyone have anything
to get off his chest?" And in his previous job he had been nicknamed,
"Hi, guys." A psychiatrist contrasted the old and new superintendents:

Dr. Smith was a very dignified, proper, distant administrator. You had
to request an appointment to see him. Dr. Lattimore is sort of easygo-
ing, friendly, informal—more a sibling than a father image like Dr.
Smith.

It is clear from the above quotations that Dr. Lattimore did *not* initiate a "surge of bureaucratic development." To do so would have run
counter to his whole style of administration. The way he did proceed to
solve the problems raised by his succession can be illustrated in part by
his relations with his medical staff.

When Dr. Lattimore arrived at the hospital, there were two clinical
directors. Both had had psychoanalytic training, and neither was especially interested in the social psychiatry or research endeavors that
formed the center of Dr. Lattimore's interests. Dr. Cheever, the senior
director, was clearly in charge of the clinical program and residency
training. He followed in a line of clinical directors who had enjoyed considerable autonomy under Dr. Smith.

Four months after Dr. Lattimore arrived, Dr. Cheever resigned. In
an interview with one of the authors he stated:

I was used to the autonomy of my department. I was used to having my decisions backed up. Under Dr. Lattimore I couldn't make a decision, nor could I get anyone else to. My views and his about community psychiatry are at opposite poles.

The last sentence of the quotation calls attention to the sharp ideological disagreement which existed between Dr. Lattimore and Dr.
Cheever.[20] Granted that difference, trouble between the superinten-

dent and the clinical director could have been predicted, regardless of the style of the successor. However, style played a crucial role in determining how the successor handled the trouble. A successor with a tight style might have done one òf several things:

1. replaced the clinical director with a man of his own choosing,
2. left the old clinical director with the autonomy he had, even though this would have meant abdicating any control over his activities,
3. increased bureaucratic measures in order to check up on the recalcitrant lieutenant and increase executive control of the organization.

Gouldner suggests the likelihood of choice (3) in the initial stages of succession, since (1) would mean moving with "unseemly haste" and (2) would mean organizational ineffectiveness from the successor's viewpoint.

With his loose style Dr. Lattimore chose none of the above alternatives. Instead, he tried to "win over" Dr. Cheever through informal contact. In the meantime, since he wanted to get things moving rapidly, he preferred to "work around" his clinical director in areas where they came into opposition. For example, Dr. Lattimore started a social-psychiatric rehabilitation program even though Dr. Cheever vehemently opposed the particular form this enterprise took. The clinical director interpreted Dr. Lattimore's activities as "meddling" and as "undermining" of his authority, and, as a consequence, resigned.

In seeking a replacement, Dr. Lattimore was strongly influenced by the remaining clinical director and several senior psychiatrists. Accepting their counsel, he appointed a psychiatrist who had formerly been at ESH for some years and was at that time in psychoanalytic training. Thus, while the replacement was regarded as "legitimate" by the old lieutenants, there was some question as to how well the superintendent and the new clinical director could work together. Perhaps in realization of this fact, the new man was not given a position as *the* clinical director—a position Dr. Cheever had held—but shared authority with the remaining clinical director and a third psychiatrist, another old lieutenant who was also promoted to clinical director. In addition, a fourth psychiatrist was added to the staff at a high level, and functioned as a clinical director. He was closer to Dr. Lattimore ideologically than the other clinical directors, but his legitimacy was questioned more and he was never fully integrated as a clinical director.

During this period, Dr. Lattimore's defenses as a successor were especially apparent. He tried to woo the existing clinical directors and other old lieutenants by exchanging ideas with them and seeking their advice. At the same time he tried to maximize his own freedom by leaving the situation ambiguous and fluid, sometimes accepting their advice, sometimes moving on his own initiative where it ran counter to their wishes. Above all, he did not *fix* the authority system in any clear-cut way. To do so along previous lines might have jeopardized the possibility of moving the hospital in the direction he thought desirable. On the other hand, if he had moved decisively in his own direction, he might have shaken the equilibrium of the organization. He wished to avoid an exodus of top psychiatric personnel because he valued the abilities of the old lieutenants, and he realized the difficulty of recruiting staff members for state hospital positions. In short, Dr. Lattimore hoped that leadership compatible with his own interests would emerge eventually, but that he could manage not to rock the boat too much in the meantime.

Nine months after the new clinical director's arrival, he resigned. He stated in an interview:

> The question is, how many clinical directors are there to be. It has varied—three, four, or five. Now the clinical directors are assigned administrative functions. Dr. Lattimore gave each a different service. He usurped, thus, the authority of the senior physicians over their services. Then the superintendent and the assistant superintendent began to deal directly with seniors, bypassing the clinical directors. . . . There is very little communication at the hospital. . . . No administration or organization.

The clinical director voiced strongly the classic complaint against the loose style—its tendency to "meddle" and to skip proper organizational levels to "deal directly" with subordinates (the "seniors"). His other complaints are also familiar: role diffusion (the assigning of administrative functions to the clinical directors), inadequate formal communication, and the lack of administrative organization.

At about this time the fourth clinical director also faded from the scene, leaving the junior clinical director from Dr. Smith's administration and the promoted old lieutenant as the two remaining clinical directors. The latter was in charge of the outpatient program while the former devoted his energies mainly to the training program; thus a modus vivendi was reached. Dr. Lattimore was continually criticized, however, for interfering in clinical areas and in the training program, formerly the exclusive provinces of the clinical directors.

The activities of Mr. Eisenberg, a nursing supervisor, provide another example of the working of a loose administrative style. Shortly after Dr. Lattimore's succession, Mr. Eisenberg established contact with the new administration, especially Dr. George, the new assistant superintendent. Mr. Eisenberg was supported by Dr. George in his controversial efforts to take over the family care program, a program involving the placement of patients in foster homes in the community. The social service department had jurisdiction over this particular program, but, lacking personnel and medical supervision, it had been able to run the program only on a very limited basis. Investing enormous energy and ignoring criticism from both his own superiors and other departments, Mr. Eisenberg increased the number of patients in this program from 29 to 60 in a two-year period, with nurses under his direction making the required weekly visits. In addition, Mr. Eisenberg established a community preparation ward and vigorously continued his work on the renovation of part of the aged North Side of the hospital.

The loose style of the administration was manifested in several ways. First, Mr. Eisenberg communicated directly with Dr. Lattimore and Dr. George, bypassing the nursing hierarchy and the senior psychiatrist in charge of the service. Second, departmental lines were crossed: The nursing service performed what was traditionally a social service function. Third, a subordinate with considerable talent was given support directly from the top in his conflicts both within his service and with other departments.

It is understandable that Mr. Eisenberg's superiors in the nursing service, the social service department, and the senior psychiatrist in charge of the North Side were all disgruntled at various times by Mr. Eisenberg's freewheeling activities and the support they received from the administration. In varying degrees, they felt bypassed, undermined, and, at the very least, uninformed.

Dr. Lattimore's loose style in rapidly implementing new programs, as illustrated by the support he gave to Mr. Eisenberg, led to considerable criticism of his methods by the old lieutenants, particularly the senior medical staff and some department heads. Dr. Lattimore argued that he used the tactics he did because he often could not get the cooperation of the person formally in charge of a given service or department. Those who were bypassed—some of whom had originally been somewhat critical of Dr. Lattimore's program—now focused their opposition on his "methods," complaining that they did not object to his goals but to the "way" he pursued them. Probably both interpretations held a degree of truth.

It is important to note that when Dr. Lattimore found a department head or service chief who moved energetically in directions of which the new superintendent generally approved, he fully respected the autonomy and authority of that person. In short, what was experienced as a loose or "undermining" style by some, was experienced as strong support by others. Indeed, a tighter administrative style might have prevented Dr. Lattimore from giving as much support to those he favored. He could bend the rules or break traditions in a way which fostered a rapid mobilization of resources for a project he wished to further. This ability to provide differential strong support was especially useful to Dr. Lattimore in recruiting, and helps to explain how he was able to persuade many psychiatrists to come to work at a State hospital.

DISCUSSION

As our discussion of administrative style implies, there are advantages and disadvantages to both the tight and loose styles. The gains and losses that accompany a loose style at the time of a succession are well illustrated by the course of events at ESH.

A successor's loose style permits him to avoid the Charybdis of premature direct confrontation with his recalcitrant lieutenants and the Scylla of institutional paralysis stemming from the resistance of the old lieutenants. To some extent he can impose his will on the organization by working around the recalcitrant lieutenants without forcing a showdown. He can do this by communicating with and supporting innovative and creative subordinates "down the line." At the same time he can try to win over or at least effect a working relationship with the recalcitrant lieutenants through a variety of informal means. He thus avoids drastic measures such as replacement, and formalizing measures such as the requiring of more reports and lengthier and more frequent meetings, which might fulfill the letter but not the spirit of his intentions.

The disadvantages of the loose style are also numerous. Department heads, already threatened by the coming of the successor, may feel even more insecure and undermined when the successor wheels and deals directly with subordinates. Resistance that was originally focused on the successor's aims can now be buttressed by criticism of the *way* he seeks to fulfill them, compounding the controversy. The loose style also may make it difficult to insure accountability, since working around a recalcitrant lieutenant may involve assigning an overlapping role to another person; determining who is responsible for any particular aspect of the job can remain a continuing source of ambiguity.

The advantages of a tight style for the successor have been clearly outlined by Gouldner. When confronted with inadequate communication and recalcitrant lieutenants, the successor with a tight style can rely upon formal methods of communication and control to impose his will upon the organization. We wish to add that in the face of the ideological and personal clashes that often accompany a succession, "going by the book" provides external criteria which cannot easily be challenged.

However, the absence of challenge does not necessarily mean the presence of commitment to the successor's plans. A disadvantage of the tight style is that the successor may be hampered by covert bureaucratic "sabotage" by the old lieutenants; at the same time, because of his style, he may be unable to mobilize support for his policies from sympathetic subordinates at lower levels of the organization. To the extent that he relies on the rules and the formal chain of command the successor limits his freedom and flexibility.

In addition to specific gains and losses at times of succession, there are general advantages and disadvantages to tight and loose styles. A tight style fosters responsibility and order in an organization, but can also lead to stagnation and rigidity. A loose style may nurture creativity and flexibility, but it can lead to chaos and irresponsibility.

Responsibility and creativity are both essential to the healthy growth of an organization. Conversely, stagnation and chaos must both be discouraged. We suggest that organizations "strike a balance" over time in these areas by means of alternating periods of tight and loose administration. We further speculate that the expansion phase of organizational growth may occur more frequently during periods of loose administration, while the consolidation phase may be associated more with periods of tight administration. These periods need not necessarily be associated with the term of a single top executive. As long as further tightening does not strangle the organization and further loosening does not result in disintegration, a leader with the same style as his predecessor may be tolerated. Some organizations may function well for an extremely long period of time or indefinitely with a particular style of administration. However, if and when the disadvantages of either the tight or the loose style accumulate and the losses accompanying a style of administration outweigh the gains, it becomes "time for a change." At such times a successor with a different style can provide a needed stimulus to the growth of an organization. We feel that this occurred in the succession which we are discussing.

At ESH there were signs that the organization was entering a period of stasis after 17 years of dynamic but tight leadership. Dr. Lattimore's "loosening" and "stirring things up" may indeed have provided a needed stimulus to the hospital. The new manager in Guest's study came to a plant characterized by an atmosphere of "obedience to orders, enforcement of rules, the exercise of power through the threat of punishment. . . ."[21] The new manager had a loose administrative style and his "freeing things up" reversed a trend toward constrictively tight administration. Those who appointed the new manager in Gouldner's study felt that there had been too much laxness at the plant under the old manager, and they expected the new manager to improve production. In their view the new manager's "tightening up" reversed a progressively deteriorating situation.

A final example of organization growth through an alternation of styles is provided by Eastern State Psychiatric Institute. ESPI is a small, university-affiliated psychiatric hospital which experienced a succession in 1958. The retiring superintendent, Dr. Rosenberg, had a loose administrative style, and under his leadership the hospital had achieved national prominence. However, it was felt by some of the medical staff that toward the end of Dr. Rosenberg's administration there was too much role diffusion and a lack of clear-cut authority in the organization. The new superintendent, Dr. Presley, had a tight administrative style and was known as a crisp decision-maker. He emphasized clear-cut lines of authority and delegated responsibility. His increase in bureaucratization took the form of new requirements for formal reports, formalization of the assistant clinical dirctor's job and role, and demands for punctuality.

Thus, in Gouldner's study and at ESPI, a successor with a tight administrative style brought an increase in bureaucratization. However, at ESH and at the automobile plant described by Guest there was no "surge of bureaucratic development." We contend that a successor's administrative style is an important factor determining his responses to the exigencies of succession. A successor with a tight administrative style may rely heavily on bureaucratic methods; a successor with a loose administrative style may be unable or willing to do so. Executives with different styles may react quite differently to problems they encounter as successors. The success of the change may depend on the fit between a successor's style and the needs of the organization at a given time.

In conclusion, we would like to suggest some areas for further investigation. We have suggested that it is helpful to describe an executive's administrative styles as either tight or loose. But are there executives whose styles are neither tight nor loose—that is, executives flexible enough to realize the advantages of both styles? (Presumably an executive who seized the disadvantages of both would not long remain an executive.) Might the styles we have delineated be described better in other terms? Moreover, our characterizations of tight and loose administrative styles are very broad. What further distinctions can be made concerning the components of these styles, and what subtypes are there within the two categories? For example, is it useful to think of a tight dominating style (along the lines of de Gaulle's) in contrast to a kind of light leadership where the top executive delegates authority with little imposition of his own wishes or conceptions?

The relationship between personality, social structure, and executive functioning to a great extent remains to be explored. For example, if the tight-loose distinction proves to be useful, what are the psychological and sociological determinants of these behaviors? To what extent can a successor's style be predicted on the basis of prior knowledge of him as an individual, and to what degree is his style determined by the exigencies of his situation on a particular organizational setting? Specifically, can a given administrative style be adopted consciously as a strategy of management? Parenthetically, with regard to psychological determinants we caution against any casual association of a tight administrative style with authoritarianism or a loose administrative style with equalitarianism. Franklin Roosevelt, for example, used a loose style very effectively to keep major decision-making in his own hands, and many subordinates found his leadership very dominating.

Finally, our speculation concerning an alternation of tight and loose styles during the course of an institution's history implies that over time the disadvantages of a particular style create the need for its opposite. Other explanations are possible, however. For example, style alternation in management succession may in part reflect the need of a successor to be *different* from his predecessor, to create his own *executive identity*.

It is our conviction that research pertaining to general issues of executive functioning, as well as to the specific problem of management succession, will both expand conceptual sociopsychological knowledge and contribute practical suggestions that may help the successor in handling his often difficult problems.

NOTES

1. Joel Kotin and Myron R. Sharaf, "Intrastaff Controversy at a State Mental Hospital: An Analysis of Ideological Issues," *Psychiatry* (1967) 30:16–29.
2. Daniel J. Levinson, "Role, Personality, and Social Structure in the Organizational Setting," *J. Abnormal and Social Psychology* (1959) 58:170–180. Richard C. Hodgson, Daniel J. Levinson, and Abraham Zaleznik, *The Executive Role Constellation*; Cambridge, Mass., Division of Research, Harvard Business School, 1965. Abraham Zaleznik, *Human Dilemmas of Leadership*; New York, Harper and Row, 1966. Daniel J. Levinson and Gerald L. Klerman, "The Clinician-Executive," *Psychiatry* (1967) 30:3–15.
3. Alvin W. Gouldner, *Patterns of Industrial Bureaucracy*; Glencoe, Ill., Free Press, 1954.
4. Gouldner writes: "A common indication of the degree and source of workers' resistance to a new manager is the prevalence of what may be called the 'Rebecca Myth.' Some years ago Daphne DuMaurier wrote a novel about a young woman who married a widower, only to be plagued by the memory of his first wife, Rebecca, whose virtues were still widely extolled. One may suspect that many a past plant manager is, to some extent, idealized by the workers, even if disliked while present." See footnote 3; p. 79.

    The most dramatic example in recent times of the operation of the Rebecca Myth emerged in Lyndon Johnson's succession to the Presidency. William Manchester (*The Death of a President*; New York, Harper and Row, 1967) has documented in considerable detail the resentment of the Kennedy staff toward Johnson and his new lieutenants. He also shows how Kennedy staff members who did move vigorously to serve the new President were accused of opportunism and disloyalty by other "old lieutenants." Perhaps more significantly, not only those close to the Presidency, but also large segments of the population were soon quick to emphasize anything they regarded as "bad" about the new President and to contrast him unfavorably with the departed and now idealized Kennedy.

5. See footnote 3; pp. 93–94. Gouldner also describes two other strategies available to a successor to increase his communication and control: "close supervision," and the use of *"gemeinschaft* techniques." Each of these, however, has considerable limitations. Close supervision of subordinates by a successor is difficult in a large organization and many arouse resentment. The use of *gemeinschaft* techniques—that is, becoming friendly with subordinates and working through the informal system—is difficult for a new man, especially if a Rebecca Myth is prevalent.

6. Robert H. Guest, *Organizational Change: The Effect of Successful Leadership*; Homewood, Ill., Irwin Dorsey Press, 1962.

7. See footnote 2; p. 249.

8. See footnote 1.

9. The names of persons and places have been altered.

10. The programs themselves plus the accompanying controversy were described previously. See footnote 1.

11. Bernard J. James, "Advanced Study for Psychiatric Administrators," *Mental Hospitals* (1964) 15:686–688.

12. Gouldner also found that promotions given to old lieutenants by the new manager were simply regarded as the "paying off" of inherited obligations; the promoted men felt they owed nothing in return.

13. See footnote 3; p. 93.

14. See footnote 2.

15. See footnote 3; p. 70.

16. "Schlesinger at the White House. A Conversation with Henry Brandon," *Harper's Magazine*, July, 1964; p. 58.

17. Hans J. Morgenthau, "Monuments to Kennedy," *New York Review of Books*, January 6, 1966; p. 8.

18. John Cumming and Elaine Cumming, *Ego and Milieu*; New York, Atherton, 1962; pp. 128–129.

19. See *Human Dilemmas of Leadership*, in footnote 2; pp. 95–96.

20. See footnote 1.

21. See footnote 6.

Management
Succession
Revisited

MYRON R. SHARAF
JOEL KOTIN

We consider ourselves extremely fortunate to have had the opportunity to study Eastern State Hospital during a crucial time in its history. The problems of studying organizations in depth are manifold. Psychiatric institutions, however, afford unique possibilities for study.[1]

In our case the idea of scientific inquiry was acceptable to the administration and we were invited into all meetings, consultations, etc., as observers. Moreover, psychiatrists, we think, may be more willing than other executives to discuss their feelings openly. Furthermore, we observed Eastern State Hospital during one of the most crucial developmental periods in its 130-year history. A strong effective leader with a commitment to particular policies whose administration had lasted 17 years, was succeeded by another strong, effective leader with a different administrative style and commitment to different policies.

We were equally fortunate in having data on a similarly pivotal succession at Eastern State Psychiatric Institute for comparison. Thus, we could observe in pure culture different strategies of coping with the succession crisis, different administration styles, and the results of these interactions throughout the organizations.

Since 1967, Eastern State Hospital has undergone far-reaching changes. (Our data in this retrospective are less systematically complete and more impressionistic than in our previous effort but there has also been less turmoil and polarization in the organization.) There have been two successions to the superintendency at Eastern State Hospital since our study—in 1967 and in 1973. Even more far-reaching, however, has been the administrative decentralization of the hospital into smaller units, each serving a geographic catchment area. This change was begun by Dr. Lattimore and continued by his successors.

These two successions have not been accompanied by as much polarization in the form of a "Rebecca Myth" as the successions we studied. Several factors may be responsible, including decentralization. This step enhanced the power of the unit chiefs and decreased the power of central administration (Superintendent and department heads), with the important proviso that the Superintendent could still hire and fire the unit chiefs.

The leader who fights for decentralization represents a paradox in several ways. For one thing, the very idea of a leader surrendering power is not usually regarded as the way a strong leader behaves and is often viewed with some suspicion—as a kind of trick—by subordinates. At the same time, it takes considerable vigor on the part of the top leader to effect decentralization. The chant "power to the people" is popular on both the political left and right. But, in fact, people who have not had responsibility are often loathe to assume it, and people who have had power under a more centralized regime are not eager to relinquish it. The leader who fights for decentralization often has to utilize his authority in decisive, controversial ways that readily arouse the criticism of "dictatorship." For example, unitization of the hospital erodes the power of department chiefs; community school boards limit the authority of the central school department and, in some instances, civil service protection for teachers and principals; impounding congressionally authorized funds (in order to protect revenue sharing as a key instrument of fiscal decentralization) is, in a real sense, an attack on congressional authority.

However, once decentralization has taken firm roots, the authority of the top leader of a large organization may in fact be considerably diminished. Moreover, the process of decentralization, with increased power for unit chiefs, may reduce the emotional salience of the top leader for many members of the organization, who now see their primary loyalty as belonging to their "local" chief. In our view, this helps explain the fact that when Dr. Lattimore resigned from Eastern State Hospital in 1967 to take a more responsible position, his successor faced a much less pronounced Rebecca Myth than did Dr. Lattimore when he replaced Dr. Smith.

If decentralization was a major factor in reducing the emotional upheaval around succession, it was not the only one. A second important factor was length of tenure. Dr. Lattimore had replaced a leader who had been Superintendent for 17 years, but he himself served for only 4 years. This difference, in itself, made Dr. Lattimore's departure a less wrenching blow to the organization. Nor was his shorter tenure idiosyncratic. Today, there is much greater career mobility for psychiatrists, and there are many more prestigious positions above the level of Superintendent than there were in the 1940s and 1950s. Moreover, leaders of urban institutions, be they mayors of cities or heads of service organizations such as Eastern State Hospital, are likely to have a shorter tenure because of the crushing pressures of the job. Relatively peaceful reigns for heads of large institutions, insulated in various ways from public controversy, seem to be a thing of the past.

Another reason for the lessening of the Rebecca Myth appears to be the fact that top leaders today are increasingly involved in dealing with other organizations. Levinson and Klerman[2] have noted that the chief executive's extensive participation in "foreign relations" means that responsibility for internal operations must be delegated to subordinates, a result—we have suggested—which also flows from the current emphasis on decentralization.

Levinson and Klerman suggest that the limitation of contact between the top leader and the people who work for him produces an increase in "transference" phenomena. However, it may also reduce the emotional salience of the top leader, even if it generates an increased mythology about what this shadowy figure is like.

It might be argued that, in the situation we are describing, Rebecca Myth phenomena are simply displaced to the unit chiefs and it is their departures and arrivals which generate emotional storms for the staff. To some extent this is the case. However, several distinctions need to be made. First, unit chiefs are likely to be younger and less established persons than top administrators of the organizations. Hence, they tend to generate less intense transference phenomena than the revered or hated "old man" who was perceived as running the whole show. Second, there is more opportunity for day-to-day contact with the chief of a small unit. This permits greater working through of transference distortions in general and, in connection with succession crises, working through the splitting of feeling between the old and new leader which contributes to the Rebecca Myth.

The trend toward decentralization has stimulated in us new thoughts concerning "tight" and "loose" styles of administration. Smaller units are more likely to permit patterns of authority which include some differentiation into levels plus the possibility of jumping echelons without too much fuss. In this structure the Chief of a unit can hear the complaints of a lower-level subordinate and at the same time bring in the subordinate's supervisor so that the latter does not feel bypassed, or, if so, only temporarily. Face-to-face contact, group meetings, and the relative accessibility of the leader offer the possibility of loosening rigid organizational barriers without abandoning such principles as delegation, supervision and accountability.

W. H. Auden once wrote that social scientists dream of systems so perfect that no one has to be good. Lest we give the impression that decentralization represents that system, we hasten to note some of *its* problems. Decentralization puts a heavy premium on "good" unit chiefs. Their capricious or destructive exercise of authority can be especially devastating because of the weakening of the line of authority that previously flowed from department chiefs. The latter often served to protect representatives of their disciplines (e.g., nursing or psychology) from the abuses of the unit leader. Close monitoring of unit performance by the top leader (and *his* aides) is necessary. Which takes us back to the issues of top management where we began.

Recognition that the pendulum swings back and forth need not induce a feeling of futility about organizational progress—the search for combining the values of "tight" and "loose" styles of administration goes on apace. There is increasing experimentation in industry, as well as in human service organizations, with small, relatively unhierarchical work groups which have considerable autonomy in arranging their organizational structure. These also encourage role diffusion, e.g., the nurse does not restrict herself narrowly to nursing nor the assembly line worker to only one small part of the total operation. Yet there is also awareness of the necessity for accountability—someone outside the work group has to take a hard look at the output (cost analysis, evaluation of treatment program, and the like).

Above all, there is growing recognition of the fact that there are no easy answers. The emphasis on traditional bureaucratic virtues (such as clearcut, objectively determined criteria for hiring and promotion) may end up in the crippling straight-jacket of many civil service regulations. On the other hand, nice sounding terms such as democratic decision-making often serve to conceal organizational confusion and irresponsibility. As William Morris put it many years ago: "Men fight and lose the battle and then the thing they fought for comes about, but when it comes it turns out not to be what they meant and others have to fight for what they meant under a different name."

Our differentiation of tight and loose styles grew out of an attempt to understand an organization's experience of succession. Seven years after our study, our feeling remains that succession has been inadequately studied. A new leader represents both a trauma and an opportunity for growth for an organization. Further studies are needed in several directions. The vicissitudes of top- and middle-management successors in various organizations could be compared, e.g., in organizations with similar goals such as mental hospitals but with different organizational structures and philosophies. Another direction would be to study succession in different social settings, e.g., when a new therapist begins treatment of an ongoing therapy group or when a school class has a new teacher.

Succession is important because it relates to profound psychological issues for the individual. These include how losses are handled, the individual's relations to authority, and the universal hope for a better tomorrow.

NOTES

1. See Hodgson, Levinson and Zaleznik, as cited in the original article.
2. Levinson, Daniel J., and Klerman, Gerald L. The clinician-executive. *Psychiatry: Journal for the Study of Interpersonal Processes,* 30(1): 3–15, 1967.

C. Board-Executive Relationships

14

Board, Executive, and Staff

HERMAN D. STEIN

A good deal has been written about boards and executives and the relationship of both to staff. With most of what has been written one can take no exception. The words of Eduard Lindeman about boards and volunteers remain as sound today as they were when he first uttered them. Records of board institutes of twenty-five and thirty years ago contain useful and important lessons.[1] More recent works like Sorenson's *The Art of Board Membership*,[2] Houle's *The Effective Board*,[3] Schmidt's *The Executive and the Board in Social Welfare*[4] and Trecker's many works on administration[5] and on board membership all contain important, sound principles for useful practice. Many journal articles offer fine material.[6] What is there to add?

Two things, perhaps. One is more prodding below the surface of the principles that have been thus far developed. The other is the raising of some nagging questions about generalizations that we may regard as self-evident.

The time has passed for mere registering of complaints and wringing of hands or, for that matter, for self-congratulation on the wonders of voluntarism. We are in a period where only the most sober and hard-headed analysis of our organizational problems will do. Social welfare, voluntary or governmental, is coming increasingly into the forefront of public attention, and our responsibilities to society are deep and serious. The inner organizational relationships among board, executives, and staff represent one facet of these problems and to the extent that further analysis can improve our operations and thus the manner in which we discharge our responsibilities, this area merits continued exploration.

My task, therefore, is to examine some of the existing realities and to raise questions about some well-established tenets and assumptions.

THE MOTIVATION OF TRUSTEES

A decade or so ago some people were shocked to learn that eminent trustees in agencies all over the country, voluntary and public, may have had as part of their motivation for becoming trustees a prestige, political or other self-interest objective. Now we realize that excellent trustees may be utterly dedicated and altruistic or may have some degree of self-interest.

Houle reports on a survey which found that 10 percent of the members of local boards of education were extremely altruistic, 36 percent apparently altruistic, 44 percent partially self-interested, and 10 percent extremely self-interested.[7] Studies of social agency boards refer to the same phenomenon, although not in statistical terms.[8] This information should be no more surprising than the fact that some social workers come to their profession completely altruistically and some with other motivations in mind. We are far more interested in the surgeon's capacity to wield the scalpel effectively than in his dedication to surgery. What his motivations are may affect his chances of selecting and being accepted for a medical career, and how good a doctor he becomes, but the test of whether he is a good doctor lies in his performance, not in his motivations. The same is true of board members, of professional social workers, and of almost everyone else.

We have no evidence to suggest that board members are any more or any less dedicated than are professionals. We should not expect board members to be angelic any more than we except staff members to be angelic. We have a right, however, to expect competence in their respective roles. What is essential to keep in mind is that the presence of some degree of self-interest among some proportion of trustees does not necessarily conflict with dedication to their work, and that a degree of self-interest does not necessarily impair the productive effort of a board member any more than it does that of a staff member.

POLICY AND EXECUTIVE;
BOARD AND EXECUTIVE

If we agree that the evaluation of board member and executive behavior should be made on the basis of performance without reference to motivation, we then have to consider what comprises the job of each. We have had many words about this, and most of them have been good words. We have been told in no uncertain terms that policy determination is the responsibility of the board alone, that policy execution is the responsibility of executive and staff, that the executive ultimately is responsible for the results of agency programs. Nearly everyone understands these points and yet boards and executives have had trouble ever since there were boards and executives.

It is not, of course, only in social work that problems arise. Every field has its own version of the same underlying concerns. Note, for example, these quotes from a manual for trustees of colleges and universities, written by a retired college president some fifteen years ago:

> Certainly, the president should feel free to suggest changes in policy and the trustees should give his suggestions careful consideration, but the fact remains that the control of policy is a function of the trustees and one of their most important functions. It is also one of which they very often lose sight. . . . When the trustees overlook their function of determining policies, they tend to become an official rubber stamp of the actions of the president. It is rather their duty to assure themselves that the president's administration conforms to the policies laid down by themselves.[9]

> A shocking percentage of the 17,000 men and women serving as trustees, directors and members of the boards controlling our American colleges and universities know little of their responsibilities and care little about their institutions, perfunctorily attend board meetings, and approve presidential recommendations without understanding or serious consideration. On the other hand, there is no finer or more valuable group of people in the country than our able, responsible college trustees.[10]

Nothing would be gained by an attempt to analyze the nature of potential difficulties by assigning the role of villain either to board or to executive. It is more to the point to suggest that there are inherent functions and relationship problems which simply have to be understood and coped with and that good will alone will not prevent difficulties from arising. Basic to these problems is the determination of what is policy and what is execution, or professional responsibility, and the way in which this decision is made.

The matter of waiting lists offers one kind of test by which casework agencies and clinics can determine whether they are attributing a policy character or a professional character to a given type of decision. Let us take a community psychiatric clinic as an example. One could drop a psychiatric clinic almost anywhere in the country and have a waiting list within a matter of weeks. It is not only that many people want psychiatric care, but that quite a number of organizations—schools, hospitals, recreational agencies—breathe a sigh of relief when a psychiatric clinic is available and automatically refer to it clients with whom they cannot deal. As Dr. Jerome Frank has pointed out, it is one facility that breeds its own public.[11] Now some psychiatric clinics grapple with their waiting list problem by making sure that everyone is seen for at least 15 minutes or so to make sure that he is in the right place and then determine whether his situation is critical or not. If he is not in the right place, he goes somewhere else. If the situation is not critical, he is left on the waiting list, in the hope that perhaps he will get better while he is waiting. These tactics have reduced waiting lists considerably. It does mean, however, that staff is engaged in seeing more people, for fewer interviews per person and with less per capita time for interviews, so as to make sure that no emergency situation is skipped. The principle here is to provide the widest spread of service for those in need.

In other clinics, the decision is that good standards must not be jeopardized, and if someone requires intensive interviews several times a week over a period of many months or years, that is what the agency will provide. If such a policy leads to a waiting list, there is a waiting list. Another factor may be that the existence of a waiting list acts as a constant source of pressure on the financial powers that be.

If the board does not determine waiting list policy, the decision is made by the executive and staff and may never come before the board as a policy issue. If, however, the board considers intake in terms of the disposition of agency resources, the matter would become a policy question on which it would have to take a formal position. Every type of agency has these borderline issues, and I submit that in the rational determination of what is a policy matter, and who determines it, lies the true test of the board's assumption of policy responsibility.

Here is where one touches the concept of "strong" and "weak" executives. Often a "strong" executive is termed such because he basically determines as well as initiates policy and makes it easy for the board to accept his position. There are really strong executives whose strength in the executive role does not lie in sapping the strength of the board, even if it prefers to be supine. The executive in this context makes it possible for the board members to exercise their prerogatives intelligently and deliberately, and if their point of view conflicts with that of the executive, there is no loss of confidence in the executive. In other words, he helps the board to carry its own responsibilities whether it wishes to do so or not.

Sometimes a board simply cannot seem to take a policy position on an informed or dispassionate basis. Short of resigning, the executive has little choice other than to lead the board to make what he considers to be the best decision and gradually to help the board members become more aware of the preparation they need in order to make decisions themselves. For an executive to accept a policy-directing function permanently, however, even with board encouragement, is to lay the groundwork for serious agency weakness.

There were dramatic shifts in board-executive roles in an old-fashioned children's agency whose board members' favorite activity was that of running the Thanksgiving programs. There was only one trained worker, and frequent turnover made it difficult to keep the position filled. About ten years ago the board expanded to more than sixty members in order to provide for continuity. The younger members continued to review cases and hire and fire personnel, but they did not like the new executive who had been hired by the old guard. He was low-salaried, stuffy, and penurious. The younger members could not get him discharged, but they nagged him by insisting that they be allowed to read records, in accordance with the time-honored practice of this agency. The poor executive had to retain some measure of self-esteem and professional pride, and so he resigned. His replacement had excellent qualifications and demanded a good salary. He quickly established his sphere of authority, acquired good staff, worked rationally and flexibly with his board, gradually got them out of their old ways, and developed a fine board whose members understood and accepted their appropriate responsibilities. They would not dream of looking at a case record, and they were far more comfortable in this pattern than in the old. Moral: Boards can change if executives make it possible.

EVALUATION OF THE EXECUTIVE

Whether an agency is a small one or a large one, it is usually the executive more than any other single individual who is assumed to represent the interests, the goals, the cultural climate, and the values of the organization. In any organization, therefore, the operating premise should be that the board supports the executive since the board supports the agency as a whole. Anything which is likely to upset the security of the executive upsets the stability of the agency and is not in its interests.

Both because this is a conscious premise and because it is a natural tendency of sympathetic board members, boards tend to lean over backward not to imperil the security and stability of the executive position. This can lead to a dilemma: how can the board support the executive and yet perform one of its key functions, namely, evaluate his work.

Again, we are interested in principles. One principle is that the board should be in a position to evaluate the executive; that means that the board, or at least its officers, should have the information that will enable it to judge executive performance. Another principle is that this evaluation should be formal, and regularized, and so carried out that the position of the executive is not made untenable. If there is a formal evaluative session with the executive—as generally there should be—it would not be held in order to discover all the weaknesses of the executive and everything that has gone wrong in the agency but to consider together what the strong and weak points have been in the past and what better might be done, where executive performance bears on agency results.

If, indeed, an executive's performance is so questionable that his position is in jeopardy, this situation would, of course, have to be handled. But a formal evaluation session makes it possible to prevent minor questions or criticisms from becoming major rumors of board opposition to an executive. It makes it possible to put all these questions together in a neutral atmosphere at an appropriate and scheduled occasion. No matter how close and warm the daily interaction between the executive and the board may be, this kind of session is most wholesome, and gives both the executive and the board an opportunity to take a careful, reflective look at past achievements and weaknesses and direct their relationship in the future.

CLIQUES AND FRIENDSHIPS

There will usually be cliques in large boards. One way to minimize the likelihood of a clique-*ruled* board is to limit the number of board members. If a board has 100 members of whom no more than 20 or 30 usually attend meetings and only 7 or 8 participate on important committees, the likelihood is that no more than the 7 or 8 will be truly influential in making board decisions. The other board members will be on the outside looking in, either attempting to participate in meetings with middling success, or giving up and staying on the board as a necessary chore or as a desultory activity until something better comes along.

Even on medium-sized boards of fifteen to twenty-five a few members will have more influence than others. There should be some delegation of authority. The chairman should be the most important member of the board, and the executive committee should be among its most influential members. Differentiation of inner board status in this sense is not a weakness.

That friendship groups exist within the board does not mean that the body itself is weakened unless these friendships control decisions before the issues reach formal channels. Here is where the board chairman has one of his greatest responsibilities. No matter what the personal relationships may be, he must see to it that board decisions are made as part of the formal activity of the board.

Moreover, a personal relationship between some board members and the executive which interferes with business-like decisions poses a severe organizational strain and constitutes a trap for all concerned. I have made my position clear elsewhere and shall simply restate it.[12] First, I am in favor of friendship. If an executive and members of the board become personal friends, there is nothing inherently wrong with this. What is important, however, is that the informal relationship be kept as distinct as possible from the formal relationship; the larger and more complex the organization, the more important this is. It should be possible for a difference of opinion to arise at a board meeting even among friends. It should also be possible if an agency matter comes up in private conversation for one party to say, "Well, this ought to be brought to the board," instead of letting it be settled outside the board meeting so that either it will never come up before the board or will appear as a *fait accompli*. It requires self-discipline and sophistication to maintain distinct roles, but it is altogether possible; for the separation of friendship and organizational roles is achieved in many agencies.

BOARD-STAFF RELATIONSHIPS

Most references in the literature represent a close relationship between board and staff as a good. In other words, the more board and staff interact, the better. Sorenson states: "It is also wise to allow other senior staff members to attend board meetings with absolute freedom. Mystery is thereby dispelled and acquaintanceship promoted."[13] He suggests that other staff members may also benefit from attending board meetings as a training device and that there should be rotations in presentations by staff members to board.

The factor of size is quite important in determining what is a useful relationship between board and staff. In a small agency consisting of the executive and two professional staff members it makes sense for all the staff to know the board, and vice versa. There should be a great deal of face-to-face contact and participation on policy and direction. Quite the reverse, however, can be true of a larger, more complex organization. If one is working with 100 professional staff members, 150 nonprofessional staff members, and a board of 40 who have many other claims on their time and energies, it is both unrealistic and unnecessary to impose close and frequent interaction between board and staff.

This does not mean that staff should never see the board or vice versa. It does mean that the occasions for such meetings would be relatively formal when, for example, the program of the entire agency is being discussed, or quasi-formal when it is a matter of becoming familiar with names and faces.

So far as participation of staff members in board meetings is concerned, the central principle is that their participation should be encouraged when it is relevant to the program of the organization—not for training purposes in how to prepare a case presentation, nor to enable the board in large organizations to know the staff. It often makes sense, when particular staff members have special competence to serve on board subcommittees, for them to do so and therefore to be in rather close association with certain members of the board. However, it should be recognized that in relatively large agencies the organization does not require one-to-one contacts between board members and staff. It is usually all the board can do to take care of its immediate responsibilities adequately with the participation of the executive, and merely going through the motions of becoming acquainted with staff members is worse than useless. Staff should, nevertheless, know who board members are, should have some general occasions to meet them outside the board meeting, and through the actual policies of the organization should develop awareness and respect for their leadership.

A problem remains, and it is a serious and difficult one. In the large organization, where hierarchical lines of authority are observed, staff have no direct access to the board formally except through the executive. When all goes well, this is fine. But if trouble is brewing between executive and staff, there may be no way for the board to know it until a crisis develops. Developing board-staff lines that bypass the executive's authority will seriously weaken the organization. Ways should therefore be found for the board to satisfy itself on appropriate staff involvement in policy and on understanding staff views expressed through formal channels. It should also be possible, particularly in the large agency, for there to be a channel from staff to board available in cases of really serious disagreement between executive and staff, a channel which the executive himself keeps open. (I am glad that Houle takes this view.[14]) Even if this device is never used, its existence attests to a basic relationship of trust and confidence, and to a democratic spirit in administrative policy.

It must not be assumed, however, that distance between board and staff constitutes a problem only with voluntary agencies. While public boards are constituted under various legal arrangements and their powers are more clearly spelled out than is true of voluntary agency boards, the remoteness of some public boards from the firing line of staff activity, and their vulnerability to local political pressures, can be troublesome. In one Western state where child care institutions are under the State Board of Education, there are also local advisory bodies. Since the board could not visit the agencies, a custodial committee did so a few times a year. The committee found one children's institution in which the superintendent was concerned only with rigid economy and the children were forlorn and regimented. Consultation was secured, and it was recommended that the home become an institution for adolescents in need of group care. A new superintendent was hired, new staff, all changes were made. The State Board went on to other things, but the local advisory board did not like the looks of the "tough" youngsters who were the new clientele. They protested to the State Board. The result was, again a new superintendent, new staff, and reversion to the former policies of narrowly conceived function and stringent economy, for the State Board felt powerless to cope with local pressure.

In a second instance, jurisdiction over a state-wide public child care agency was shifted from the board of Child Welfare to another board with different policies. The staff, who had visited their clients by means of agency cars they could garage at home, now found themselves restricted, in the name of economy, to an agency pool to which they had to come each morning. The results were fewer home visits, time unnecessarily spent each morning and evening to pick up and deposit cars, and considerable loss of morale by a devoted staff who wanted to use their time productively for their clients rather than for ferrying agency cars, and who often in the past had worked many more hours than were demanded of them. Here the distance between staff and board was so great, and so little provision was made for staff reaction and participation in policy changes, that what seemed to be a minor administrative change brought serious impairment to an entire agency service.

One of the anachronisms of modern agency life is a hangover from bygone days. In many agencies, the executive must have a trustee cosign every check; in others, only trustees can sign checks, and often two signatures are required. In one of the oldest family agencies in the country both the executive director and a member of the board had to be consulted before a staff member could grant an emergency loan in excess of $100. In one instance, when neither one could be reached, the agency was forced to call upon the Salvation Army to help a family in an overnight crisis. It might be well for agencies to reexamine how much professional responsibility is really accorded by these practices (that no business could abide), and their implications in terms of the confidence really placed by the boards in their executives and staffs.

BOARDS AND SOCIAL WELFARE ISSUES

The relation of voluntary agency boards to major issues in social welfare has been receiving well-merited attention.[15] The voluntary agency and the public agency differ in a number of respects. Not the least of these is the higher visibility of the public agency, and its greater vulnerability to pressure and intrusion. By contrast, the voluntary agency is far more protected, less readily called to account, its policies and practices less likely to be presented to the public gaze by the mass media even when, as is true of many children's agencies, the bulk of their operating funds come from government sources.

I shall comment on only one of the ramifications of this state of affairs: the responsibilities of voluntary agency boards to be informed of, concerned with, and actively related to, relevant social welfare issues. For the heart of the matter lies in the ease with which boards of voluntary agencies can keep themselves removed from the fierce currents of controversy in social welfare, from the attacks on those in need of social services as well as on the services themselves. From all we can observe, this strange aloofness has a frequent if not uniform pattern, with many outstanding exceptions. Indeed, in many agencies board members have taken leadership in developing new and imaginative agency policy in advance of staff thinking and despite staff trepidations. The impression many voluntary agencies convey, however, is that the Newburgh phenomenon and the attacks on ADC and on public welfare provisions generally are really none of their concern. To what do we owe this phenomenon? To a number of things:

- apathy,
- ignorance of the facts,
- ideological sympathy with the attacks,
- absence of initiative in bringing the issues to attention.

Apathy is understandable, if not acceptable. There are many competing demands on time and energy and interest of board members. It is natural that attention would be given first to matters of immediate agency concern. The task here is to make it clear that some of these issues *are* of immediate agency concern, that no social agency in this day and age should be regarded as a privileged and autonomous sanctuary, unrelated to the entire pattern of social welfare in the country.

Ignorance is likewise understandable particularly if there is apathy, but hardly excusable as a basis for unconcern. Board members have a social responsibility to be informed, not only about the purpose and operations of their own agency, but about the social welfare context in which their agency exists.

Many a loyal and devoted board member of a family agency, community center, or even of a school of social work, may feel quite sympathetic with the position taken by Newburgh's City Manager Joseph Mitchell, with New Orleans's action on ADC, with the great concern about welfare "chiselers," with the feeling that public welfare "weakens the moral fibre"—with any or all and more of these. Now, holding such positions is any citizen's right. But something is clearly amiss if a dedicated board member does not see that the agency he supports is carrying on its work on ideological premises quite opposed to his. What is amiss in such a case is not necessarily the board member's lack of awareness, but the fact that there is nothing within the operation of the agency, the work of its staff, or, mainly, the performance of the agency's executive that leads him to feel there could possibly be an inconsistency in his point of view.

One cannot place the onus for the apathy, the ignorance, or the inconsistent point of view solely at the door of board members. It belongs as well to executives who take no initiative in bringing crucial social welfare issues to the attention of their boards, who do not realize that the much-vaunted function of "educating the board" includes education on such matters. There are three chief reasons for this lack of initiative:

1. They do not wish to rock the boat. Why raise questions that may induce board friction and conflict? The executives feel that they have enough trouble without adding to it unnecessarily.
2. They do not see such matters as relevant to the board or to the agency. "If we gave our attention to every social problem we would never get our work done."
3. They are not sufficiently convinced of the merits of the social work side of the case. This feeling is honest, if rare, but does not preclude raising the issue anyway.

None of these reasons is good enough, and it is time we placed part of the responsibility for the inaction of our lay leaders on ourselves, those of us who are in a position to work with trustees as executives, senior staff, consultants, or teachers.

I am not recommending that boards necessarily take a stand identical with that of the official social work community. We take our chances with democratic process, with the intelligence and objectivity of board members. Moreover, let us concede that if they disagree with formal social work positions, they may sometimes be right. I am simply recommending that the social work case be heard and understood.

I am not suggesting either that every agency has to be concerned with every social welfare issue at all times. Obviously, this is impossible and undesirable. On some issues information is sufficient, others call for discussion. There would have to be clear determination of relevance before the board takes a public position, and on many issues trustees may prefer to speak as private citizens rather than in their capacity as board members. It would be expected that agencies dealing with immigrants would be more concerned with immigration laws than would psychiatric clinics; settlement houses would be more concerned with delinquency than would hospital social service departments, and so forth. One could hope that across-the-board onslaughts on public welfare clients and attacks on basic decency in welfare management, however, would be considered the moral concern of all agencies.

I am not suggesting that no criticism of our public agencies should ever be made. On the contrary, all of us recognize that there is not only room for improvement, but for considerable change. But we have to earn the right to be critical, by supporting those general objectives which we all share, by identifying ourselves with these objectives and lending our strength to public agencies that are unfairly under attack, by recognizing that all of social work is being attacked when the public agencies are under fire.

Board members of voluntary agencies are vital in this conflict. They are assumed to have a special right to speak because they are social agency board members and therefore are both knowledgeable and public-spirited; their names carry weight in the community. Legislatures which hear no opposition to punitive welfare measures from agency board members would have every reason to feel that no responsible or at any rate significant opposition exists. Moreover, voluntary agencies can carry on their special functions—innovation and experimentation, for example—only by the grace of the existence of government-supported social welfare. Board members may take any position they wish on any given issue—whatever the position, it is better than apathy—but none should be unaware of this fact of life in American social work. Nor should they be unaware of the views held by our professional associations, notably the National Association of Social Workers, so that they can have some notion of the positions likely to be held, by the very social work staff in which they take pride. No greater bond can exist between board and staff than that of genuine mutual concern on fundamental matters of principle.

American society has accepted the proposition that issues of war and peace are too important to be left to the military. We seem to be arriving at the decision that policy on medical care is too serious to be left to doctors. It may therefore not be amiss to suggest that matters of social work policy are too vital to be left to social workers. As our profession moves into a position of greater authority, our need for a system of checks and balances increases. One essential element in making such a system work is to see to it that the laymen who serve on boards and presumably control policy are prepared, as many fortunately are, to exercise their responsibilities with informed intelligence and devotion to the general welfare of our society as well as to the well-being of their own agencies.

This is not to say that social workers should not contribute in the development of social policy or move toward constructive social change. On the contrary, our contribution should be stronger. We cannot and should not wish, however, to control policy. It may be fair to note that in the governmental sector of social work, the profession is generally over-controlled, more checked than balanced. The reverse is more true of the voluntary agency field, where social work executives can have undue control, when there are weaknesses in board structure, process, commitment, or competence. These imbalances should be redressed so as to enhance the rational operation of our programs and, more basically, to enable us to be more effective and more responsive to the needs of those who require our services most, and to spur the development of needed change in organizations and policies.

As social workers, we should expect respect for our professional competence and brook no trespass. We should make our voices heard clearly on issues of social welfare. We should take leadership in the formulation of social policy. To help insure this respect, to strengthen our voices, we must have support, ideas, effective communication, and, above all, assumption of genuine responsibility by those who serve as trustees for the common good—even if we have to spur them to assume this responsibility. To those hundreds of board members who meet these expectations, we owe a great debt, whether or not they and we always see eye to eye.

NOTES

1. E.g., *The Board Member* (New Haven, Conn.: New Haven Council of Social Agencies, 1936).
2. Roy Sorenson, *The Art of Board Membership* (New York: Association Press, 1951).
3. Cyril O. Houle, *The Effective Board* (New York: Association Press, 1960).
4. William D. Schmidt, *The Executive and the Board in Social Welfare* (Cleveland: Howard Allen, Inc., 1959).
5. E.g., Harleigh B. Trecker, *New Understandings of Administration* (New York: Association Press, 1961).
6. Notably, Elinor K. Bernheim and Irving Brodsky. "The Realities of Board-Executive Relationships," *Journal of Jewish Communal Service*, XXXVII (1961), 381–89.
7. Houle, *op, cit.*, pp. 19–22.
8. E.g., Solomon Sutker, "The Jewish Organizational Elite of Atlanta, Georgia," *Social Forces*, XXXI (1952), 136–43.
9. Raymond M. Hughes, *A Manual for Trustees of Colleges and Universities* (Ames, Iowa: Iowa State College Press, 1945), p. 13.
10. *Ibid.*, p. 167.
11. Jerome Frank, *Persuasion and Healing: a Comparative Study of Psychotherapy* (Baltimore, Md.: Johns Hopkins Press, 1961).
12. Herman D. Stein, "Some Observations on Board-Executive Relationships in

the Voluntary Agency," *Journal of Jewish Communal Service*, XXXVII (1961), 390–96.

13. Sorenson, *op. cit.*, p. 81.
14. Houle, *op. cit.*, p. 95.
15. E.g., James R. Dumpson, "Public and Voluntary Agency Partnership Responsibilities," *Child Welfare*, XLI (1962), 2–9; Joseph Walker, "Have Board Members Been Silent Too Long?" *ibid.*, XLI (1962), 168–71. Mr. Walker, president of an agency board, answers in the affirmative.

15

The Board-Executive Relationship Revisited

HERMAN LEVIN

The state of board-executive relationships in voluntary social agencies is not well. The current situation has been long in the making, evolving in tandem with the professionalization of the social welfare enterprise —particularly, with the development of professional social work— and the increasing governmental dominance over social welfare matters. The latter severely aggravated the situation, raising questions about the continuing functional viability of administrative volunteers and about the future necessity for voluntary agencies. Today's "crisis" in board-executive relationships may be viewed simply as one of a series of periodic eruptions of a longtime struggle over functional responsibilities. But there is peril in doing so because, with the implementation of the social service provisions of Title XX of the Social Security Act, the context of the struggle has changed markedly. Although this article focuses on the board-executive relationship, it seems increasingly clear that improvements in this relationship must not only await the resolution of functional conflicts, but probably the resolution of governmental-voluntary agency relationships as well.[1]

HISTORICAL BACKDROP

Awareness of deterioration in the dominance of laymen over social agency operations appeared earliest in the two areas of social agency activities first subject to professionalization: fund raising and direct service delivery. In 1921, the president of Buffalo's Charity Organization Society took cognizance of the extent to which the rise of federated financing and·the hiring of paid community organizers had "deprived boards of directors and governing committees of what was formerly their main function." With so important a task gone, he asked, "What is there for them to do? How shall they direct? And how shall their interests be enlisted and their abilities kept at work?"[2] The last was a particularly pertinent question because the concomitant evolution of professional helping and, starting as early as 1916, the proliferation of professional associations of social workers had also relegated volunteers to the performance of nonspecialist, frequently meaningless, service activities.

The exigencies of the depression of the 1930s exhausted the resources of professional social workers and required the use of volunteers "to render once more tasks that were gradually assumed by the professional group to be too technical for volunteer effort."[3] This new working relationship was uneasy at best, and, writing for *The Survey Midmonthly*, one board member was quite ready to admit to the antagonisms that exist between laymen and professionals and to give voice to the accusation that "the trained worker [had] taken over the board member's job."[4] Challenging the skepticism with which the use of volunteers was viewed, she continued, "I believe there is almost no type of service in which the trained, effective board member . . . cannot share directly. . . ."[5]

In the course of events, the delivery of direct, that is, casework, service did not evolve as a fruitful area of volunteer activity. The emergence of public programs, especially after the passage of the Social Security Act in 1935, required a redefinition of voluntary agency function and expertise and led to a reemphasis of highly skilled counseling services that were deemed by social workers as the exclusive province of professionals. In 1940, *The Survey Midmonthly* again called on a board member to describe the relationship of volunteer and professional. What she saw was a professional standing "between the one who is helped and the one who does the helping." Almost in desperation, she wrote that the board member "must have something important and interesting to do."[6]

Executive vs. Board Member

By the 1960s, differences that had previously been defined as antagonisms between lay people and professionals were more specifically seen to reside in the relationship of board member and executive. At issue were the tasks belonging to each, as well as the power to determine the nature of those tasks. In 1963, the statement of one executive demonstrated that the balance, perhaps irretrievably, had swung toward the latter: "Today it is thought desirable to restrict the administrative function of boards. . . . In an organization that is structured on an executive leadership model, board members who fail to understand this distribution of functions may seriously disrupt. . . ."[7]

Nevertheless, the struggle endured. Two studies appearing in 1964 attest to the continuing deterioration of board-executive relations and indicate the response of board members to the organizational "realities" of social service agencies. E. Elizabeth Glover found such relationship crises to result from functional confusion "twice as frequently as from any other condition." Glover found the board member responsible for each instance of confusion cited and, in each instance, the board member had attempted to engage in activities considered the professional responsibility of the executive. The implication was that board members did not view their own assignments with satisfaction.[8]

Henry Klein, in a Philadelphia study, examined the board memberships of seventy-nine persons found to "represent the real power and prestige of the community."[9] Among the sixteen social welfare organizations listed were the United Fund, the Health and Welfare Council, and twelve of their member agencies. Leading the list, the United Fund had garnered twenty-two "power and prestige leaders" as board members. The findings in regard to direct service agencies were dismaying. In a city where voluntary child welfare is preeminent, only two child welfare agencies were able to attract any representation of these community leaders. One boasted two as board members, the other only one. None of these leaders was to be found on the boards of the local family agencies, again despite national and historical prominence. Thus, the United Fund, having relieved its member service agencies of the admittedly burdensome task of raising funds, had, simultaneously, commanded the lion's share of community leadership. Whatever their degree of professionalization, centralized planning, fundraising, and fund allocation organizations offered opportunities for decision-making activities whose significance continued to capture the imagination and interest of administrative volunteers. Simultaneously, centralized planning agencies offered the administrative volunteer disengagement from potential conflict with service agency executives.

THE CURRENT SITUATION

Indications are that the administrative volunteer's demand for meaningful activity in return for participation on service agency boards will contribute to further, perhaps increasing, tension in their dealings with executives—assuming that volunteers do not entirely withdraw from posts in direct service agencies. A recent study of role expectations among the personnel of twenty agencies documents the continued existence of disturbing tensions.[10] Based on a survey of the literature on the management of voluntary social agencies, the study hypothesized that a failure of board, executives, and staff to observe "the primary functions of each division" could create conflict in agency administration. Data collected indicated that "boards of directors, staff members, and executive directors in voluntary social agencies are moderately clear about their roles and functions."[11] Years of experience made for some improvement in role clarity on the part of executives and staff but not in the performance of board members. The findings disclosed a lack of effort at helping board members attain and sustain functional clarity: "Based on the literature, the researchers assumed that training sessions for board members would include a discussion of the appropriate functions of a board member as distinct from those of the executive director and the staff. Analysis of the content of the training sessions indicated that this assumption was incorrect."[12] For executives, too, an alternative to increased tension may be disengagement.

PUBLIC MONEY AND PRIVATE ALLEGIANCE

The voluntary social agency sector's growing dependence upon public dollars seems to complicate potential solutions to board-executive relationship problems. Particularly critical are the purchase-of-service regulations stemming from the provisions of Title XX of the Social Security Act. For many voluntary agencies, the sudden availability of Title XX funding has been life-sustaining, but, however necessary, there are risks to autonomy and to the essential nature of voluntarism attendant upon the acceptance of governmental payment for service to persons considered public agency clientele.

The dependence of voluntary agencies on governmental funding is well documented. For example, the Child Welfare League of America's special report on the funding of its voluntary agency members, 1960–1975, showed that 56.6 percent of the support of the agencies covered by the study came from government in 1975. In that same year, federated (voluntary) funds were providing only 14.7 percent of their income.

In 1975, merged family and children's agencies received 31.3 percent of their support from government sources; federated funds provided 46.1 percent of their income. In 1960, these merged agencies had received only 8.5 percent of their income from governmental sources, 67.2 percent of their support from federations.[13] Such heavy reliance upon government—no matter what the risks—may be unavoidable in view of the fact that United Ways are themselves urging the search for "other than" federated dollars. This encouragement derives not only from the growing costliness of meeting demands for agency services, but also from the move on the part of United Ways themselves toward funding selected, time-limited programs rather than agencies per se.[14]

Arrangements for the purchase of service, whether by governments or by United Ways, threaten control over program decisions. Service agencies are especially vulnerable to purchases by governmental entities because of the relatively huge amounts of money involved. In either instance, however, the actual and potential loss of control over program and money decisions may lessen further the possibility of providing meaningful activities to engage the interests of volunteer board members. Of equal importance is the possibility that executives may see less return from (and less need for) board participation. First, the skills required for proposal writing and for meeting the service and accountability objectives of purchase-of-service contracts portend the further professionalization of administrative tasks. Efforts to provide volunteers with sufficient knowledge to participate effectively may seem to be fruitless. This may well be, if the allegiance of executives shifts from their boards and from the communities represented by their boards to their funding sources.[15] As for commitment to the notion of voluntarism, the history of social welfare is replete with instances of philosophy waiting upon money. Executives may be even more sorely tempted now when the difficulty of finding quality and influential board members is aggravated by the rapid move of women into the labor force. Be that as it may, the likelihood of resolving board-executive relationship difficulties seems unfortunately remote at this moment when lay participation—especially the participation of poor people—in social welfare has become so vital a concern for people generally and for social work in particular.

IMPLICATIONS

The seemingly dismal picture outlined here in no way negates the importance of resolving functional conflicts between boards and executives, nor is improvement of their working relationship impossible. Nevertheless, it must be realized that the future strength of voluntary social service agencies and of voluntary social welfare is at stake and is worthy of concern. For board members and for executives, a process of change for the better can begin with a reaffirmation of the historic significance of voluntary social welfare and of voluntarism for a democratic society: "Citizen participation on policy-making boards of voluntary agencies fosters the democratic process. . . . This . . . may, indeed, be the major contribution of voluntary agencies. . . . For while governmental bureaucracy continues to provide the majority of social welfare services, the principle of citizen participation is being kept alive through a voluntary movement in which lay leadership is central."[16] If this were more than rhetoric, if it were integral to the beliefs of board members and executives, the seemingly larger problem of confused voluntary-governmental agency relationships might fade.

It seems that much of the responsibility for the start of a change process must rest with the executive. He or she is the professional, with all that promises of knowledge about individual and societal needs, with all that promises of skill to bring together those components that can construct an effective social service system. An executive cannot use this knowledge and skill positively without prior conviction about the value of a strong board:

- That an active, "in control" board makes for strong administration, that is, for a strong executive.
- That a knowledgeable board asks crucial questions about the agency's conscience and professional wisdom—and relays informed responses to the community for community support.
- That a representative board speaks for the community and rightfully comments on its behalf.
- That a strong board assures the executive of a concerned and involved, yet independent, lay group worth talking to—"a window on the world."[17]

Inherent in implementing an executive's conviction about the value of the board is the development of opportunities and time for board members to engage in meaningful, contributive activity. Board members "must have something important and interesting to do." More than thirty-five years later, the statement still holds true. And patience wears thin.

NOTES

1. The reality of the urgent need for resolution was demonstrated during preparations for an Institute on Management offered jointly for twenty-five voluntary family and children's agencies by the School of Social Work and the Wharton School of Finance, both of the University of Pennsylvania, during June, 1977. When asked to order priorities among a list of twenty-nine topics proposed as institute content, the executives gave third preference to executive-board relationships. The topic was again included in the course content of two similar institutes offered in April and May, 1978.
2. Ansley Wilcox, "The Board Member—What is He? What are His Responsibilities? How Can He be Made Efficient," *Proceedings of the National Confer-*

ence of Social Work, 1921 (Chicago: University of Chicago Press, 1921), pp. 406–07.

3. Robert W. Kelso, "Why Is a Board of Directors," *The Survey Midmonthly* 67 (October 1931): 77.

4. Lillian L. Strauss, "Is It Trained Worker vs. Board Member?," *The Survey Midmonthly* 67 (December 1931): 301.

5. Ibid., p. 303.

6. Helen C. Baker, "Grandma Called it Charity," *The Survey Midmonthly* 76 (November 1940): 316.

7. Chester A. Nemland, "Current Concepts and Characteristics of Administration," *Child Welfare* 42 (June 1903): 276.

8. E. Elizabeth Glover, "Crises in Board-Executive Relationships in Social Agencies" (D.S.W. diss., University of Pennsylvania School of Social Work, 1964), p. 144.

9. Henry Klein, "The Anatomy of Power, II," *The Greater Philadelphian* 56 (November 1965): 59.

10. Vernon R. Weihe, "Role Expectations Among Agency Personnel," *Social Work* 23 (January 1978): 26–30.

11. Ibid., p. 29.

12. Ibid.

13. Barbara L. Haring, *Special Report on Funding of CWLA Voluntary Agency Members: 1960–1975* (New York: Child Welfare League of America, 1977).

14. For a discussion of Plan Y, the proposed purchase by local United Ways of high priority services from voluntary agencies, see Volunteer Leaders Conference, Chicago, Illinois, 6–7 May 1974, *Proceedings, Planning and Allocations Sessions* (Alexandria, Va.: United Way of America, July, 1974).

15. The possibility is suggested by the Pennsylvania State Department of Welfare's practice of permitting executives of voluntary agencies to "sign off" for purchase-of-service contracts. Cosigning by a designated officer of the board is not required.

16. Peter M. Glick, "Why Voluntarism?" *Social Casework* 55 (December 1974): 631.

17. The list provided above is paraphrased from Peter Drucker, "The Bored Board," *The Wharton Magazine* 1 (Fall 1976): 19–25. It is interesting that such a delineation of the values of a board should come from an author whose expertise is in the area of administration in private enterprise and who, in this reference, is writing about private enterprise boards.

D. Minority and Female Executives

16

The Minority Administrator: Problems, Prospects, and Challenges

ADAM W. HERBERT

The first National Conference on the Role of Minorities in Urban Management and Related Fields was held in Washington, D.C., on June 10 and 11, 1973. The significance of this conference was three-fold:

1. It was the first organized national meeting of non-elected minority public administrators and educators held to discuss the problems, education, responsibilities, and needs of minority public sector professionals.
2. It represented a symbolic acknowledgement that the quest of minority groups for more responsive government must, and does now include a sophisticated concentration on the political and administrative affairs of government.
3. Its theme suggested, quite appropriately, that minority administrators do have an important and unique role to play in the public man-

agement field, which they must accept if the plight of minority (if not all) people in America is to be improved.

Since this Conference, a number of major developments around the country suggest that minority administrators, however small in number, are increasingly gaining positions from which they can respond to the universal cry for more responsive government. Five cities as diverse as Compton, California, and East Lansing, Michigan, have selected black city managers to administer their governments. Black elected administrators are leading 108 cities in all regions of the nation, including Los Angeles, Atlanta, Raleigh, and Detroit. Another 62 serve as vice mayors.[1] Data from the 1973 State and Local Information Survey (EEO-4) reveal that 18.2 percent of the total labor force in state and local governments represent minority groups (Blacks, Spanish-Surnamed Americans, Asian, American Indian, and Other). While only 6.8 percent of this group is labeled "Professional," on the surface these figures do suggest growing influence on local government policy implementation and formulation.[2]

Recent federal employment data as reflected in Table 16−1 reveal that despite the continued decline in total federal employment, minority employment has continued to increase. Total minority employment (20.4 per cent of the federal work force) expanded 1.9 per cent for the period May 1972−May 1973.[3] While the increase in the number of GS 14−15, and supergrade administrators is not significant, current hiring practices will result in greater opportunities for minorities to make inputs into agency decision-making and policy execution.

Although there has been a conscious movement toward equal employment opportunity and affirmative action in the field of public administration since the late sixties, the nature of these public sector efforts continues to be questioned in many circles. Indeed a major finding of the aforementioned Conference was that:

Minority persons are still skeptical about the willingness of governmental systems to accept them as trained professionals with the knowledge and ability to perform in administrative positions of increasing responsibility and authority.[4]

This finding appears to coincide with several conclusions reached by the Civil Rights Commission in its 1969 survey of cities in seven SMSAs. While employment rates have improved for minority group administrators since this 1969 survey, some of the Commission's conclusions are worth mentioning, particularly in light of the skepticism felt by many minority group members relative to the good will of government agencies. The Commission found that:

TABLE 16–1. Net Change in Employment Under the General Schedule and Similar Pay Plan, by Grade Grouping from May 31, 1972 to May 31, 1973

Grade Grouping	Total Employment Change	Minority Group Employment Change					
		Total Minority	Negro	Spanish Surnamed	American Indian	Oriental	All Other
Total, General Schedule, or Similar	− 173	+ 11,210	+8,756	+ 1,913	+200	+341	− 11,383
GS 1–4	+9,159	+ 3,704	+2,797	+ 869	− 45	+ 83	+ 5,455
GS 5–8	−6,906	+ 3,952	+3,538	+ 348	+ 48	+ 18	− 10,858
GS 9–11	−4,298	+ 2,169	+1,518	+ 434	+ 130	+ 87	− 6,467
GS 12–13	+ 1,133	+ 961	+ 697	+ 173	+ 45	+ 46	+ 172
GS 14–15	+ 805	+ 416	+ 199	+ 84	+ 24	+ 109	+ 389
GS 16–18	− 66	+ 8	+ 7	+ 5	− 2	− 2	− 74

Source: U.S. Civil Service Commission, *Minority Groups Employment in the Federal Government* (Washington, D.C.: U.S. Government Printing Office, 1973).

Minority group members are denied equal access to State and local government jobs.

(a) Negroes, in general, have better success in obtaining jobs with central city governments than they do in State, county, or suburban jurisdictions and are more successful in obtaining jobs in the North than in the South.

(b) Negroes are noticeably absent from managerial and professional jobs even in those jurisdictions where they are substantially employed in the aggregate. In only two central cities, out of a total of eight surveyed, did the overall number of black employees in white-collar jobs reflect the population patterns of the cities.

(c) Access to white collar jobs in some departments is more readily available to minority group members than in others. Negroes are most likely to hold professional, managerial, and clerical jobs in health and welfare and least likely to hold these jobs in financial administration and general control.

(d) Negroes hold the large majority of laborer and general service worker jobs—jobs which are characterized by few entry skills, relatively low pay, and limited opportunity for advancement.[5]

Related to these conclusions (particularly point "C") are data from the aforementioned EEO-4 survey which indicate that while minorities do hold a number of administrative positions outside *social* agencies, most continue to work in these areas. Table 16–2 provides a summary of current local government hiring practices by functional areas. As the Civil Rights Commission indicated in 1969, minorities continued in 1973 to be assigned primarily to departments that have a "social" orientation. It is particularly significant to note that police and fire departments continue to employ significantly lower percentages of minority group people than do other governmental agencies. Financial administration also continues to be an area in which minority people have been unable to make significant inroads, although employment rates in this area are higher than in police and fire departments. It is also important to note that with the exception of housing, the percentage of professionals and officials/administrators (white collar jobs) continues to be low in all functional areas.

At the federal level, a similar pattern of minorities being hired by some agencies at much higher rates than others is evident, as reflected in Table 16–3. Three distinguishable groups of agencies seem to be evident with reference to the percentage of minority group members em-

TABLE 16–2. Federal Government Minority Group Employment Rates, 1972–1973

Group		Per Cent Non-White Employment	Officials/ Adminis- trators	Pro- fessionals
I	Sanitation and Sewage	38.8	12.4	8.9
	Housing	34.6	20.7	24.2
	Hospitals and Sanitariums	30.4	9.1	18.6
II	Public Welfare	23.6	11.0	15.4
	Utilities and Transport	22.7	9.4	10.6
	Other	18.9	7.9	10.0
	Employment Security	18.7	8.2	13.5
	Corrections	18.7	9.8	14.7
	Health	17.8	3.2	11.6
	Natural Resources	15.9	6.2	8.9
	Community Development	15.1	7.9	13.2
III	Streets and Highways	11.8	3.8	6.0
	Financial Administration	11.4	5.3	7.9
IV	Police	9.3	4.4	5.5
	Fire	5.0	2.2	2.8

Source: Compiled from data cited in the Equal Employment Opportunity Commission, *State and Local Government Information, EEO-4, National Statistical Summaries* (Washington, D.C.: EEOC, Office of Research, 1974).

Agencies	Total Employment Rates of Agency GS 9–18	Total Minority Employment of Agency GS 9–18	Percentage Minority Employment			
			Percent of Total GS9–18	Percent of Total GS9–11	Percent of GS 12–15	Percent of GS 16–18
OEO	1234	385	31.2	46.3	26.6	40.9
ACTION	946	220	23.3	30.3	19.6	18.8
State	2491	456	18.3	32.2	8.5	2.5
Labor	7568	1336	17.6	27.3	14.3	6.8
HEW	40178	5796	14.4	18.0	10.9	9.3
HUD	9912	1304	13.2	15.9	11.0	9.4
OMB	383	47	12.3	22.1	10.0	9.0
Interior	27883	2646	9.5	12.7	5.9	3.2
Commerce	16108	1434	8.9	11.7	7.3	2.3
Treasury	45133	3004	6.7	8.3	5.0	2.1
Defense	262726	16797	6.4	8.2	4.2	1.1
Transportation	46337	2578	5.6	7.9	4.3	7.0
Justice	20041	1109	5.5	7.4	3.6	3.3
Agriculture	41725	2110	5.1	6.2	3.3	2.4

TABLE 16–3. Federal Government Minority Group Employment Rates, 1972–1973

Source: Compiled from data cited in the U.S. Civil Service Commission, Minority Group Employment in the Federal Government (Washington, D.C.: U.S. Government Printing Office, March 1974).

ployed. The first group contains four agencies, three of which—Action, OEO, and Labor—might be labeled as "traditional." The presence of the State Department in this first group reflects a deviation from the usual governmental pattern related to minority employment. The Office of Economic Opportunity and ACTION stand out above all other federal agencies as the employers of both the greatest percentage of minority professionals at the GS 9 levels or above, and the greatest percentage of supergrade administrators. The Departments of State and Labor also have relatively high rates of minority employment overall, and particularly at the GS 9–11 levels. At the super grade levels, however, both departments have much lower minority employment rates.

The second cluster of agencies contains three departments, two of which might be labeled as "social" or "traditional" in the sense referred to by the Civil Rights Commission—Health, Education, and Welfare; and Housing and Urban Development. To some observers it may be surprising to note the presence of the Office of Management and Budget in this second group. The OMB employment figures are especially significant because of that agency's overall importance in the governmental process.

The third cluster of agencies includes Interior, Commerce, Treasury, Defense, Transportation, Justice, and Agriculture. None of these agencies are usually regarded as being social service agencies; as a consequence, the lack of substantial minority employees is not surprising. It is significant that at the federal level, as in the case of state and local governments, the percentage of minority employees decreases rapidly as decision-making responsibility (GS level) increases. The one exception to this trend is the Office of Economic Opportunity, where the percentage of supergrade administrators (40.9 per cent) is at a level comparable to those at the GS 9–11 levels (46.3 per cent) within that agency.

Although we in the public affairs field have given little attention in our literature to these data and the resulting debate, it is important to recognize that, as the number of minority professionals and administrators at all levels of government increases, the expectations of minority people for more responsive government will probably expand simultaneously. As will be argued later, the powers possessed by minorities employed in the public sector in most cases seldom are adequate to meet these expectations. As a consequence, short of a commitment on the part of administrators generally (white and non-white) to become responsive to the needs of "all" citizens, governmental agencies will continue to address on a priority basis the demands of the more powerful and affluent in our society. Where public agencies do not manifest a change in programmatic efforts which might be interpreted by minority communities as being more responsive to their needs, the tasks of minority administrators within those agencies, particularly at the local level, will become increasingly more difficult.

These difficulties will arise, in part, because of the collective perception that minority administrators understand the nature and magnitude of the problems confronting those from lower socioeconomic backgrounds. Indeed, whether one is black, brown, or red, the visible presence of an administrator with whom he/she can identify causes at least greater initial security that someone is listening who can understand the needs, realities, and perceptions being described, and who will help if at all possible.

Another factor creating the expectation among minority groups that the system will change as a result of greater "integration" of public agencies is the belief that many of these positions were made possible through community efforts. It is expected, therefore, that minority administrators and professionals will be spokesmen for other minorities out of an inherent *obligation* to speak out in their best group interest.

Perhaps the most critical factor, however, relates to bureaucratic promises made as the number of minority group members working for an agency or jurisdiction increases. In far too many cases, hiring practices are utilized to demonstrate efforts to be responsive to minority community needs. Because many agencies or governmental jurisdictions equate programmatic commitment or effort with the employment of a large number of minorities, governmental employees from those groups can become convenient targets of protest when expectations and/or promises to the community groups are unfulfilled.

These and many other related demands and expectations create a number of major dilemmas for minority administrators to which most agencies are insensitive. In some respects many of the dilemmas and forces mentioned in this article confront all administrators, but the minority administrator seems to be subject to their weight more than most. For ultimately, every minority administrator and professional must consciously or otherwise respond to two basic and difficult questions:

1. "What responsibility do I have to minority group peoples?"
2. "What role should I attempt to play in making government more responsive to the needs of all people?"

ROLE DETERMINANTS

In addressing these questions, it is useful to consider six forces which confront the minority administrator, and which influence significantly his/her potential effectiveness and perhaps perceptions of responsibility to both the governmental agency and minority peoples more generally. Graphically these forces might be viewed as indicated in Figure 16–1.

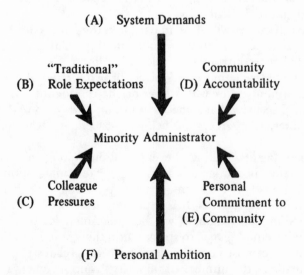

(A)   System Demands

"Traditional"   Community
(B)   Role Expectations   (D) Accountability

Minority Administrator

Colleague   Personal
(C)   Pressures   Commitment to
                                              (E) Community

(F)   Personal Ambition

FIGURE 16–1. Role demands on minority administrators

A. System Demands

The first force, "system demands," refers to those expectations of public employees that a governmental system reinforces through a range of sanctions and rewards. Bureaucratic systems are perpetuated because they demand and receive obedience to orders. The traditional model of hierarchy as described by Weber suggests that decisions are made at the top and implemented by those at lower levels within the organization. For political appointees, a failure to respond to demands made by those at the top may mean harassment, dismissal, and embarrassment. Similarly, in a civil service system, pressures are applied "to do as ordered." In cases where the civil servant "bucks" authority, intensive pressures and/or sanctions are applied (e.g., the Fitzgerald vs. Department of Defense case, as well as political pressures recently applied on the IRS, CIA, and FBI).

With regard to blacks, the system has successfully enforced its demands through a careful "weeding out" process. Only the "very best" minority group members could advance as illustrated in Sam Greenlee's novel, *The Spook Who Sat by the Door*. The techniques utilized by agencies to assure the hiring and advancement of these "outstanding" and, as Greenlee suggests, "safe" minority group members include: high education requirement, experience, oral examinations, performance tests, arrest records, probationary periods, general requirements related to residency, etc. Again, if the minority administrator is able to meet these requirements, the ongoing test that remains is that of the willingness to respond to the demands of higher-ups *without question*. Because of their historical difficulties in obtaining employment, some minority public administrators placed job security over program content or impact, and thus have become impediments to efforts to address the needs of their communities.

B. "Traditional" Role Expectations

A conventional wisdom in public administration has been that certain people do particular kinds of jobs well. Tables 16–1 and 16–2, as well as the aforementioned Civil Rights Commission report, revealed that a large percentage of minority administrators work in specialized areas. The Civil Rights Commission noted that:

> Access to white-collar jobs in some departments is more readily available to minority group members than in others. Among the seven metropolitan areas studied, the same general pattern of employment in white-collar jobs was discernable in both the North and the South. Negroes were most likely to hold jobs in health and welfare and least likely to hold them in financial administration and general control.[6]

The Commission went on to point out that:

> In addition to the "old traditional jobs" for Black Americans, "new traditional jobs" appear to be emerging. These are usually jobs as staff members of human relations councils, civil right commissions, or assistants to ranking administrators. They are status jobs carrying major responsibilities and usually bring excellent salaries. But they remain almost exclusively related to minority group problems.[7]

Many of the jobs given minority administrators at both the federal and local levels have been "flack-catching" positions. As Tom Wolfe has indicated in *Radical Chic and Mau-Mauing the Flak Catcher*, during the 1960s in particular, black and brown administrators were often placed in their positions only to become sacrificial lambs in the face of community unrest.

With regard to the future, it is important that minority group members not be herded into "traditional" departments only, nor should they blindly allow themselves to be so directed. Important decisions which affect minority people are made in agencies throughout a governmental jurisdiction or agency. Minority group participation and contributions in all these decision-making processes are becoming increasingly more critical.

C. Colleague Pressures

One of the greatest dangers to the quest for governmental responsiveness remains the pressures imposed by one's peers. Peter Maas' recent book and the adopted movie, *Serpico*, clearly document the pressures which can and frequently are brought to bear on public administrators. The pressures on minority group members take many forms:

1. The minority group policeman who wants to be accepted by his peers may be forced to "bust heads" to gain acceptance, and promotions.
2. The minority welfare worker may be forced to "get tough" with welfare recipients to be regarded as a competent professional.
3. The minority school teacher is placed in the position of "blaming the victims" of the educational process to retain a place of acceptance among his/her colleagues. It is not allowed that these professionals begin to question the quality of the educational experiences of the children supposedly being served, or the unions which represent them in the quest for working conditions which may not be in the best interest of the children.

As social animals, we desire to be accepted as peers by our colleagues. It is difficult, therefore, to ward off these peer pressures.

Clearly the task for the minority administrator is that of placing such col-legial pressures into a perspective that does not allow them to over-shadow broader program objectives and community needs.

D. Community Accountability

In recent years we have heard growing demands for greater community control, coupled with a cry for more minority group professionals who will be responsive to the needs of their people.[8] The problem histori-cally confronting black communities in this latter regard is well de-scribed by Piven and Cloward:

> Much Negro leadership exists largely by the grace of white institutions: white political parties and government agencies, white unions and busi-nesses and professions, even white civil-rights organizations. Every-thing in the environment of the Negro politician, civil servant, or pro-fessional makes him attentive to white interests and perspectives.[9]

The demand is clear. Minority people want and need administrators who will listen to them, who can communicate with them, who care about them. If this is not manifested, community control becomes the ul-timate demand, and perhaps a necessity.

E. Personal Commitment to Community

Of critical importance in this context is personal commitment to the community. The degree to which the administrator feels that there are obligations to fulfill and a role to be played which only he/she can fulfill can make a critical difference in public policy discussions, decisions, and ultimately, service output. It is my belief that as the number of minority administrators increases, commitment to addressing community needs will increase if only because there is more security in numbers. Equally important is the fact that a growing number of committed young minor-ity administrators are gradually assuming more responsible positions in public agencies. They appear able to address the difficulties of balancing agency objectives with client expectations and their own personal ambi-tions far better than many of those who have preceded them.

F. Personal Ambition

People want to advance their careers. It is my belief that all administra-tors weigh important decisions not only in terms of possible program-matic consequences, but also with regard to implications for their own careers. As employment opportunities for minority group people have expanded, personal ambitions among this group have also increased.

Until the early 1960s, the bureaucratic system was very effective in minimizing this desire for advancement, basically because it was clear that
few opportunities for promotions into professional positions existed. As
positions became more available in the 1960s, the initial result was
greater competition for an apparently large but actually limited number
of high-level appointments. Although employment opportunities have
expanded, as mentioned above, it is still argued by some that most agencies do place limits on the numbers of minorities who will fill these positions. The challenge to minority administrators is that of seeking personal security, while simultaneously manifesting a commitment to urge
greater efforts to meet governmental responsibilities more effectively.

DILEMMAS OF THE MINORITY ADMINISTRATOR

In light of the above discussion, several dilemmas stand out as being of
particular significance for the minority administrator. The effective minority administrator will be one who can respond to the challenges of
leadership in the quest for more responsive government in light/in spite
of these obstacles:

• Governmental role expectations of minority administrators do not
  necessarily coincide with the minority administrator's own perceptions, goals, or expectations;
• Unresponsive public policies put minority administrators in extremely tenuous positions vis-à-vis the agency, himself/herself, and
  the community of which he/she is a part;
• Frequently the minority administrator is put into flack-catching
  positions without the capacity to make meaningful decisions, but is
  expected to accept the responsibilities of programmatic failures
  and "keep the natives calm."
• Advancement within the governmental system is generally a function of adherence to established organizational norms; one of
  these norms historically has been that one need not be concerned
  about the needs or priorities of minority communities.
• Informal pay and promotional quotas still seem to exist for minority administrators; moreover, it is assumed that they can only fill
  certain types of positions, usually related to social service delivery
  or to communication with other minority group members.
• Minority communities sometimes expect much more of the minority administrator than he/she can provide; and in most cases demand a far faster response to their demands than these administrators have developed the capacity to deliver.

- Agencies seem to search for the "super" minority administrator, and even these are frequently hired as show pieces. In other cases there has been evidence of agencies hiring individuals who clearly would be unable to do a job with the intent of showing that an effort was made but "they just can't do this kind of work."

While other dilemmas might be identified, this brief listing seems to reinforce the argument that the task of being a minority administrator within public agencies is not an easy one. Moreover, in the short run the challenges reflected in these dilemmas may become greater in magnitude as governments at all levels fail to address in a meaningful fashion such quality of life problems as hunger, health, housing, etc.

CONCLUSION

For almost two centuries, minority groups have been systematically excluded from making inputs into the administrative processes of government as both decision makers and policy implementors. In the final analysis, it is now the responsibility of governmental leaders generally to expand opportunities for the perspectives of minority administrators to be articulated and acted upon. This responsibility derives not only from executive orders and congressional mandates, but also from the reality that there frequently is a minority perspective on public problems which policy makers should understand if public programs are to be truly responsive and effective.

Schools of public affairs also have a major charge to educate more minority administrators to assume these critical positions. The frequently criticized decrease in foundation monies previously utilized to provide financial assistance to these students must not be utilized as a cop-out to explain away lack of effort in this regard. The minority academic also has a role to play in supporting these efforts to provide the kind of professional training essential to the development of the number and caliber of top-flight minority administrators so critically needed in public agencies. They must also begin to work more closely with both minority elected officials and administrators in continuing education, and in policy research and analysis if some of the major problems facing minority group communities are to be effectively described, understood, and attacked.

Finally, to the minority administrator goes the challenge of accepting the obligation of working for the development and operation of public programs which more effectively meet the needs of *all* people. In some cases this may require an advocacy position. It may demand that the minority group perspective on public policy questions be researched, developed, and articulated. It will frequently demand the capacity and willingness to discuss policy options, directions, and needs with those who have expressed a lack of faith in the governmental process. It will demand a rejection of the argument that administrators are/must be value free and completely neutral in implementing policy decisions. Simultaneously, however, there exists the reality that public employees do work within a bureaucratic context with established procedures, job requirements, and program objectives. These neither can, nor should be ignored. Nor should minority public administrators be *expected* to present minority views, or be given positions solely because they are black, red, or brown. Public agencies, however, must begin to recognize and accept the reality that, in light of the problems confronting our society, it is in the public interest that minority administrators not forget who they are, or from whence they have come.

NOTES

1. Joint Center for Political Studies, *National Roster of Black Elected Officials* (Washington, D.C.: the Joint Center, April 1974).
2. Equal Employment Opportunity Commission, *State and Local Government Information EEO-4 National Statistical Summaries* (Washington, D.C.: Office of Research, 1974).
3. U.S. Civil Service Commission, *Minority Group Employment in the Federal Government* (Washington, D.C.: U.S. Government Printing Office, March 1974), pp. i, ii.
4. *Summary of the First National Conference on the Role of Minorities in Urban Management and Related Fields* (Washington, D.C.: Metropolitan Washington Council of Governments, 1973), p. 19.
5. U.S. Commission on Civil Rights, *For All The People . . . By All The People* (Washington, D.C.: U.S. Government Printing Office, 1968), p. 118.
6. *Ibid.*, p. 2.
7. *Ibid.*, p. 3.
8. For a representative sample of the literature describing these attitudes, see: Alan Altshular, *Community Control* (New York: Pegasus, 1970); Charles E. Wilson, "Year One at I.S. 201," *Social Policy* (May/June 1970), pp. 10–17; Sherry R. Arnstein, "Maximum Feasible Manipulation," *Public Administration Review*, Vol. XXXII (September/October 1972), pp. 377–390; and Mario Fantini and Marilyn Gittell, *Decentralization: Achieving Reform* (New York, Praeger, 1973).
9. Francis Fox Piven and Richard A. Cloward, "Black Control of Cities," in Edward S. Greenburg, et al. (eds.), *Black Politics* (New York: Holt, Rinehart and Winston, Inc., 1971), pp. 128–129.

17

The Sex Dimension of Organizational Processes: Its Impact on Women Managers

ROSLYN H. CHERNESKY

The problem of getting women into management and the difficulty around moving women up the managerial ladder has received a great deal of attention over the past few years (Terborg, 1977; Chernesky, 1980). There is now a greater understanding of the factors that account for the under-representation of women in management, and an appreciation of both the organizational barriers as well as the personal constraints that act as obstacles to women's entrance and upward mobility (O'Leary, 1974; Kanter, 1976). While attention and efforts to help women overcome these obstacles have focused on moving women into and up in management (Pierson, 1982), the issue of what happens to women who have obtained managerial status has been relatively neglected.

An increasing concern today is that women's ability to manage, even if they are given the opportunity to do so and have the necessary skills and competence, may be adversely affected by the experiences encountered within organizations (Forisha & Goldman, 1981). Is it not likely that women in administrative positions will face obstacles in their attempt to be effective managers just as they did in their efforts to become managers? And, is it not likely that these obstacles will also stem from organizational barriers and personal constraints, and will also result from the complex interaction of organizational discrimination and the behaviors of individual men and women?

There is growing evidence that women managers continue to find themselves in situations encumbered by stereotypes, role traps and sexism which prevent them from performing at their full competence (Johnson, 1976; Kanter, 1977; Bayes & Newton, 1978; Curlee & Raymond, 1978; Kanter & Stein, 1979; Massengill & DiMarco, 1979; Rowe, 1981). Therefore, there is a need to better understand the experience of women inside organizations (Forisha, 1981). The focus of this article is on the sex dimension of organizational processes and is concerned with how differences in sex along with the resulting differences in expectations, treatment and behavior, influence the organizational experience of women.

EXISTING KNOWLEDGE: AN OVERVIEW

The existence of sex differences in work organizations and in work behavior is neither well documented nor fully accepted despite considerable interest in the phenomenon (Snyder & Bruning, 1979). Evidence is now available that shows that dysfunctional behaviors such as poor performance, absenteeism, turnover, job strain and isolation can be related to one's experience in a work organization, and that women are more likely than men to be in situations and positions which result in these negative consequences (Acker & Van Houten, 1974; Miller, Labovitz, & Fry, 1975; Kanter, 1977).

Women in management positions not only face organizational constraints that affect their functioning but, it is hypothesized in this paper, women who may be competent and qualified managers can be rendered ineffective depending upon the situation in which they are placed. Since some situations will be more conducive to women managers while others will be less so, an examination of women managers in the context of their organizational environment should be useful if we are to understand the behavior of women managers.

Three situations in which women managers may find themselves have been selected to illustrate how the organizational experience can have a differential impact on men and women:

1. task oriented or work group situations,
2. situations in which there is only one woman manager or it is rare to be one, and
3. situations in which the woman's leadership style is neither accepted nor respected.

Although other examples could similarly demonstrate how the experience of women managers can be affected by situational variables, these three have been the focus of a good deal of research and inquiry by women, and thus there are substantial findings to draw upon. It is important to note, however, that this research has serious limitations. First, there are actually no comparative studies of male and female managers upon which we can base our discussion. Second, sex differences in organizational behavior are not readily open to study since comparing or controlling for sex eliminates the very difference that is hypothesized to influence the male and female administrative experience, and should therefore constitute the basis of study. Third, most studies of the situations discussed here have been conducted in a lab rather than in the field which is more likely to result in distorted data overstating the influence of sex (Osborn & Vicars, 1976; Terborg, 1977).

TASK ORIENTED OR WORK GROUP BEHAVIOR

As part of their jobs, managers frequently participate in a variety of task oriented group situations. Differences between men and women in activity, influence and task orientation depending upon the sex composition of the groups have been observed in both lab and field studies for a number of years. More recent studies of sex differences in group behavior (Eskilon & Wiley, 1976; Lockheed & Hall, 1976; Meeker & Weitzel-O'Neill, 1977; Fennell et al., 1978) have supplemented earlier research on small groups that found clear differences in roles between men and women in mixed-sex task oriented groups. Several generalizations can be drawn from these studies:

1. Men are more verbally active than women; they are more talkative and take the initiative more often than women.
2. Men are more influential than women; men are less likely to yield to a woman's opinion, and women are more likely to defer to a man's point of view.
3. Men spend a higher proportion of their group participation in task oriented categories of behavior; women's contributions to the group, in contrast, give greater emphasis to social-emotional-expressive activities such as agreeing, expressing approval, and encouragement.
4. Contributions of women, or those attributed to women, are less likely to be accepted and will be evaluated less positively than those of men.
5. Men are more likely than women to be perceived by other group members as leaders, and to emerge as leaders.

Differences in male and female group behavior were initially explained by role differentiation theory. Any viable small group supposedly required some members to perform the role of instrumental leader or task specialist, and others to serve as expressive leaders. Men were considered to be appropriate instrumental leaders while women were seen as suitable expressive leaders because of innate characteristics and/or differences in sex role socialization. Recently this hypothesis of sex differences in group behavior has received little support. Questions have been raised as to whether task behavior and social behavior in groups are incompatible thus requiring leadership in the two arenas to be held by separate individuals. In addition, there has been a lack of reliable evidence to indicate that women were more inclined to the expressive role in contrast to men who were thought to be more inclined to the instrumental role (Meeker & Weitzel-O'Neill, 1977).

It is now widely recognized that factors such as status characteristics and expectation states among group members more fully explain sex differences in group behavior (Berger et al., 1972; Lockheed & Hall, 1976; Fennell et al., 1978). Briefly summarized, the theory postulates that when a group is working on a valued task, when some competence is necessary for successful completion of the task, and when individuals involved differ in perceived or real status, all the group members will expect the high status individual(s) to be more competent at the task and to assume positions of leadership, power and prestige. High status members therefore get more opportunities to participate, initiate more actions, receive more positive feedback, have greater influence, and are less likely to defer to low status members.

Gender apparently continues to function as a status characteristic in our society, in organizations, and in work groups. Because male status is more highly valued than female status, men take on and are given leadership roles in task oriented mixed-sex groups. Thus, without intent and without the group's knowledge, the group experience inhibits, restricts and channels women's activity and the nature of their participation. As a result, not only does the group fail to reap the full benefit of women's contributions, but women fail to emerge as viable and competent leaders thereby confirming the stereotypes regarding women's leadership capacity.

Deliberate efforts to intervene in this process are necessary if men, because of their real or perceived higher status, are not to continue to dominate. The most effective way to bring about situations in which sex differences in group behavior disappear is to assure that information is provided to and accepted by all group members that the male status characteristic is not relevant. This may be done by explicitly delegating to women leadership positions and the authority that accompanies them. When women group members are placed in leadership positions and are aware of their rights and expected behaviors, and it is made known that the authority of the leader will be supported, they are less likely to be treated in the same manner as women otherwise have been. Invariably, when individuals with low status are placed in situations where leadership is legitimated by organizational authority, effective leadership performance is more likely to emerge (Eskilon & Wiley, 1976; Lockheed & Hall, 1976; Parcel & Cook, 1977; Fennell et al., 1978). Women, once legitimated, can then demonstrate the kinds of activity, influence and task orientation in mixed-sex task groups that have traditionally been associated with men and with competent and effective management.

THE SOLO PROFESSIONAL

Because women are relatively new to management and are still a rarity at high level administrative positions, women managers may find themselves in situations where they are the only professional women or the rare one in an otherwise all male group or setting. This experience may also have negative consequences for women although the results are somewhat different from those associated with the dynamics of task oriented mixed-sex groups.

Studies of work groups with only one woman member suggest that the dynamics in groups with so skewed a sex distribution are likely to result in the woman being stereotyped, isolated or ignored (Wolman & Frank, 1975; Ruble & Higgins, 1976; Frank & Katcher, 1977; Kanter, 1977). In groups with a greater number of women, these tendencies are much less likely to surface, although they are never totally absent. Should the woman assert herself and try to either influence the group or change its course, she is unlikely to be successful and, the same studies show, may make the situation even more intolerable for herself. Wolman and Frank (1975) found, for example, that women who persisted in taking on leadership roles after having been ignored either continued to be ignored or received a kind of coordinated reaction that is typical of the way groups handle deviants and isolates. They also found that women's efforts to resist or get out of the sex role stereotypes in which they were placed were usually interpreted with sex role stereotypes thereby increasing women's differences and isolating them further. If the solo woman deals with the situation by acting friendly, she is thought to be flirting; if she appears weak or appeals to the men, she is infantalized or treated as a little sister rather than a peer; if she becomes angry, she is seen as competitive or incapable of taking it like one of the "boys." Regardless of what she may do to counteract the situation, and irrespective of whether she intentionally provoked the situation, the solo woman will more than likely be subjected to intense pressure to assume subordinate behavior.

In trying to explain this group phenomenon, Wolman and Frank draw upon theories that suggest that all male peer groups engage in bonding and in a variety of behaviors that are disrupted by the very presence of a woman. The lone woman is therefore resented. She may not even be aware that she is trespassing nor appreciate how her desire to be fully accepted as a group member must be dealt with by the male group. What therefore appears to be a deliberate process to exclude women can be seen as an instinctive reaction in order to preserve the all male group. Most importantly, it is carried out in a manner that is within the boundaries of group dynamics and generally considered to be legitimate by society.

An alternative explanation has been offered by theorists such as Kanter (1977) who suggests that much of what the lone woman encounters is experienced by anyone whose social type is rare among the social composition of the membership. Men, blacks, and ethnic minorities, for example, can just as easily as women be in situations where their number points them out as different. Placed in such a situation, the lone individual is given token status and consequently takes on the characteristics associated with that position. The attitudes and behaviors of the solo professional therefore can best be understood as situational responses to the pressures placed on people in token positions.

Among the characteristics Kanter (1977) hypothesizes are associated with people whose type is represented in very small proportion are the tendencies to:

- be more visible, be "on display,"
- feel more pressure to conform, to make fewer mistakes,
- try to become "socially invisible," not to stand out so much,
- find it harder to gain "credibility," particularly in high uncertainty positions,
- be more likely to be excluded from informal peer networks,
- have fewer opportunities to be "sponsored,"
- face misperceptions of their identity and role in the organization and hence, develop a preference for already established relationships,
- face more personal stress.

The solo woman manager is thus isolated from the mainstream of group interaction which in itself can preclude the establishment of relationships critical for effective performance. In addition, the pressures on the solo woman engendered by the situation, no matter how subtle, require her to focus considerable energy on efforts to overcome the stereotypes and isolation, energy that ought to be directed toward her work. Moreover, it has been found that women tend to use underachievement or overachievement strategies in response to the dilemmas of tokenism, both of which operate to the detriment of women (Spangler, Gordin, & Pipkin, 1978). A woman manager who is the only one, or one of the few, among men managers may not be able to function at the level of her skill and competency because of the situation, thereby confirming the organization's decision not to hire any more women managers.

Counteracting this situation invariably involves increasing the numbers of women in management positions and the numbers of women participants in groups, a strategy strongly advocated by Kanter (1977). Ruble and Higgins (1976) suggest that by altering the sex composition of the group, the dispositions and attitudes of each member of the group may be altered. Frank and Katcher (1977) advise, however, that increasing the numbers and proportion of women will not necessarily lead to changes in men's negative perception of women's leadership ability. As Curlee and Raymond (1978) point out, female administrators who experience sexist role casting may feel they are in a no-win situation.

Efforts must be undertaken to remind women that they personally are not to blame when cast in sex role stereotypes or are isolated but that both are a consequence of being a token. Because of the powerful group forces that occur in face of the lone woman, women might be best off not trying to intervene in the process but instead bide their time, temporarily accepting the situation. Accommodation or submission by the solo professional will not change the situation and will incur costs to both the individual involved and the group or setting which will not have the advantage of a fully participating member.

LEADERSHIP STYLE

Women managers may find themselves in a third situation—settings in which their style of leadership is incongruent with the prevailing male managerial model and consequently is neither accepted nor respected. Identification of and comparison between male and female leadership styles have been a focus of much attention, producing generally contradictory and inconsistent findings (Chapman, 1975; Chapman & Luthans, 1975; Osborn & Vicars, 1976; Bartol, 1977).

Despite the absence of reliable evidence to support a relationship between the sex of the manager and effectiveness or to demonstrate whether one style of management is more effective than another, the leadership style that has traditionally been associated with the masculine sex role stereotype continues to be considered effective, that is, "decisive, direct, rational, authoritarian, logical, aggressive and impersonal" (Pearson, 1981). On the other hand, women's approach to management is viewed as weak and ineffective, that is, cautious, conciliatory and subjective (Rosener & Schwartz, 1980; Pearson, 1981). Not surprisingly, any deviations from the male managerial model by women are likely to be devalued, thereby devaluing women managers as well.

Studies of male and female communication, for example, clearly demonstrate how sex differences in the style of presentation, both oral and written, are subject to interpretation to the advantage of men and disadvantage of women (Baird, 1976; Baird & Bradley, 1979; Goldman, 1981; Pearson, 1981).

A review of the more recent research on differences in male and female communication styles suggests the following:

1. Women generally communicate more openly than men; they are more willing to reveal information about their attitudes, beliefs and concerns;
2. Men and women produce messages that differ in content; whereas men tend to be task oriented in their communication, women tend to be socially oriented;
3. Women exceed men in expressing emotion, showing concern, being attentive and encouraging, and exhibiting warmth, helpfulness, sensitivity and affiliation;
4. Men exceed women in dominance, in being quick to challenge others, in directing the course of conversation, and in holding the conversation floor;
5. Women favor greater use of questions, modifiers and qualifiers, and hedging constructions; they are more likely to answer questions with questioning intonations, add questions on to the end of statements, make personal references, and are reluctant to generalize from their experience.

Analysis of writing style also shows a difference between men and women. Goldman (1981) compared the professional writing appearing in journal articles of men and women and found that all, or almost all, of the difference in the way language was used stemmed from greater hesitancy and tentativeness at making definite statements on the part of women.

The way women communicate has been explained as a strategic response to powerlessness, to being in an inferior position, or to having outsider status, all of which involve signals of deference, compliance, dependence and support that may be found in the communication pattern of all persons so situated (Kotker, 1980; Pearson, 1981). Because the style is so closely associated with women, it has been referred to as feminine rhetoric.

Some women may use the rhetoric unknowingly having successfully learned to survive as a subordinate in a society dominated by men. Others may choose to communicate in this manner because they believe the feminine style, typified by a climate of openness, concern, receptiveness and the like, is a more appropriate and effective approach for managers than the male model of administration (Baird & Bradley, 1979; Hauptman, 1981). In either case, a negative stigma is attached to the style and the women using it are likely to be evaluated as not meeting organizational needs nor being effective managers.

Style of communication is just one aspect of managerial behavior that appears to differentiate men and women. Sex differences in the use of power (Johnson, 1967; Wagner & Swanson, 1979), and in the perception of authority (Neuse, 1978) have recently been found. Given the popular interest in identifying additional areas of difference, it is likely that an increasing number of findings will similarly be interpreted in terms of sex role stereotypical behavior. Consequently, as with communication, whatever behavior is associated with women will be viewed as less valuable and effective than what men do. Despite a lack of evidence to suggest that the male leadership style is in fact better or more successful, and despite theories and data that indicate location in an organization is a more accurate predictor of organizational behavior than gender, women's styles will undoubtedly continue to be judged negatively and the women will be perceived of as ineffective.

To solve this problem, the burden of change tends to be placed upon the women who are in situations where they are neither accepted nor appreciated for what they bring to their managerial role. They are expected to overcome what are considered to be deficiencies that stem from their socialization. And, women are expected to adopt and enact the male model, thereby disregarding feminine values and orientation. Women may also be advised to seek out those organizations where their styles will be appreciated. Unfortunately, solutions such as these fail to recognize the value of differences or build upon women's strengths. In the long run these solutions deprive organizations of the contributions women can make to their administration (Hooyman, 1978; Forisha & Goldman, 1981).

Another approach to the problem is to help organizations and their current leadership to tolerate and support a variety of styles, including the feminine style, which may lead to more effective management. Steps in this direction have yet to be taken.

SUMMARY

The three situations discussed here were selected from among a large number which would illustrate how experiences within organizations can adversely affect women managers. The discussion is based upon three assumptions:

1. Competence and qualifications are not sufficient for effective management.
2. Effective management and leadership require a conducive situation.
3. Women are likely to find themselves in situations which may be conducive for effective management for men but present serious obstacles to the performance of women.

The emphasis has deliberately been upon situations in which no one is at fault. Instead, the dynamics of group or organizational processes constrain women managers. Only through close and careful examination of these processes can we expect to gain the insight necessary in order to counter them.

REFERENCES

Acker, J., & Van Houten, D. R. Differential recruitment and control: The sex structuring of organizations. *Administration Science Quarterly*, 1974, 152-163.

Baird, J. E. Sex differences in group communication: A review of research. *Quarterly Journal of Speech*, 1976, *62*, 179-192.

Baird, J. E., & Bradley, P. H. Styles of management and communication: A comparative study of men and women. *Communication Monographs*, 1979, *46*, 101-111.

Bartol, K. M. The sex structuring of organizations: A search for possible causes. *Academy of Management Review*, 1978, *3*, 805-815.

Bayes, M., & Newton, P. M. Women in authority: A sociopsychological analysis. *The Journal of Applied Behavioral Sciences*, 1978, *14*, 7-20.

Berger, J., Cohen, B. P., & Zelditch, M., Jr. Status conceptions and social interaction. *American Sociological Review*, 1972, *37*, 241-255.

Chapman, J. B. Comparison of male and female leadership styles. *Academy of Management Journal*, 1975, *18*, 645-650.

Chapman, J. B., & Luthans, F. The female leadership dilemma. *Public Personnel Management*, 1975, 173-179.

Chernesky, R. H. Women administrators in social work. In E. Norman & A. Mancuso (Eds.), *Women's issues and social work practice*. Itasca, IL: Peacock Publishers, 1980.

Curlee, M. B., & Raymond, F. B. The female administrator: Who is she? *Administration in Social Work*, 1978, *39*, 307-318.

Eskilon, A., & Wiley, M. G. Sex composition and leadership in small groups. *Sociometry*, 1976, *39*, 183-200.

Fennell, M. L., Barchas, P. R., et al. An alternative perspective on sex differences in organizational settings: The process of legitimation. *Sex Roles*, 1978, *4*, 589-604.

Forisha, B. L. The inside and the outsider: Women in organizations. In B. L. Forisha & B. H. Goldman (Eds.), *Outsiders on the inside*. Englewood Cliffs, NJ: Prentice-Hall, 1981.

Forisha, B. L., & Goldman, B. H. (Eds.). *Outsiders on the inside: Women and organizations.* Englewood Cliffs, NJ: Prentice-Hall, 1981.

Frank, H. H., & Katcher, A. H. The qualities of leadership: How male medical students evaluate their female peers. *Human Relations,* 1977, *30,* 403-416.

Goldman, B. H. Women, men, and professional writing: Signature of power? In B. L. Forisha & B. H. Goldman (Eds.), *Outsiders on the inside.* Englewood Cliffs, NJ: Prentice-Hall, 1981.

Hauptman, A. R. Styles of leadership: Power and feminine values. In B. L. Forisha & B. H. Goldman (Eds.), *Outsiders on the inside.* Englewood Cliffs, NJ: Prentice-Hall, 1981.

Hooyman, N. Roots of administrative styles: Modes and models. In E. Wattenberg (Ed.), *Room at the top.* Minneapolis: University of Minnesota, 1978.

Johnson, P. Women and power: Toward a theory of effectiveness. *Journal of Social Issues,* 1976, *32,* 99-110.

Kanter, R. M. The impact of hierarchical structures on the work behavior of women and men. *Social Problems,* 1976, *23,* 415-427.

Kanter, R. M. *Men and women of the corporation.* New York: Basic Books, 1977.

Kanter, R. M., & Stein, B. A. The gender pioneers: Women in an industrial sales force. In R. M. Kanter & B. A. Stein (Eds.), *Life in organizations.* New York: Basic Books, 1979.

Kotker, Z. The "feminine" behavior of powerless people. *Savvy,* March 1980, 36-42.

Lockheed, M. E., & Hall, K. P. Conceptualizing sex as a status characteristic: Applications to leadership training strategies. *Journal of Social Issues,* 1976, *32,* 111-123.

Massengill, D., & DiMarco, N. Sex-role stereotypes and requisite management characteristics: A current replication. *Sex Roles,* 1979, *5,* 561-570.

Meeker, B. F., & Weitzel-O'Neill, P. A. Sex roles and interpersonal behavior in task-oriented groups. *American Sociological Review,* 1977, *42,* 91-105.

Miller, J., Labovitz, S., & Fry, L. Inequities in the organizational experience of women and men. *Social Forces,* 1975, *54,* 365-381.

Neuse, S. M. Professionalism and authority: Women in public service. *Public Administration Review,* 1978, *38,* 436-441.

O'Leary, V. E. Some attitudinal barriers to occupational aspirations in women. *Psychological Bulletin,* 1974, *81,* 826-890.

Osborn, R. N., & Vicars, W. M. Sex stereotypes: An artifact in leader behavior and subordinated satisfaction analysis? *Academy of Management Journal,* 1976, *19,* 339-449.

Parcel, T. L., & Cook, K. S. Status characteristics, reward allocation and equity. *Sociometry,* 1977, *40,* 311-324.

Pearson, S. S. Rhetoric and organizational chance: New applications of feminine style. In B. L. Forisha & B. H. Goldman (Eds.), *Outsiders on the inside.* Englewood Cliffs, NJ: Prentice-Hall, 1981.

Pierson, J. *Moving women up: A manual for breaking down barriers.* Washington, DC: NASW, 1982.

Rosener, L., & Schwartz, P. Women, leadership and the 1980's: What kind of leaders do we need? In C. Steele (Ed.), *New leadership in the public interest.* New York: NOW Legal Defense and Education Fund, 1980.

Rowe, M. The minutiae of discrimination: The need for support. In B. L.
     Forisha & B. H. Goldman (Eds.), *Outsiders on the inside.* Englewood Cliffs,
     NJ: Prentice-Hall, 1981.
Ruble, D. N., & Higgins, E. T. Effects of group sex composition on self presenta-
     tion and sex-typing. *Journal of Social Issues,* 1976, *32,* 125-132.
Snyder, R. A., & Bruning, W. S. Sex differences in perceived competence: An
     across organizational study. *Administration in Social Work,* 1979, *3,* 349-358.
Spangler, E., Gordon, M., & Pipkin, R. Token women: An empirical test of
     Kanter's hypothesis. *American Journal of Sociology,* 1978, *84,* 160-170.
Terborg, J. R. Women in management: A research review. *Journal of Applied Psy-
     chology,* 1977, *62,* 647-684.
Van Wagner, K., & Swanson, C. From Machiavelli to Ms.: Differences in male-
     female power styles. *Public Administration Review,* 1979, 66-72.
Wolman, C., & Frank, H. H. The solo woman in a professional peer group.
     American Journal of Orthopsychiatry, 1975, 45 (1).

18

The Latina Social Service Administrator: Developmental Tasks and Management Concerns

ERMINIA LOPEZ RINCON
CHRISTOPHER B. KEYS

Compared to women in general, the Latina is a latecomer to the world of work, and in particular to male-dominated occupations. A recent search in several data bases yielded no research respective to the Latina in administrative or executive positions in the social service field. One could hypothesize that her emergence into these fields has been slower than that of other women because she has three handicaps. She is oppressed as a female, as a member of a minority group within the mainstream culture, and finally, as a female within the Hispanic culture. As such, she is in the uniquely awkward position of fighting for and against her male Hispanic counterpart. While she struggles with him to liberate their subculture and to improve conditions for Hispanics, she struggles to free herself from the confining position in which she has been kept by Hispanic males. Intuitively, because of this triple handicap, Latinas may experience more stress in positions of authority than non-Latinas.

The authors thank Rose E. Ray for her valuable comments in reviewing the manuscript.

The purpose of this paper is twofold. The first is to offer a conceptual framework for looking at the professional development of Latinas. In order to develop and to succeed professionally, a Latina must accomplish three tasks, namely, transcend her culture, develop a sense of personal identity, and adopt a professional role. The second purpose is to discuss specific difficulties, related to the tasks, the Latina may face in the course of carrying out the duties and responsibilities associated with positions of authority. The senior author's experience as the only female director in a network of approximately 100 social service agencies provided the material for this paper. The agencies were established nationwide to provide services to Hispanics and minorities.

TRANSCENDING THE CULTURE

In order to grow, one must first be able to set oneself apart from his/her origins (Forisha, 1978). The Latina who wishes to change traditional patterns must remove herself from the influence of her culture insofar as sex roles are concerned. The Hispanic woman, typically, is held fast to passive and submissive behaviors by the Hispanic male—father, brother, or husband. To illustrate: Argentina's Claudia Casablanca, 17, while competing for the tennis title at the Southern Open Tournament in Chicago, was grabbed and slapped soundly by her father on the court in full view of three thousand spectators (Belnap, 1978). Presumably, Claudia's father did not agree with her decision to use her talent publicly. Miss Casablanca left the court but was subsequently encouraged by her supporters to resume the match. She did so unsuccessfully. Claudia may have been intimidated and humiliated by her father's callous action and lost the will to win.

Usually, unless she breaks the cultural pattern, the Latina's script is written. She will continue in the inferior, passive, and submissive role culturally ascribed to Hispanic females (Geyer, 1970; Gonzalez, 1975), and under the rule of the often exploitative and dominative Hispanic male (Boulette, 1976; Duarte, 1979).

Rarely is a Latino supportive of a Latina's career aspirations. Even those Latinos in positions of influence seldom assist their Hispanic counterpart by violating the rigid cultural code. Generally, Latinos who refuse to consider qualified Latinas for administrative positions justify their behavior by claiming that the community prefers a male in these positions because leadership is a man's role (Aguilar, 1977; Nieto, 1974).

Paz, a vocal adversary of the macho personality (male chauvinist), contends that the sexist attitudes of Latinos produce confusion and are destructive to the growth of healthy male/female relationships. The efforts of Paz and others who would change the existing attitudes are thwarted by Latinos and by professional, non-feminist Latinas alike

(Gonzales, 1979). Hypothetically, the latter resist change becuse change is accompanied by conflict and fear of losing "the known self, the known place, and the known environmental supports" (Forisha, 1978).

The Latina who resists her culture's norms is strongly motivated to avoid the Hispanic woman's lifestyle. Her motivation begins with her ability to imagine her future within the Hispanic culture. Through cognitive representation of future outcomes, one is able to generate current motivators of behavior to bring about change (Bandura, 1977). However, without reinforcement, the Latina's motivation cannot maintain the strength needed to effect the changes she must make in her life and to cope with the psychological stress associated with change.

A SENSE OF PERSONAL IDENTITY

In freeing herself from the constraints of her culture, the Latina has taken the first step in developing a vital characteristic of professionals and executive—a sense of personal identity. She recognizes that she can act independently in making decisions that affect her life and in matters that concern the organization. For example, it would be inappropriate for a female executive to have to obtain her spouse's or parents' permission to work late. Indeed, an argument often used for not considering women for executive positions is that they are limited by family commitments (Williams, 1977).

The traditionally subordinate status of women coupled with strong socialization in feminine roles is likely to produce women who have low levels of self-esteem, autonomy, and adjustment (Bardwick, 1971; Davis, 1971). Such women tend to over-value the personalities and performances of males and to devalue themselves. Two factors make the Latina particularly vulnerable to feelings of inadequacy and self-doubt.

The first factor concerns the Hispanic culture. Hispanic mothers tend to be over-protective and tend to offer ready solutions to tasks confronting a child (Steward & Steward, 1973). Further, the restrictive control of Hispanic parents, particularly the father, over the activities of their daughters can discourage a child from engaging in competitive, rigorous interactions with others (Padilla & Ruiz, 1974). Social comparison theory holds that most people evolve their own standards for personal success and failure out of the implicit comparison of themselves with the performance of others whom they regard as peers or equals (Festinger, 1945). Hence, the consequence of Hispanic parental practices is that the Latina is not likely to have direct experiences of success and failure so that she can develop standards by which she might evaluate herself.

On another level, the Latina's efforts to see herself as a distinct person may be hampered by a prevailing Hispanic notion—that a woman is either good (virgin-like) or bad (the fallen woman). In either case, the Latina must deny a part of her humanness, making it virtually impossible for her to be a whole person. And, neither of these models is compatible with professional or executive roles. The task for some Latinas, then, may be to accept facets of themselves contained in the two models and to create an identity that is closer to reality than the dichotomous identities handed to them by their male counterparts.

The second factor, which compounds the first, is the second class status of Latinos in the mainstream culture (Gonzalez, 1975; Nieto, 1974), and the stereotype of the Hispanic women held by members of the dominant group (Escobedo, 1980). It is likely that the negative attitudes held by Anglos are internalized by Latinas in much the same fashion that women in general have internalized the negative attitudes of the dominant sex toward them. Indeed, members of minority groups typically show low levels of self-esteem and feelings of inferiority (McDavid & Harari, 1968). Such feelings reveal themselves even among Hispanic dignitaries when confronting prominent members of the dominant culture (Newsweek, Oct. 1, 1979; Eder, 1980). Gonzales (1979) stated that the greater the physical and psychological defeats of a people, the greater the oppression of the female members of the group.

The implication of the second factor is that a climate that can promote self-hatred among Latinas exists (Frieze, et al., 1978). Conceivably, the climate is nurtured by the low status of her ethnic group in the mainstream culture, its effect on male Hispanics, who, in turn, may vent their frustrations on Latinas in the form of exploitation and domination.

A sense of self should serve as a means of creating and strengthening expectations of personal efficacy—a belief that one can successfully execute the behaviors required to produce desired outcomes (Bandura, 1977). A strong sense of self can provide the Latina with the psychological strength not to fall apart in crisis situations which often confront executives. It can promote objectivity so that unfortunate events are not taken personally and that she not act defensively upon receipt of criticisms and complaints. These are problem areas for many women (Williams, 1977). The Latina may be particularly vulnerable in these areas and also vulnerable to manipulation and domination by others.

ADOPTING THE EXECUTIVE ROLE

Williams (1977) stated that in order to succeed as an executive, a woman must feel equal to men and that this expectation of equality must be an integral part of the woman's personality. Women must imagine themselves as executives, feel comfortable in that role, and be confident they can do the job. Specifically, women must learn new ways of behaving.

According to social learning theory, an effective method for learning new patterns of behavior is by observing others whom one might wish to emulate (Bandura, 1977). A recurring theme in the literature on women's issues is that women's success as executives is inhibited by a dearth of female role models (Frieze, et al., 1977; Williams, 1977). The Latina is less likely than non-Hispanic women to have the benefit of role models whose behavior she could emulate, or peers from whom she might obtain support while advancing her education (Escobedo, 1980). Respective to the latter, until recently, few Latinas continued their education beyond high school.

Admittedly, for the Latina, and for most women, the process of adopting an executive role is likely to be attended by strain, tension, insecurity, and periodically, the temptation to revert to familiar female behaviors. These behaviors, however, are forces that can hinder any would-be executive. Also, seductive behaviors, which a female may have learned as a means of manipulating others to gain desired outcomes, are likely to work against her in managerial or professional positions (Williams, 1977).

If the Latina's sense of identity is weak, the hurtful experiences she is bound to encounter in an executive capacity may reinforce her passive conditioning even as it undermines newly acquired self-confidence and feelings of self-worth (Boslooper & Hayes, 1973). The Latina cannot shield herself from these experiences. Executives must be visible and willing to receive complaints, a difficult feat without self-confidence (Chernesky, 1979).

Assuming it is inevitable that traces from the past will surface at crucial moments, the task of the developing Latina is to recognize them and to accept them for what they are—residuals—and try to move past them.

The three developmental tasks discussed in this section were approached with the Latina in mind; however, women in general may find themselves identifying with the issues raised. The process of rejecting the traditional female role and becoming an achiever in male-dominated fields is stressful but rewarding. In setting herself apart from her culture, the Latina is free to pursue personal growth. In developing a sense of personal identity, she becomes aware of herself as a distinct entity, able to say, "I am I" (Fromm, 1965). In adopting the executive or professional role, she succeeds in perceiving herself as an able person and in reducing the inequality between males and females.

CONCERNS

In addition to the three developmental tasks discussed above, the Latina administrator may have a number of concerns. These include:

1. assertiveness,
2. susceptibility to manipulation by others,
3. showing weaknesses/characteristics considered feminine, and
4. isolation on the job.

These concerns are not mutually exclusive. Also, the Latina may have to guard against two related possibilities:

1. viewing authority figures, primarily male, in her new environment as destructive and prohibiting forces (Henry, 1949); and
2. allowing anger toward members of the dominant sex and dominant culture, who denied her opportunities for growth in the past, to spill over into her relations with these persons in the present.

Assertiveness

Typically, women trained in assertiveness tend to be much tougher on each other than they are towards men (Brodsky, 1979). Megaree (1969) found that when high dominant women were paired with low dominant males, the women were reluctant to assume overt leadership—they deferred to the male. Also, when department heads, who differed little on factors such as power and assertiveness, were compared on the basis of gender, both genders rated the departmental climate lower when departments were headed by women than when they were headed by men (Roussell, 1974; Hansen, 1974).

Respective to the Latina, the material available generally consists of self-reports. For example, Martinez (*Chicago Tribune*, Aug. 17, 1978) was "very forceful" in order to be effective as a lawyer. Yet, she stated that often it was necessary for her to establish her competence because she is a woman and a Mexican-American. Rodriguez, a Puerto Rican once labeled a "slow learner," became a doctor and subsequently the director of a pediatrics department (Cabezas, 1977). Boulette's (1976) years of clinical experience with women of Mexican descent showed lack of assertiveness to be a frequent characteristic among these women.

There are numerous situations requiring the Latina executive to behave assertively. Three of them, and suggestions for solutions, are cited here. These situations required that the Latina exercise some form of power in order to be heard and to have her requests granted. Six power bases (e.g., reward, coercion, referent, legitimate, expert, and informational) have been identified (French & Raven, 1959). It may be difficult for women to use effectively any of these power bases because they conflict with the stereotypes of women (Frieze, et al., 1978). It was the experience of the senior author that informational power proved to be effective in each case.

Situation 1. Speaking up to males in authority. It is difficult for most women to make demands on their own behalf (Williams, 1979). A demand might include asking a male-dominated board for a raise or requesting that the Board increase her power (e.g., asking for authority to hire personnel, which often rests with the Board).

The question of salary could be handled by writing a letter to the Board chairman pointing out that her salary is not commensurate with the demands of the job, experience, and educational background. The matter of hiring could be addressed at a Board meeting. It could be pointed out that Board hiring of staff delays filling vacancies, hence: a) services to clients is disrupted, b) staff is burdened needlessly, and c) unused funds revert to the prime sponsor. Further, it places a burden on the members whose time is limited. In the present case, the Latino Board members responded positively to objective arguments.

Situation 2. Defense of women. The Latina may find herself the only female at Board meetings. Negative remarks about women are likely to surface. For example, Latino women may be blamed for the rising delinquency among Hispanic youth because they are beginning to work outside the home and are not available to supervise their children.

In defense of women, it could be pointed out that there are other forces contributing to the rise in juvenile delinquency, namely, the growing militancy among Hispanics, the general rise in delinquency in the schools, the increased permissiveness in society in general, and so forth.

Situation 3. Demanding accountability. One example of this from the senior author's experience occurred because of misappropriation of funds at the county level resulting in closure of the agency by order of the Federal government. Neither the Federal agents nor the county officials wanted to assume responsibility for the unpaid wages for staff, stipends for program participants, and vendor bills incurred shortly before and after the closing of the agency. Appeals by letter and personal contact with individual members of both groups to approve payment of these obligations failed. Consequently, the director brought the issues before a public hearing of the county commissioners. The incident received newspaper coverage, and shortly thereafter monies were made available to the director for disbursement to the appropriate parties.

Needless to say, success in this endeavor was crucial to the director's self-esteem and her relations with her employees. The employees' personal losses in the matter may have prompted some to overlook the power politics involved. Failure may have been viewed as a sign of weakness.

However difficult being assertive may be for the Latina, it is better to risk disapproval for atypical sex role behavior than to remain quiet and seethe when confronted with situations such as described above.

Susceptibility to Manipulation
and Antipathy from Others

There are two possible reasons why women in managerial capacities may be vulnerable to manipulation by and antipathy from others. First, in comparisons with men on most levels, women are least favored (Constantini & Craik, 1972; Deaux & Enswiller, 1974; Mischel, 1974; Haefner, 1977). Second, women who enter business or the professions are subject to role conflict (Frieze, et al., 1978; Terborg, 1977). These two factors may predispose women to lack self-confidence, doubt themselves, and feel uncertain or ambivalent about their status. As a result, women's self-esteem may be low, which may make her susceptible to the manipulative influence of others (McDavid & Harari, 1968). Further, because of these forces, self-hatred among women and jealousy toward successful women may prevail (Frieze, et al., 1978; Kiesler, 1973; Williams, 1977).

Lack of substantial empirical data precludes making definitive statements about the Latina's level of self-esteem. However, Boulette's (1976) clinical study showed that low-income Mexican-American women think poorly of themselves. Clearly, because of her sex and ethnicity, coping with manipulative efforts may prove difficult for the Latina low in self-esteem. Again, several situations may help to illustrate this point.

Situation: Female employees. Female employees may attempt to undermine or sabotage a female director's efforts to manage the agency in a professional manner. Some strategies used may be refusing to carry out assigned duties, refusing to cooperate with other employees, taking unverified sick leave during crisis periods, making outright charges to the director that she is incompetent, and comparing the director's performance with that of a male.

Williams (1977) proposed that if a female employer is supportive to female employees, they are not apt to harbor resentment toward her. This is not always the case. The Latina executive's closeness to the difficulties many Latinas experience presents a paradox. While the director can be particularly empathic and understanding, this sensitivity may also make her vulnerable to attacks by jealous Latinas. The executive may be a reminder to the employee of her inability to transcend the Hispanic culture to the point where she could be her own person. The employee may be in a cultural bind. She may feel pressure from her desire to work, on the one hand, and from her husband and family's expectations for her as wife and mother, on the other. Hence, she may resent the director's achievements and use the director as a scapegoat for her internal problems. Indeed, an increase in the director's helpful treatment of the employee was met with increased hostility on the part of the employee. It is also likely that the employee may have internalized some sexist assumptions and think that a female employer is weaker, less able, and easier to manipulate than a male one.

In the end, the director may be faced with the distasteful task of firing an employee who persists in being insubordinate and antagonistic. If firing the employee becomes necessary, the director must be prepared for and expect an appeal through all levels of hierarchy: Board, State Employment Service, Department of Labor, and the County Compliance Officer. Thus, it is imperative that objective documentation of the events that lead to an employee's dismissal be maintained so that decisions on the appeals will be in the director's favor.

Showing Weaknesses: Characteristics Considered Feminine

According to the finds of researchers, men and women alike are of the opinion that women are not likely to succeed in business or management because they manifest behaviors considered feminine, e.g., crying, emotionality, passivity (Frieze, et al., 1978; O'Leary, 1974; Terborg, 1977). Williams' (1977) extensive interview study of successful women showed that women are penalized for behaving in typically feminine ways. While some women may find it difficult to control these behaviors, there is evidence that they are happier and more satisfied when they are more potent, supportive, and unemotional than when behaving "femininely" (Gordon & Hall, 1974). Furthermore, crying in response to problems on the job is uncomfortable for the actor and the observer.

Boulette (1976) discussed the difficulty of helping Latinas of Mexican descent become assertive. Among the factors inhibiting the use of assertiveness were: compliance rather than assertion was reinforced by their culture, fear of provoking violence, fear of being deserted, fear of their own inadequacies. Conceivably the Latina administrator has outgrown these fears. However, she may have to cope with the social unease that being in the company of Anglos sometimes arouses (Bayard, 1978; *Newsweek*, Oct. 1, 1979). She may have to guard against feeling intimidated and reacting with passivity and compliance.

Situation 1. Interactions with Anglos. Limited resources in social services often prompt agencies to look to business and industry for help. In many cases, the director must hold and preside over meetings with a committee of Anglo executives. The Latina may approach the task with anxiety attributable in part to sex and ethnic differences and in part because of her inexperience as an executive. There may be self-doubt as to whether she can preside over the meeting with poise and self-confidence. The Latina executive may question first, will they attend, and second, will she be heard.

Ideally, having a mentor available would ease these situations, but this is unlikely (Boulette, 1976; Escobedo, 1980; Williams, 1977). Some board members will be supportive. Even if they are not supportive, the director should keep in mind that she knows her agency and its programs and she should not be afraid to use this knowledge (informational power) to her advantage in making the agency's needs known to the group.

Situation 2. Interactions with governmental administrators. There is some similarity between Hispanic female role-expectations and characteristics found among Federal employees—passivity and submissiveness (Kilpatrick, Cummings, & Jennings, 1964) and between the authoritarian orientation of the Hispanic culture and the organizational hierarchy of the Federal government. Hence, relatively passive and submissive Latinas may experience less conflict relating to Federal officials. Conversely, a more active, dominant Latina may have to deal with resentment, frustration, and powerlessness that is likely to surface when faced with the officials' dogmatic approach and unyielding positions. When Federal officials are on the scene, it is often difficult to react with behaviors other than passivity and compliance. Sometimes a Latina must curb her resentment and passively yield to those in power.

Situation 3. Attacks on integrity. Discrediting an executive by casting suspicion on his/her handling of funds is not an uncommon practice. A letter to this effect may initiate an investigation without advance notice to a director. Angered, hurt, and humiliated by unfounded charges, a Latina's first impulse may be to permit the investigation. However, she should ask herself what influences the choice she makes in so doing—her ethnic/female status which makes her falter in the face of authority, inexperience as a director, the surprise element, or all three. The alternative, of course, is not to allow the investigation until explicit information concerning the charges is provided to her in writing in advance.

Assuming the investigation is allowed, and a follow-up letter is not forthcoming, the Latina should demand a letter from the parties involved concerning the outcome of the case so that her staff can be informed.

Isolation on the Job

Women who abandon stereotypic roles to enter male-dominated fields often fight a battle of loneliness and isolation (Brodsky, 1979; Terborg, 1977; Williams, 1977). Escobedo (1980) discussed the plight of Latinas in university settings. Socializing with female employees is not recommended because it can be a source of conflict later when dealing with problems arising from failure by female subordinates.

Situation 1. Minority of one. Some non-traditional Latinas' encounters with Hispanic males may be few. Hence, being the only female at Board meetings where all are Latinos may be a new experience for her and a source of discomfort initially. She cannot know how closely they adhere to their culture's norms. Hypothetically, the closer the Hispanic male is to his culture, the more sensitive he may be to having to interact with a woman on an equal basis. Business meetings are set up so that a mutual exchange of information can take place. In this setting, the input of the Latina may be stifled.

The position of a Latina amidst a group of Latinos is paradoxical. If she has not mastered the tasks identified earlier, she may revert to passivity. Or, if she is fearful that she may be kept in "her place," she may manifest aggressive and dominative behaviors. Neither of these alternatives is effective. In the former, the advances she has made in her development as a professional may be in jeopardy, and in the latter, she may be committing political suicide within the organization. It may be difficult to establish a close working relationship and open channels of communication with board members, who can assist her with agency problems, creating new programs, and providing moral support.

Situation 2. Relaxation alone. Being the only female in a group of male directors may subject the Latina to social isolation. Conferences away from one's home base provide opportunities to explore new places and to relax after hours. Neither the choice of accompanying her associates nor the choice of being alone is without possible negative effects. If the Latina opts to socialize with her peers, she may put herself in a vulnerable position or she may invite criticism if her behavior deviates from "feminine" behaviors.

On the other hand, if she chooses isolation because she is acutely aware of Hispanic male/female relationships and is uncertain about the Latinos' expectations of her, or because she has not achieved the tasks above, she puts a limit on the amount of information she can bring back to the agency. In protecting herself, she may be limiting both her and the agency's growth. And, her feelings of isolation and loneliness may be intensified because she may be excluded from discussions centering on the informal gatherings.

SUMMARY

Women who enter male-dominated fields experience hardship. This review of three developmental tasks and related issues suggests that the Latina's triple handicap (i.e., oppression as a female within two cultures and as a member of a minority group within the dominant culture) intensifies the difficulties for her. This statement is yet to be confirmed empirically.

The conceptual framework and issues discussed raise interesting research questions. If a difference exists in the negative experiences of women in male-dominated fields, is the difference a matter of degree, due to ethnicity, or some other factor? Are Hispanic female employees harder toward Hispanic female employers than they are toward Anglo female employers? Are Anglo males more accepting of females in nontraditional roles than are Hispanic males?

In another vein, the topics discussed can be of use to persons who wish to understand potential socializing problems of Hispanics and to develop programs for Latinas.

REFERENCES

Aguilar, L. The Chicana and unequal opportunity. *La Luz*, 1977, *6*, 29-30.

Bandura, A. Self-efficacy: Toward a unifying theory of behavior change. *Psychological Review*, 1977, *84*, 111-125.

Bardwick, J. *The psychology of women: A study of biosocial conflict.* New York: Harper & Row, 1971.

Bayard, M.P. Ethnicity, family and mental health. In J. M. Casas and S. F. Keefe (Eds.), *Monograph 7*, 1978. Spanish Speaking Mental Health Resource Center.

Belnap, D.F. Latin machismo dies hard. *Sun Times*, March 16, 1978.

Boslooper, T, & Hayes, M. *The femininity game.* New York: Norton & Co., 1973.

Boulette, T.R. Assertiveness training with low income Mexican-American women. In M. Miranda (Ed.), *Psychology with the Spanish-speaking: Issues, research and service delivery.* Monograph 3, 1976. Spanish Speaking Mental Health Resource Center.

Brodsky, A.M. The consciousness-raising group as a model for therapy with women. In J.H. Williams (Ed.), *The psychology of women.* New York: Norton & Co., 1979.

Cabezas, D. Manana is not good enough. *Nuestro*, 1977, *16*, 18-19.

Chernesky, R.H. A guide for women managers: A review of the literature. *Administration in Social Work*, 1979, *30*, 91-97.

Constantini, E., & Craik, K.H. Women as politicians: The social background, personality, and political careers of female party leaders. *Journal of Social Issues*, 1972, *28*, 217-236.

Davis, E.G. *The first sex.* New York: G.P. Putnam's Sons, 1971.

Deaux, K., & Enswiller, T. Explanations of successful performance on sex-linked tasks: What is skill for the male is luck for the female. *Journal of Personality and Social Psychology*, 1974, *29*, 80-85.

Duarte, P. The post-lib tango: Couples in chaos. *Nuestro*, 1979, *3*, 38-40.

Eder, R. For the writer Carlos Fuentes, Iran crisis brings *deja vu*. *The New York Times*, January 9, 1980.

Escobedo, T. Are Hispanic women in higher education the nonexistent minority? *Educational Researcher*, October 1980, 7-12.

Festinger, L. A theory of social comparison processes. *Human Relations*, 1954, 7, 117-140.

Forisha, B.L. *Sex roles and personal awareness*. Morristown, NJ: General Learning Press, 1978.

French, J.R.P., Jr., & Raven, B. The bases of social power. In D. Cartwright (Ed.), *Studies in social power*. Ann Arbor: Institute for Social Research, 1959.

Frieze, I.H., Parsons, J.E., Johnson, S.B., Ruble, D.N., & Zellman, G.L. *Women and sex roles: A social psychological perspective*. New York: Norton & Co., 1978.

Fromm, E.H. Humanistic psychoanalysis. In W.S. Sahakian (Ed.), *Psychology of personality*. Chicago: Rand McNally, 1965.

Geyer, G.A. *The new latins*. New York: Doubleday, 1970.

Gonzales, S. La Chicana: Malinche or virgin? *Nuestro*, 1979, *3*, 41-45.

Gonzalez, E.M. Sisterhood. *La Luz*, September-October 1975.

Gordon, F.E., & Hall, D.T. Self-image and stereotypes of femininity: Their relationships to women's role conflicts and coping. *Journal of Applied Psychology*, 1974, *59*, 241-243.

Haefner, J.E. Sources of discrimination among employees: A survey investigation. *Journal of Applied Psychology*, 1978, *62*, 265-270.

Hansen, P. Sex differences in supervision. Paper presented at the APA, New Orleans, September 1974.

Henry, W.E. The business executive—the psychodynamics of a social role. *American Journal of Sociology*, 1949, *54*, 286-291.

Kilpatrick, F., Cummings, M., & Jennings, M. *The image of the federal service*. Washington, DC: The Brookings Institution, 1964.

Kiesler, S.B. Prejudice: Women's bias toward other women. *Intellect*, March 1973.

Lifestyle, *Chicago Tribune*, August 17, 1978, Section 5, p. 8.

McDavid, J.W., & Harari, H. *Social psychology: Individuals, groups, and societies*. New York: Harper & Row, 1968.

Megaree, E.J. Influence of sex roles on the manifestation of leadership. *Journal of Applied Psychology*, 1969, *53*, 377-382.

Mexico's new muscle. *Newsweek*, October 1, 1979, 26.

Mischel, H.N. Sex bias in the evaluation of professional achievements. *Journal of Educational Psychology*, 1974, *66*, 157-166.

Nieto, C. The Chicana and the women's rights movement. *La Luz*, 1974, *3*, 10-11, 32.

O'Leary, V.E. Some attitudinal barriers to occupational aspirations in women. *Psychological Bulletin*, 1974, *81*, 807-826.

Padilla, A.M., & Ruiz, R.A. *Latino mental health*. Rockville, MD: National Institute of Mental Health, 1974.

Roussell, C. Relationship of sex of department head to department climate. *Administrative Science Quarterly*, 1974, *19*, 211-220.

Steward, M., & Steward, D. The observation of Anglo-, Mexican-, and Chinese-

American mothers teaching their young sons. *Child Development*, 1973, *44*, 329-337.

Still more room at the top. *Newsweek*, April 29, 1974, *74*, 79-80.

Terborg, J.R. Women in management. *Journal of Applied Psychology*, 1977, *62*, 647-664.

Williams, J.H. *The psychology of women*. New York: Norton & Co., 1979.

Williams, M.G. *The new executive woman*. New York: New American Library, 1977.

19

Participatory Management: An Alternative in Human Service Delivery Systems

KENNETH P. FALLON, JR.

Social service administrators have been incorporating into practice a number of methods and systems developed by business administration. These management systems have offered the agency administrator new approaches to making maximum use of scarce resources for effective service delivery (Bradburd, 1967). Such tools as Program Evaluation Review Technique, Planning Program Budgeting System, and Management by Objectives have all had their impact upon social service administration. The accountability demanded of social service management by legislators, private boards, and consumers alike has been facilitated by these tools. Nevertheless, the greatest resource of management remains the personnel within the organization. Berliner (1971, pp. 562–563) suggested the benefits of full utilization of staff resources: "Happy is the administrator who has learned the virtues of, and techniques for, sharing of his power. Sharing of power leads to high staff morale, organizational effectiveness, and on-the-job education of a generation which inevitably must succeed him."

Argyris (1955, pp. 1–7) reported in the *Journal of Business:*

Studies show that participative management tends to 1) increase the degree of 'we' feeling or cohesiveness that participants have with their organization; 2) provide the participants with an overall organizational point of view instead of the traditional more 'now' departmental point of view; 3) decrease the amount of conflict, hostility and cutthroat competition of participants; 4) increase individuals' understanding of each other, which leads to increased tolerance and patience toward others; 5) increase the individual's free expression of his personality, which results in an employee who sticks with the organization because he (i.e., his personality) needs the gratifying experiences he finds while working there; and 6) develop a 'work climate' as a result of the other tendencies, in which the subordinates find opportunity to be more creative and to come up with the ideas beneficial to the organization.

Likert (1967, p. 46) reported studies that indicated that "those firms or plants where System 4 (participatory management) is used show high productivity, low scrap loss, low costs, favorable attitudes, and excellent labor relations. The converse tends to be the case for companies or departments whose management system is well toward System 1 (exploitative-authoritative management)."

Participatory management implies that staff will have a voice and a vote in those management decisions that affect their work. Employees who participate in this management style feel more highly motivated and tend to incorporate the organization's goals more readily than employees working in management organizations that are autocratic or consultative in nature. Participatory management encourages people to stay in the organization and improve their role performance (Likert, 1961, 1967; Litterer, 1967).

The writer was introduced to participatory management principles at the Alaska Children's Services, a multiservice agency in Anchorage. In the summer of 1972, the writer introduced participatory management to the North Idaho Child Development Center. In both agencies, the participatory management proposal was presented by the executive directors as a management alternative, and was adopted by vote of all staff members. Both agencies were fairly new. The staff of both agreed that participatory management practices would facilitate developing programs responsive to clients' needs.

DETAILS OF PARTICIPATORY MANAGEMENT

The proposal adopted by both staffs mandated that participatory processes be applied to all major decision-making tasks, and include all elements of the staff. Democratic decision making required that decisions that affect the work of any segment of the staff be made by them. Decisions were generally to be made by voting, except in smaller staff areas, where more liberal process (consensus) applied. The process required that, if possible, proposals to staff groups be made in writing and be available in advance to the staff.

Limitations of the Process

Limitations of the democratic process include:

1. No segment of the staff is empowered to make any decision that affects the work of another segment. (Example: A group home staff may not make a decision affecting staff in a residential treatment center.)
2. Democratic process may not invade areas that are a matter of designated expertise of specific staff members. (Example: Speech therapists may not make decisions affecting psychometric tests used by psychologists.)
3. The competence or performance of staff is not subject to the democratic process except as applied to elected staff representatives. (Example: The professional expertise of a speech therapist must be evaluated by a speech therapist, whereas the performance of an ad hoc committee, elected by the staff to study a budget question, may be subject to democratic process.)
4. Staff may not make decisions that require expenditure of funds not under their authority. (Example: Child care workers may decide how to use recreational funds available to their particular cottage, but not how recreational funds are to be used by another cottage.)
5. Agency policy decisions are reserved for the board of directors in the case of the Alaska agency, or the administrator of the Department of Environmental and Community Services in the case of the North Idaho agency. (Example: Decisions to develop a new group home, halfway house, etc., were reserved for the board of directors of the Alaska Children's Services. Decisions regarding contracts with local school districts to develop an educational program for older retardates rested with the administrator of the Department of Environmental and Community Services in the case of the North Idaho Center.)

Basil summarized these constraints: "There is one firm rule regarding participation of subordinates in the decision-making process: that the prerequisites for participation must be ability and knowledge. Participation in decision making must be restricted to individuals with ability to comprehend what is required and the knowledge to contribute to the position" (1970, p. 159).

254   PARTICIPATORY MANAGEMENT

Levels of Decision Making

Examples of decisions to be made by each level in the agency were as follows:

The board of directors or the administrator:

1. agency policy decisions,
2. selection of a director,
3. determinations of basic program direction, with input from the community the agency serves, the board or advisory board, and the staff.

The administrative group (composed of designated members of each program unit, usually those with responsibility for major program supervision):

1. recommendations concerning coordination of services;
2. new service recommendations to the board of directors or the administrator;
3. preparation of proposals to various segments of staff.

Ad hoc agency committees (elected by the program units to deal with specific agencywide issues):

1. all staff recommendations to the board of directors or the administrator;
2. inservice training content;
3. budget review for priorities;
4. personnel practices such as regulations, and salary recommendations to all staff and the board of directors.

Program units:

1. program changes within a unit;
2. staff schedule;
3. intake into unit;
4. transfer, referral, and discharge from the service;
5. unit budget decisions;
6. changes in use of staff and of staff patterns;
7. unit routines and rules.

Cross-unit staff:

1. exchange or sharing of staff for special team projects;
2. some kinds of inservice training that may pertain to specific disciplines, programs, etc.

IMPLEMENTATION OF THE PROCESS

Determination of Client Need

In October 1972 the North Idaho Child Development Center held 14 meetings for professionals, consumers of service (parents and children), and interested citizens in eight communities to determine needs of children and families in those communities, and services the community felt would be responsive to those needs. In each meeting, the participants were requested to identify needs without establishing priority. Subsequently, the participants set up priorities and identified services that could be developed in response to the needs. Staff participated as resource persons but did not take part in identifying needs or service responses.

The staff reviewed the data gathered at these meetings, as well as other available data, and wrote proposals regarding program services. The proposals were summarized and sent to all participants in the community meetings. The participants were asked for their response by a community representative elected at the community meetings to represent them at a staff-community representative retreat. In November 1972 the staff proposals were considered at the 3-day retreat. Programs affecting all staff were voted upon. Three new programs required funds not then available: a preschool program for handicapped children in two rural communities, a life skill acquisition program for 13- to 21-year-old retardates, and a parent training program in communication skills and infant stimulation. The community representatives set the priorities for the programs; the staff had no vote on this.

Since November all of the programs have been put into operation. The first priority, the life skill acquisition program, was funded through a contract using money available through the public schools and 4-A money available to the North Idaho center. The second priority, the preschool programs for handicapped children in two rural communities, used money made available to the communities through a Title VI grant written by the Child Development Center on behalf of the school district. The third program, parent training in communication skills and infant stimulation, was developed through reallocation of existing resources within the Child Development Center and participation of AFDC recipients in infant stimulation through a special WIN program.

Full use of the participatory decision-making process allowed the North Idaho Child Development Center to develop an effective programming budget in the five-county region of North Idaho from $400,000 in fiscal 1973 to over $800,000 in fiscal 1974.

Staff Response

The initial response of staff to the participatory management practices was one of suspicion and ambivalence. As opportunities arose for the invoking of the process, staff became more committed to it. Most of those staff members who had doubts about the participatory process became committed through involvement in budget development. The give-and-take in staff's wrestling with the onerous task of developing a budget with limited funds was gratifying to both staff and management. Also, the evidence from both agencies suggests that staff are more responsible in managing their budget when they are involved in its development.

Staff are also aware that, like any other management method, democratic decision making is only as good as the administrator's intent to uphold its principles. One writer has indicated manipulatively: "An intelligent manager will, therefore, at times appoint a committee to come up with a recommendation or decision on a matter in which group deliberation is not necessary, a matter he has already decided or to which there is but one good answer. By skillful leadership or by the sheer force of facts, the group can be brought to a foregone conclusion. If the manager can avoid the appearance of 'railroading,' he is likely to obtain a stronger motivation toward acceptance in successful prosecution of a plan than if he had announced it to his subordinates without their participation" (Koontz & O'Donnell, 1968, pp. 382–383).

It is unlikely that staff could long be so deluded. As Basil stated: "When a manager has already made a decision, he should never ask his subordinates to participate. The subordinates will soon recognize that the executive has made the decision and is merely attempting to placate them by discussion of alternatives" (1970, p. 159).

A method for determining what management style is current within an organization and what the staff would desire the management style to be was made available by Likert. He devised a questionnaire on organizational performance and characteristics of different management systems (1961, pp. 223–233; 1967, pp. 14–24).

This management orientation questionnaire, as modified by Comanor (1973), was administered to the staff of the North Idaho Child Development Center in June 1973. The purpose was to elicit from the staff where they thought the center was in management orientation and where the staff desired the center to be. The results of the questionnaire are shown in Figure 19–1.

The respondents were 13 nonsupervisory staff and four supervisory staff. There are some parallels in the spikes and valleys in the figure between supervisory and nonsupervisory staff. In general, the nonsupervisory staff perceive the center's management system as more toward

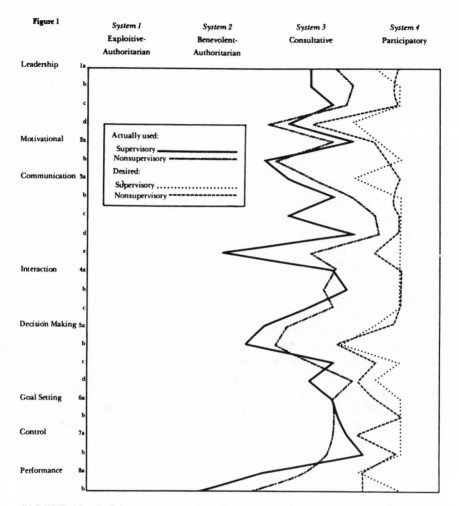

FIGURE 19–1. Management system used and desired by North Idaho Child Development Center prior to June 1973, as seen by supervisors and nonsupervisors

the participatory model than supervisory staff. Those areas where the spikes infringe in the benevolent-authoritarian area indicate problem areas to be overcome by management and staff, with management by participation as the goal.

The questionnaire was also broken down into responses by discipline and office location. This was useful in providing management with additional data in identifying specific areas where participatory management was working well and where problems existed.

The figure indicates that basically the management system at the center was consultative. It also indicates a strong desire by staff that the management be participatory.

DISCUSSION

Two months before the questionnaire was administered, the agency's former umbrella agency—the Idaho Department of Social and Rehabilitation Services—was merged by the Legislature on April 1 with the Department of Environmental Protection and Health. The new agency was named the Department of Environmental and Community Services. Its overall goal is to provide an integrated, comprehensive human service delivery system in a community-based service model. There was anxiety subsequent to the merger that the Child Development Center would lose its autonomy, and the participatory management system that had been operating in the agency might be lost to a less responsive, bureaucratic autocracy.

The staff was aware that even at best an agency that operates under the regulations of local, state and federal governmental agencies has difficulty in fully implementing a participatory management system. "When the top management of an enterprise is committed to System 2 (benevolent-authoritarian) and seeks to use it throughout the company, it is extremely difficult for a manager to learn System 4 (participatory management) and to shift to it" (Likert, 1967, p. 190). Participatory management requires a commitment in practice by management, which will also be the watchdog and guarantor of the participatory process. If that commitment is lacking or if upper management uses an authoritarian or benevolent-authoritarian management practice, middle management will have great difficulty in implementing a participatory management system in specific areas.

The staff of the Child Development Center reaffirmed commitment to the participatory management system at a staff meeting in September 1973. At a subsequent retreat (involving representatives from the Department of Environmental and Community Services in the five northern counties of Idaho), they won unanimous adoption of a participatory management proposal affecting all staff of the newly formed department. The proposal was similar to the one adopted by the Child Development Center staff the previous year.

REFERENCES

Argyris, Chris. Organizational leadership and participative management, *Journal of Business*, XXVIII, 1, January 1955.

Basil, Douglas C. *Managerial Skills for executive action.* American Management Association, 1970.

Berliner, A. K. Some pitfalls in administrative behavior, *Social Casework, LII,* 9, 1971.

Bradburd, A. W. The relationship of systems work to administration, *Public Welfare, XXV,* 4, 1967.

Comanor, Al. Program management workshop. Paper presented at Child Welfare League of American Northwest Regional Conference, Edmonton, Alberta, 1973.

Koontz, Harold, & O'Donnell, Cyril. *Principles of management: An analysis of managerial functions,* 4th edition. New York: McGraw-Hill, 1968.

Likert, Rensis. *The human organization: Its management and value.* New York: McGraw-Hill, 1967.

———. *New patterns of management.* New York: McGraw-Hill, 1961.

Litterer, Joseph A. *The analysis of organizations.* New York: John Wiley & Sons, 1967.

20

Client Participation in Mental Health Service Delivery

LOUIS E. KOPOLOW

Client participation in the direction, evaluation, and priority-setting of treatment programs in community mental health centers (CMHCs) is an extremely controversial issue, with special and broad significance for the entire mental health system. In the past many mental health clients accepted the role of passive recipients of care, but today increasing numbers are demanding that their human and legal rights be respected and that they be given greater autonomy in controlling their own lives and resolving their own emotional problems.

GOALS AND THEORY

A number of factors have limited the role that present and former mental health clients can have in their own or other clients' treatment. These factors include the historic reliance on mental health profession experts as administrators of mental health services, the prejudice and stigma associated with any present and former client who has been labeled "mentally ill," and the lack of resources or organization by which ex-patient groups could establish viable alternatives to traditional services or collaborate effectively with existing programs.

While some mental health professionals would support increased former client participation in the mental health service delivery system, relatively few would endorse the concept of totally independent patient-run alternatives. This objection to independent patient-run programs rests on the fundamental question of the nature of mental illness as a disabling condition. Mental health professionals view mental disability as an illness or disorder requiring treatment from experts. These experts acquire their status as a result of special training, education, and work experience. With the status of expert comes the power to set priorities and direct programs, and the responsibility to assure that one's clients are receiving appropriate and quality care (Lieberman, 1970).

Although former clients may have had direct experience in the workings of the system, their views are generally discounted. Former patients must contend not only with the limitations placed on them by their disability (which at times limits their ability to communicate their perspectives effectively), but with an even greater obstacle resulting from the stigma associated with the label "mental patient" (Armstrong, 1980). The prejudices against present and former patients held by much of society make it extremely difficult for them to assert their rights and take an appropriate role in aiding their fellow citizens with emotional problems.

Members of the ex-patient movement in recent years have become increasingly vocal in demanding changes in society's behavior toward those labeled mentally ill and especially in mental health professionals' treatment of this population. Individual ex-patient groups differ in strategies (some favor the complete abolition of the existing mental health system; others feel that major changes in staff attitudes and more responsive services are the best approaches to follow), but they share a common opposition to forced treatment and a belief in the value of patient input and direction of mental health services.

Such input and direction have been, unfortunately, rare occurrences in the United States, although model programs (which are discussed below) exist right across the Canadian-American border in Vancouver, British Columbia. Among the obstacles faced by ex-patients in trying to set up patient-run alternatives is the very serious problem of the difficulty in obtaining adequate funding. Insurance programs for mental health services funded by public as well as private sources generally require sophisticated accounting and management procedures, organizational systems, licensed mental health professionals, and traditional types of mental health services. These specifications are often too inflexible for many self-help programs, which, with their loose organizational structure and innovative style, rarely qualify for such funding (Chamberlin, 1979).

Although client involvement in the mental health system and in the creation of alternative services is barely in its infancy, the potential benefits from such activities deserve much broader recognition and closer scrutiny than they have received. There are several potential benefits:

1. *Increased sense of self-esteem.* Through participation in self-help programs, clients recognize that they can help themselves and others, rather than being merely compliant recipients of services.

2. *Increased optimism about recovering.* This optimism can be gained through seeing former patients functioning and working as effectively as staff. A former patient has pointed out that almost all of the former clients that a person in a treatment program sees are those who are readmitted as a result of treatment failure (Lovejoy, 1980). It is important for clients to see that mental illness does not inevitably lead to chronicity and hopelessness.

3. *Development of innovative programs more responsive to the needs of clients.* Many former clients have argued persuasively that mental health professionals frequently underestimate the capacities of clients to behave in autonomous fashion. Just as former drug addicts and alcoholics have been extremely useful in development of strategies and treatment for their disorders, it seems equally likely that former mental patients can provide useful insights into responding to treatment problems of other patients.

4. *Decreased cost.* The use of clients and ex-patients to perform some of the functions otherwise done by more costly professional staff will significantly diminish the cost and increase the availability of services.

5. *Creation of a community-based force of advocates for improved mental services.* By encouraging active involvement of clients in treatment programs, the mental health system will be relinquishing some of its power in directing programs but gaining allies in the struggle to ensure adequate and responsive services.

6. *Provision of services to underserved populations.* Some patients, upon discharge, wish nothing further to do with the organized mental health systems. Such clients, while in need of follow-up services, at times refuse to avail themselves of conventional services because of the stigma associated with continued treatment, fear of rehospitalization, or dislike of traditional treatment. Creation of patient-run alternatives can help fill the gap and provide needed services to individuals who would refuse them if offered by organized mental health care.

7. *Improved public image of the mentally ill.* Former patients can help in battling against the stigma of mental illness by showing that they can not only overcome their problems, but can help others with their difficulties. Rather than being seen as helpless or frightening individuals, clients and former clients can take an activist role of promoting the welfare of their fellow citizens.

CURRENT CMHC PRACTICE

Self-help programs frequently tend to be innovative and nonconventional in approach to mental health treatment. It is, therefore, not surprising that conventional definitions and categories are not always helpful in describing model self-help programs. The problem is made even more difficult by the tendency of mental health planners and biometricians to exclude ex-patients or ex-patient groups as a category of staff in mental health service delivery, either within conventional professional operated agencies or separate ex-patient treatment programs. The National Institute of Mental Health, for example, in its annual inventory of community mental health centers, asks for no information concerning the number of ex-patient staff working at Centers or ex-patient programs affiliated with Centers (National Institute of Mental Health, 1978). Even alcohol and drug treatment programs, which are frequently run or heavily influenced by ex-patients, fail to collect direct information pertaining to scope of patient and ex-patient input into treatment programs, priority setting, program design, or services evaluation.

The lack of routinely collected data about ex-patient involvement in service delivery makes it necessary to rely upon direct contact with staff of CMHCs, self-help programs, and regional offices to obtain information about what is happening in this area. From these sources, one realizes that only a relatively few ex-patient programs exist. Of this number, less than a handful are presently affiliated with CMHCs. The potential for mutually beneficial association, however, exists and would be logical for centers to explore further.

Ex-patient groups have been ambivalent in their attitudes toward professional treatment. They often have adopted the strategy of dealing independently with the problems of their fellow citizens. Only recently have they begun to try to collaborate with more traditional programs.

The following description of three major types of ex-patient operations (independent self-help programs, collaborative projects, and advocacy programs) makes clearer the scope of activity of self-help groups.

Independent Self-Help Programs

An independent self-help program can be defined as any organized group of people and programs run by present and former patients for the benefit and assistance of those individuals whose behavior, beliefs, or felt problems are considered by society to reflect mental illness. Many former patients reject the concept of mental illness as a medical condition. Instead, they prefer to view unusual behavior or attitudes as alternative life-styles influenced by social causes. Programs created by the ex-patient movement, therefore, offer support, friendship, and tolerance in lieu of psychotherapy, medication, or a structural milieu (Chamberlin, 1979).

Many individuals after treatment at a mental health facility still feel the same fear, vulnerability, and anxiety about their ability to cope with stresses that they felt when they started treatment. In traditional treatment programs, they may have gotten support from understanding and sympathetic mental health professionals, but they also would have been taught that their problems come from an illness within themselves that could be resolved only by acknowledging their problems and relying upon outside help and treatment. Thus, dependency and self-doubt far too often become a price individuals pay for mental health treatment.

To offset this liability resulting from dependency, ex-patient groups have sprung up in all regions in the country. Most consist of loose-knit organizations. Groups such as Emotions Anonymous, Recovery, Dawn Treaders, etc. have meetings from once to several times a week. They are not dependent on professionals or on a budget to keep themselves going. The people who participate in such programs are volunteers using donated space in churches, libraries, or schools. Their goal is to help others to survive in the community and stay out of hospitals. Some programs such as Project Release, in New York, have embarked on more ambitious activities than a regular meeting program. This ex-patient organization, in addition to trying to expose problems of inadequate housing of former patients and low-quality care in various hospitals, established a community center in which there were no distinctions in membership between those who would traditionally be viewed as staff and those who would be considered clients. Each member of the Project was required to serve on one or more committees (fund raising, community center, newsletter, etc.) that were necessary to keep the operation going. The basic philosophy of this group is stated as follows:

> In the informal program of Project Release, members seek to extend acceptance and cooperation, letting each individual set his or her own pace in tasks and responsibilities. Project Release feels that this form of self-help is a strong antidote to the anxiety of isolation and helplessness induced by society and psychiatry. [Project Release, undated]

Unfortunately, because of funding problems, Project Release no longer exists.

Like Project Release, which divided its efforts between political activism and provision of support services, the Mental Patients Association of Vancouver, British Columbia has worked to develop a model alternative to traditional mental health services. Through fortuitous circumstances, including the award of a Canadian Government grant for local projects, the Mental Patients Association of Vancouver was established in 1971. This organization of ex-patients operates a seven-days-a-week drop-in center and five cooperative residences, all on the principle of participatory democracy. All decision-making powers are in the hands of the membership and are expressed by votes taken at weekly business meetings. The viability of this group illustrates that ex-patients can formulate and run services in which the needs of clients can direct and facilitate the priorities and structure of program.

Because many ex-patient groups feel a high degree of distrust and suspicion of the activities of the mental health system, CMHCs may find it extremely difficult to develop relationships with completely independent self-help programs. Since fear of co-optation is a continuing worry for the leaders of the ex-patient movement, centers need to be sensitive to their concerns when dealing with self-help programs. Centers may, however, assist such programs to obtain funds to locate drop-in centers and, when appropriate, may refer clients for aftercare or participation in self-help programs.

Collaborative Programs

Although centers may need to keep some distance from self-help programs that adopt a philosophy of complete independence, such a response is both unnecessary and inappropriate when dealing with ex-patient groups interested in pursuing joint projects. Cooperation between ex-patient groups and CMHCs can be mutually beneficial. For CMHCs, working with ex-patient groups can be invaluable in assuring continuity and responsiveness of care provided. Such collaboration could provide CMHCs with allies in the community to fight prejudice and stigma against the mentally ill and to assure that adequate resources are available to treat those wishing assistance.

The benefits to ex-patient groups come in the form of public recognition that their programs can fill a serious gap in the aftercare system by providing an opportunity for discharged clients to be with each other for mutual support. Collaboration with a CMHC will also enable ex-patient programs to obtain the funds to provide such services and provide alternatives to existing clinically run aftercare programs. Some risks also result from such collaborative ventures. Ex-patient groups find themselves tempted to alter their programs in order to obtain increased funding or to tone down their political activism to avoid losing their support. Centers, on the other hand, may face some embarrassment from funding controversial and activist programs no matter how responsive such programs might be to clients' needs.

One of the most successful collaborative projects is presently being funded under contract by the South County Community Mental Center in Loxahatchee, Florida. This project run by the Mental Patients' Rights Association of Lake Worth, Florida consists of a small, patient-run, drop-in program and hotline service. This unusual program enables the center to serve a population in the catchment area that is unwilling to accept traditional mental health services or supports, but, nonetheless, needs assistance (Zinman, 1980). The success of this program is largely

the result of the commitment of the local center to be responsive to the
needs of its community and the willingness of an ex-patient group to accept the challenge of working with a portion of the mental health system
that it is trying to alter.

Another example of collaboration between ex-patients and traditional mental health services is found at the San Fernando Valley Community Mental Health Center, Van Nuys, California. This center makes
extensive use of volunteers, including ex-patients, and has established a
number of self-help groups and friendship clubs. These nonprofessional programs have been found, according to Lila Berman (1980), Director of San Fernando Valley CMHC, to be extremely valuable to clients in encouraging them to take responsibility for their lives.

Advocacy Programs

The third type of patient self-help activity, which has possibly the greatest impact on the mental health system, is advocacy. Advocacy, in its traditional sense, means a call to plead another's cause. Its present-day
adversarial connotation of predominant reliance on legal procedures is
not inherent in the term's basic meaning, but rather reflects the way
some advocates pursue a client's goal. All advocates should share a common loyalty to their clients and adherence to the mission of assisting the
clients in obtaining all the rights and entitlements to which they have a
claim. As long as the advocates clearly represent the client's perspective,
advocates may be mental health professionals, former patients, parents,
attorneys, or concerned citizens. The advocate serves as an extension of
the client—a force striving to assure that the client's perspective, priorities, and needs are addressed.

Clients, present and former, have often taken an active advocacy
stance and in this fashion have influenced the availability, quality, and
manner in which mental health services are delivered. Ex-patient advocates have directed their efforts in four main directions:

1. increased public understanding of the concerns of those labeled
   "mental patient,"
2. protection of the legal rights of clients and assurance of their entitlements under existing federal, state, and local programs,
3. raising clients' consciousness, and
4. mutual support programs for present and former patients.

The following brief examples help clarify how each type of group pur-
sues its advocacy activities:

Increasing public understanding. Project Overcome in St. Paul, Minnesota, under the direction of Marcia Lovejoy, is a prime example of a pro-

gram aimed at increased public understanding of patient concerns. This program has an active speakers' forum that helps the community meet and talk with former patients in the effort to dispel stigma and prejudice (Lovejoy, 1979).

Protection of legal rights. The Mental Patients Liberation Front, in Boston, not only has an excellent program of visiting patients in various public mental hospitals and informing them of their rights, but also has worked closely with attorneys in preparation of evidence for *Rogers vs. Okin* (1979). This court case has resulted in significant clarification of the patient's right to refuse treatment.

Raising clients' consciousness. An example of activities aimed at raising the consciousness of clients concerning their rights and options as provided by the programs of the Network Against Psychiatric Assault, based in San Francisco, California. This organization promotes communication among ex-patient groups through publication of *Madness Network News* (Hirsch and others, 1974). The articles in this newspaper cover the gamut of issues, including exposés of client rights violations, description of effects and potentials of psychotropic medications, letters describing personal histories, diatribes against forced treatment and physical and psychological abuse. The publications also include poems and stories about the "patient experience."

Mutual support. In the crucial area of mutual self-help and support, the Washington Network for Alternatives to Psychiatric Dependency meets regularly to help its members cope with the isolation, frustration, and anger that so often follow hospitalization (Feinberg, 1979). By sharing experience, assessing the effectiveness of various solutions to problems, and by evaluating from the client's perspective the various psychotherapists and treatment programs in the area, this group provides a service that exists nowhere else.

CRITICAL EVALUATION AND SUGGESTIONS

The potential benefits of increased client involvement in CMHC service delivery are only beginning to be recognized. Clearly, increased client input could lead to more responsive services, diminished cost of center operation, improved outreach, and the development of more collaborative and less paternalistic treatment regimens. A price, however, will need to be paid for these benefits—the sharing of some power and authority.

Center staff may resist increased client participation in service delivery because of the possibility of losing power or status. Ex-patients may also be reluctant to collaborate for fear of loss of independence or autonomy. Ex-patients remember the authority of mental health professionals during their periods of treatment and, therefore, hesitate to put themselves in the position where they can be dominated by experts. A second worry is that they will be co-opted by the system. Co-optation means that the dedication, independence, and zeal of an individual or group becomes diminished or altered as a result of compromises necessary to maintain collaboration and dialogue. The benefit to ex-patient groups of accepting contracts and associated relationships with CMHCs would make it harder for them to criticize or protest practices that might neglect or violate clients' rights.

Although collaboration between CMHCs and organized ex-patient programs may be difficult for both, such efforts need to be initiated. Centers can do much more to help establish self-help programs in their communities, encourage ex-patients to return to the CMHCs to help other clients, establish grievance procedures and advocacy operations to make the clients' perspectives heard and reflected in programs.

Not all center activities directed at increasing client participation in services will require writing contracts, establishing new programs, or expending new funds. Some changes can be implemented simply by adding ex-patients to advisory and governing boards and including them on committees concerned with program development and evaluation. Such actions would be preventive measures aimed at helping to eliminate grievances before they occur.

CMHCs could also assist ex-patient organizations by helping in grant writing or simply by letting them use copying machines, telephones, secretarial assistance, etc. As noted previously, most ex-patient groups operate on either a tiny budget or no budget, so that even the offer of copying machines might make the difference between the ex-patient group meeting to provide support for other ex-patients or cancelling an activity because there was no advance notification or publicity about the event.

Increasing client involvement in mental health service programs will not be easy. Many obstacles, resistance, and unfounded fears will need to be overcome, but through creative and persistent effort CMHCs can be at the vanguard of a national effort aimed at the recognition of the capacity of clients to help themselves.

REFERENCES

Armstrong, B. Stigma: Its impact on the mentally ill. *Hospital and Community Psychiatry*, 1980, *31*, 343–346.

Berman, L. (San Fernando Valley Community Mental Health Center, Van Nuys, Calif.) Personal communication, 1980.

Chamberlin, J. *On our own.* New York: McGraw-Hill, 1979.

Feinberg, A. (Fairfax, Va.) Personal communication, 1979.

Hirsch, S., et al. (Eds.) *Madness Network News* reader. San Francisco: Glide Publications, 1974.

Lieberman, J. *The tyranny of the experts.* New York: Walker Publishing, 1970.

Lovejoy, M. Project Overcome. *Advocacy.* 1979, *1*, 32–33.

Lovejoy, M. Unpublished comments at Services Advisory Group Meeting, National Institute of Mental Health, 1980.

National Institute of Mental Health. *Provisional data on Federally funded community mental health centers, 1976–77.* Division of Biometry and Epidemiology, 1978.

Project Release. A statement of purpose. Undated.

Rogers vs. Okin trial. Cit.: 478F. Supp. 1342 (B. Mass. 1979).

Zinman, S. (Mental Patients Rights Association, Lake Worth, Fla.) Personal communication, 1980.

21

Participatory Management in Public Welfare: What Are the Prospects?

RICHARD A. WEATHERLEY

The Department of Social Services (DSS, fictitious name) was created in 1970, when the state legislature brought under a single administrative umbrella the previously separate Departments of Health, Institutions, Public Assistance, the Division of Vocational Rehabilitation, and the Veterans Rehabilitation Council. In May 1976, a two-day meeting was convened of sixty frontline social service staff from local offices throughout the state to consider the declining morale among their ranks.

Staff complaints at the 1976 meeting included an inability to secure definitive clarification of the frequently changing policies they administered, an unclear command structure, the outdated and consequently useless policy manual, poorly defined performance criteria, burgeoning paperwork requirements, and the frequent policy initiatives sent down from above with little sensitivity to the realities of their work situations and no opportunity for comment. The DSS social service managers responded to these concerns by developing, with the initial assistance of two staff committees, what was termed the Consolidated Social Service

The author expresses his appreciation to Claudia Byrum Kottwitz, Denise Lishner, Kelley Reid, Grant Roset, Norman Wacker, and Karen Wong, who served as research assistants for the study, and to Michael Austin, James Christian, Ronald Dear, Richard Elmore, Cathie Martin, Katherine Mason, Lawrence Northwood, Rino Patti, Hy Resnick, and Walter Williams, for their comments and suggestions.

System, or CSSS. CSSS incorporated several procedural reforms under-taken by a number of state public welfare departments following the federally mandated separation of income maintenance from social services in 1973.

Some of these changes had been under consideration by DSS management at the time of the May 1976 meeting, and it seemed opportune to press forward in implementing them as a response to the concerns raised by the workers at the meeting. The major objectives of the new system included the review, revision, and consolidation of forms; introduction of goal-oriented case recording; consolidation of various vendor payment procedures into one simplified and automated system; the development of service and workload standards; revision of the social service manual incorporating program standards; service priorities, outcome expectations, and expected response times; and reorganization of service units to minimize the fragmentation of services to clients.

The administrators most directly responsible for CSSS were professionally trained social workers who had moved up through the ranks. They deliberately pursued a participatory strategy in developing and implementing CSSS to engender a sense of staff ownership of its components and to insure its relevance for staff and clients.

In addition to the initial May 1976 meeting, the following measures were taken to secure frontline participation in CSSS:

1. Committees comprised of frontline staff worked on forms reduction and simplification, and studied the feasibility of establishing a consolidated vendor payment system.
2. The major components of CSSS were developed and tested in a pilot project involving most of the social service staff in one local office. The payment system was tested in another office.
3. A statewide CSSS advisory committee was established with representation from frontline social service staff as well as regional and local office administrators. This committee was consulted at key stages in the development of CSSS, and changes were incorporated reflecting suggestions from this group.
4. Several frontline casework staff were temporarily assigned to Department headquarters to assist the CSSS project director.
5. More than 100 field staff participated in developing the policy and program standards for the social service manual, and many of their written comments were incorporated in the final draft.
6. Union representatives were routinely consulted about project components.
7. Reports on various project components were circulated for comment to the six regional offices and to headquarters administrative staff.
8. The actual implementation of the system was to be conducted in

272 PARTICIPATORY MANAGEMENT IN PUBLIC WELFARE

phases, region by region, to permit maximum administrative support at the time of conversion, and to facilitate the early correction of any problems. Regional and local office staff committees were to have a major role in training and implementation.

9. Arrangements were made for an independent assessment (by this investigator) of frontline reactions to CSSS immediately before its implementation so that any needed adjustments could be made without undue delay.

While these measures fall short of some ideal standard of workplace democracy, they represent a quantum leap from the authoritarian decision-making norms then prevalent in the Department. As one research division staff member commented, major decisions were often made on the spur of the moment by a few highly placed individuals with little regard to long range consequences and with no effort to consult subordinates.

THE FRONTLINE RESPONSE

We interviewed social service staff in four local offices, serving two urban and two rural areas. This constituted 14 percent of the state's frontline social service work force, and 19 percent of their immediate (i.e., firstline) supervisors.

Workers and supervisors alike were inclined to view most policy and procedural changes undertaken prior to CSSS with skepticism. The changes were described as irrelevant, ineffectual, superficial, disruptive, and motivated by budgetary or political concerns rather than client or worker interests. When asked to cite examples of both constructive and nonconstructive changes, 40.3 percent of the workers and 35 percent of the supervisors could not name a single constructive change. Furthermore, 73.9 percent of the workers and 70 percent of the supervisors agreed that the policy changes of the past few years had made their jobs more difficult.

There was unanimous agreement among workers and supervisors that frontline workers should be consulted about policies and procedures which affect their jobs. The primary explanation given was that they are the ones most aware of what is going on, and that their views would be practical and useful.

WORKER ATTITUDES TOWARD CSSS

In view of the strong worker sentiment advocating frontline consultation, I expected CSSS to be viewed much more positively than other policy changes which had been undertaken with little or no effort to involve social service staff. Surprisingly, this was not the case. Despite the considerable effort to involve frontline staff, factual knowledge about CSSS was limited and skepticism about its intent and probable effects was widespread. Our interviews were conducted about 18 months after the official debut of the project. Considerable effort had been made early on to publicize the project through periodic memos, through the distribution of a CSSS coloring book, development of a film strip, and use of a special CSSS logo, as well as through more conventional channels. Almost 90 percent of the caseworkers interviewed and all of the supervisors had heard of CSSS; however, about one-third of the caseworkers (32.8 percent) did not know its purpose.

Half of the caseworkers and supervisors expected some negative consequences from CSSS—more restrictions on client service or transition problems. The reasons for staff apprehension about CSSS despite strong efforts to inform and involve them become more apparent when we consider staff perceptions of their participation. We asked caseworkers and supervisors about opportunities to participate in CSSS planning and about their own and their colleagues' actual participation. The responses are shown in Tables 21–1 through 21–5.

As March and Simon (1958) have observed, the perception of participation may be even more crucial than actual participation in influencing the acceptance of managerial decisions:

> Certainly most studies suggest that the more the *felt participation in decisions*, the less the visibility of power differences in the organization, and that the latter, in turn, lessens the evocation of organizationally disapproved alternatives. Moreover . . . (provided the deception is successful) the perception of individual participation in goal setting is equivalent in many respects to actual participation. The greater the amount of felt participation, the greater the *control of the organization* over the evocation of alternatives; and therefore the less the evocation of alternatives undesired by the organization. [p. 54, emphasis in the original]

As the data show, both actual and perceived participation were limited. Only 8.4 percent of the caseworkers and 25 percent of the supervisors reported having had an opportunity to participate in the design of CSSS (Table 21–1), and only 6.7 percent of the workers and 20 percent of the supervisors said they had actually done so (Table 21–2). The general perception of frontline involvement was somewhat higher, but still not overwhelming. Thirty-one percent of the caseworkers and 40 percent of the supervisors believed that there had been some frontline involvement in CSSS; however, 68.9 percent of the caseworkers and 60 percent of the supervisors reported either "no involvement" or gave a "don't know" response (Table 21–3).

The ratings of degree of involvement in CSSS (Table 21–4) dif-

TABLE 21–1. Responses to Question, "Have You Been Given the Opportunity to Participate in the Design or Implementation of CSSS?"

Response	Caseworkers		Supervisors	
	No.	Percent	No.	Percent
Yes	10	8.4	5	25
No	85	71.4	15	75
Don't know/no response	24	20.2	–	–
Total	119	100	20	100

TABLE 21–2. Responses to Question, "To Date, Have You Participated in the Design and/or Implementation of CSSS in Any Way?"

Response	Caseworkers		Supervisors	
	No.	Percent	No.	Percent
Yes	8	6.7	4	20
No	14	11.8	1	5
Don't know/no response	97	81.5	15	75
Total	119	100	20	100

TABLE 21–3. Responses to Question, "To Your Knowledge, Have Frontline Staff Had Any Involvement in the Design of Any Aspects of CSSS?"

Response	Caseworkers		Supervisors	
	No.	Percent	No.	Percent
Yes	37	31.1	8	40
No	67	56.3	10	50
Don't know/no response	15	12.6	2	10
Total	119	100	20	100

TABLE 21–4. Ratings of Degree of Frontline Involvement in CSSS

Degree of Involvement	Caseworkers[a]		Supervisors[b]	
No involvement	1 _____	(54)	1 _____	(11)
	2 _____	(18)	2 _____	(5)
	3 _	(6)	3	
	4 __	(7)	4	
	5_	(2)	5 __	(1)
	6_	(3)	6 __	(1)
	7		7	
	8_	(3)	8_	(1)
	9		9	
Maximum involvement	10		10 __	(1)

Frequency	20	40	60	Frequency	4	8	12

[a] For caseworkers, N = 93, Mean = 2.02, (26 caseworkers did not respond or gave "don't know" responses.)
[b] For supervisors, N = 20, Mean = 2.5.

TABLE 21–5. Ratings of General Frontline Involvement in Policy and Procedural Revisions

Degree of Involvement	Caseworkers[a]		Supervisors[b]	
No involvement	1 _____	(44)	1 _____	(6)
	2 _____	(36)	2 _____	(6)
	3 _____	(15)	3 _____	(4)
	4 ___	(8)	4 __	(2)
	5 ___	(5)	5 __	(1)
	6		6 __	(1)
	7 _	(3)	7	
	8_	(3)	8	
	9		9	
Maximum involvement	10 ___	(5)	10	

Frequency	20	40	60	Frequency	4	8	12

[a] N = 119, Mean = 2.63
[b] N = 20, Mean = 2.45

fered only slightly from the rating of general frontline involvement in policy and procedural changes (Table 21–5). In both instances, responses were clustered on the noninvolvement end of the scale. In other words, *the sustained efforts of midlevel managers to consult with and involve frontline staff through mass meetings, pilot projects, advisory committees, and work groups yielded a frontline perception of their involvement not much different from when the usual top-down implementation procedures were employed.* It can be argued that the participatory efforts were well justified by the practice wisdom which was indeed incorporated in the CSSS components through the involvement of frontline staff. However, one can safely predict that irrespective of its quality and relevance, CSSS is likely, in the absence of new interventions from management, to encounter the same kind of cynicism and resistance with which frontline staff customarily greets new policy initiatives.

CONSTRAINTS TO A PARTICIPATORY IMPLEMENTATION STRATEGY

Why was it that the participatory measures were generally unnoticed and unappreciated by frontline staff? This analysis suggests a number of reasons why a participatory strategy may be difficult to carry out in a public welfare bureaucracy.

ORGANIZATIONAL TRANSIENCE

State departments of human resources like DSS operate in a highly volatile policy environment, subject to constantly shifting and often conflicting pressures from federal agencies, the governor and state legislature, clients, staff, service vendors, and a myriad of special-interest groups. They draw much attention from competing political interests and are subject to frequent changes in leadership and policy.

During the three-year period from the initiation of CSSS planning in mid-1976 to 1979, there were three agency directors, a major structural reorganization, three CSSS project directors, and a 100 percent turnover of CSSS project staff. The Office of Family, Children, and Adult Services, in which the project was originally lodged, had several different chiefs before it was abolished and its responsibilities, including CSSS, transferred elsewhere.

COMPETING INNOVATIONS

CSSS was not the only policy change undertaken during this time. In addition to the almost routine changes in policies and procedures affecting foster and day care, nursing home, chore and homemaker service payments and procedures, the Department began implementing controversial new juvenile and civil commitment laws, and also initiated an administrative decentralization plan. Policy changes, particularly those initiated by DSS management, are most often launched with a kind of patriotic fervor, possibly to catch the attention of a staff jaded by innovation overload. Anthony Downs (1976) calls the tendency for newly appointed administrators to put their mark on an agency through new policy initiatives, "The Law of Compulsive Innovation" (pp. 87–100). The periodic turnover of agency leadership ensures a steady outpouring of new management schemes on top of those almost routine changes resulting from federal and state legislative initiatives.

LIMITED COMMAND OF RESOURCES

Because of the inability to control the requisite resources, a project director may not always be able to deliver on commitments made to lower-level planning participants or follow their recommendations. As Chester Barnard (1968) observed,

> . . . coordination of action requires repeated organization decisions "on the spot" where effective action of organization takes place. . . . It is at these low levels, where ultimate authority resides, that the personal decisions determining willingness to contribute become of relatively greatest aggregate importance." [p. 192]

The writing of the manual, the revision of forms, and the development of the payment system required the cooperation of several different staff units, as well as that of outside subcontractors. CSSS project staff had no direct authority over the various program bureaus or staff units such as data processing, whose cooperation was absolutely crucial. From the perspective of these other organizational units, CSSS was not a high priority.

ORGANIZATIONAL COMPLEXITY

The size and complexity of the agency creates another kind of problem. Even while CSSS was being developed, decisions were being made in other parts of the agency—the generation of new forms and planning for implementation of the new juvenile code, for example—without consideration of their impact on CSSS. The project director must attempt to coordinate the development of project components with other units, and in the process must accommodate to some extent the needs of these other units. This negotiation process takes time and inevitably results in changes in the thrust of the project. However, frontline participants may be aware only of the changes and not the process, and may consequently believe their recommendations are being ignored.

CONFLICTING INTERESTS AND PERSPECTIVES

Management and frontline workers have differing concerns reflecting their respective roles and positions in the organizational hierarchy. It is not surprising that in discussing CSSS, management should stress accountability, while workers are more concerned about service to clients and effects on their own work routines (Lipsky, 1980). The involvement of frontline workers may sensitize them to the pressures for accountability felt by administrators, and administrators in turn may become more aware of how accountability measures may be perceived by frontline staff and affect their attitudes and behavior. To the extent that these concerns are taken into account in project planning and implementation, the participation may be deemed successful, yet there is bound to remain some tension between the goals of accountability and service which no amount of participation can reconcile completely.

CONFLICTING DEFINITIONS OF PARTICIPATION

The term "participation" has many meanings. It can apply to a wide range of activities, thus contributing to potential miscommunication about what is in fact intended. To the worker, it may suggest increased autonomy, more control over resources, and greater collaboration with peers in designing work activities. To the manager, participation may mean nothing more than consultation on matters of minor importance, or from the worker's perspective, co-optation and tokenism. To avoid misunderstanding, it is incumbent upon managers to offer potential participants a clear operational description of specific measures to be taken, and the consequences that will ensue.

TIME

A further consequence of the size, complexity, and transient nature of public welfare agencies is that policy initiatives usually take far longer to implement than anticipated. It is difficult to sustain frontline staff interest in an impending change over a period of several years. The involvement of frontline staff itself adds to the complexity and slows down the implementation process. The original momentum may be lost as other projects come along to compete for the limited resources and staff interest, and as participants move on to other activities or other jobs.

AN UNFAVORABLE COST/BENEFIT RATIO

The costs of worker participation are quite clear and calculable, but the benefits are not. Managers can accurately estimate the number of person-hours required and the delays to be anticipated when introducing a change using participatory techniques. However, the benefits of participation are less tangible and more difficult to measure. Studies have linked participation with increased job satisfaction, reduced stress and absenteeism, and increased acceptance of change; yet it is impossible to predict that a specific increase in participation will yield a measurable increase in satisfaction, compliance, or productivity, or for that matter, a better product or improved procedure.

THE LIMITATIONS
OF PARTICIPATORY MECHANISMS

In addition to those constraints inherent in the organization and structure of public social service bureaucracies, there are also limitations to the participatory mechanisms themselves which are illustrated by the study.

1. *The Sampling Problem.* Relatively few of the social service workers reported any kind of direct personal involvement in CSSS development. Only 8.4 percent said they had had an opportunity to participate in the design or implementation of CSSS, and only 6.7 percent had actually done so. From the perspective of Department management, this number is evidence of considerable participation; for the frontline worker who was not among the participants, it suggests tokenism.
2. *The Skills Problem.* To be successful, participatory management requires considerable skill on the part of both administrators and workers. Not only are such skills difficult to acquire, they can also be positively dysfunctional in bureaucracies organized along traditional hierarchical lines. Techniques for active listening, paraphrasing, giving and getting feedback, and reaching consensus must be learned and practiced in a supportive environment. Yet managers and workers are generally socialized from an early age to adapt to hierarchical settings.

3. *The Cynical Worker and Manager Problem.* The data show considerable frontline cynicism toward most changes within the agency. Workers expect any new change to affect them adversely and expect to have little or no involvement in planning these changes. Information that a serious participatory strategy is being pursued may be dismissed unless the worker has firsthand evidence that this is indeed the case. The obverse may also be true. Managers may hold biased views about the capability of workers and fear that their judgments will be personally motivated and of low quality, and may consequently dismiss the suggestions of frontline subordinates without consideration of their substantive merit.

4. *The Problem of Locating the Frontline.* Management and frontline staff may have divergent definitions of where the frontline begins and ends. Seen from Department headquarters in the state capitol, anyone from a regional or local office is in a sense at the front line; from below, anyone above the social service worker is part of management. The CSSS project advisory committee was comprised of representatives from several different organizational levels. Frontline workers could view this group as dominated by administrators, although that was clearly not intended when the committee was established.

DISCUSSION

As this study suggests, the political conditions under which public welfare services are provided reinforce an essentially authoritarian management posture. Advocates of workplace democracy should look elsewhere for a more nurturing environment.

This is not to say that participatory mechanisms should not be promoted. The instrumental benefits are well documented (Bernstein, 1976; Jenkins, 1973; Pateman, 1970; Zwerdling, 1978). Many of the problems identified in this study could be addressed by more aggressive efforts to give visibility to the participatory mechanisms used, and greater acknowledgement to participants for their involvement. The representation problem could be alleviated through more formal mechanisms for frontline staff to themselves select participants from among their ranks, and hold them responsible for soliciting frontline views and reporting back results. Management could make more creative use of internal surveys and techniques like Delphi and nominal group process to involve subordinates and keep in touch with frontline sentiments. More direct and open processing of conflict might at least serve to bring differences between management and workers into the open where, if they cannot be resolved, they can be better understood and appreciated. For any of these mechanisms to work, however, the interest and commitment of top management is absolutely essential.

The growth in size and complexity of public welfare agencies over the past two decades, exacerbated by the trend toward state level consolidation of human services, has contributed to a reliance on technically competent but substantively deficient managers to implement new accountability measures (Austin, 1978; Patti, 1975). They have supplanted an older generation of social service administrators whose professional training and work experience in the human services offered a more sensitive and sympathetic orientation to workers and clients. Governors, legislators, and citizens want welfare programs "brought under control." Managers laboring under pressure to achieve fast results inevitably invoke hierarchical controls antagonistic to a participative philosophy. The political unpopularity of the programs they administer induces many of these managers to invoke a kind of managerial machismo in which their "toughness" is directed at both public welfare workers and clients who serve as convenient scapegoats for deficiencies in the distribution of income and provision of services. As long as these conditions remain, we can expect continued turnover in management and staff, alienated workers, active resistance to change, and increased efforts to impose more and improved hierarchical controls—hardly the best conditions for expanding the role of frontline worker in designing and implementing services.

REFERENCES

Austin, D. The politics and organization of services: Consolidation and integration. *Public Welfare*, 1978, *36*, 20-28.

Barnard, C. *The functions of the executive*. Cambridge, MA: Harvard University Press, 1968.

Bernstein, P. *Work place democratization: Its internal dynamics*. Kent, OH: Kent State University Press, 1976.

Downes, A. *Urban problems and prospects*. Chicago: Rand McNally, 1976.

Jenkins. D. *Job power: Blue and white collar democracy*. New York: Doubleday, 1973.

Lipsky, M. *Street-level bureaucracy: Dilemmas of the individual in public services*. New York: Russell Sage, 1980.

March, J., & Simon, H. *Organizations*. New York: John Wiley & Sons, 1958.

Pateman, C. *Participation and democratic theory*. London: Cambridge University Press, 1970.

Patti, R. The new scientific management: Systems management for social welfare. *Public Welfare*, 1975, *33*, 23-31.

Zwerdling, D. *Workplace democracy*. New York: Harper & Row, 1978.

PART IV

Organizational Conflict and Change

Editor's Introduction

Conflict and change are persistent themes in the organizational and administrative literature. In many ways they are two sides of the same coin—change leads to conflict, and conflict leads to change. Organizations live in a force field frequently buffeted in a turbulent environment. Although organizations strive for stability and growth, internal and external pressures rarely permit the existence of a static equilibrium.

Social service organizations, like all organizations, are dynamic, evolving social systems, composed of interrelated units concerned chiefly with the attainment of specific goals. Organizational life tends to be characterized in part by pervasive processes of conflict and change, some planned, some unplanned. Among the major functions of administrators is their role in the management of these processes.

Change in organizations is endemic, propelled by both internal and external pressures. Social agencies inevitably respond to the impact of changing social circumstances which define new social needs and new client potentials growing out of the new or elaborated social problems to which their goals are directed. Such factors as demographic shifts, technological developments, developing social pathologies, and structural inequities, among others, create an agenda for social response that calls for organizational adaptation and innovation. Since the sociocultural, political, and technological environment of social practice constantly undergoes modification, both social planning and intervention are pressed to respond in novel ways. They create an ethos and ambience for social development, and determine the ebb and flow of policy, resource allocation, and program development.

As social agencies respond to new social tasks and incorporate new technologies, they move from one steady state to another, and in the process tend to upset an established equilibrium. Any disruption of the reward system, organizational "turf," status, or power tends to lead to resistance and frequently to conflict. The interdependence of change and conflict has often been noted in the literature, and this interrelation is reciprocal—change leads to conflict, and conflict often powers the change process.

The many and diverse constituencies of the social agency project a multiplicity of interests and needs that are sometimes contradictory and sometimes antagonistic. Conflict between and among these interest groups creates a force field within which administrators function. It is their responsibility so to manage these conflicts that the service goals will not be compromised, and the organization's strength will not be impaired. Administrators are well advised to anticipate conflicts within the staff, between staff and trustees, within the board, and between their organizations and others upon which they depend and with which they interact.

The literature on planned organizational change and the conception of social practitioners as change agents is substantial. The rhetoric of change is even more pervasive. Experience suggests, however, that engineering change in organizations is extremely difficult. Constraints even on executive authority need to be recognized. Change and conflict require political insight, that is to say, they must be viewed in terms of the dynamics of power and influence. Perhaps the appropriate metaphor would suggest the "power steering" function of the administrator.

The selections which follow analyze relevant concepts that inhere in these processes of conflict and change, providing clues for the development of strategies for their management. Slavin reviews the potential values and functions served by conflict, identifies a series of key concepts essential for its understanding, and catalogues four sets of strategies available to practitioners in responding to conflict situations. He develops a typology which suggests the essential conditions under which one or another response is appropriate. The key here is the relationship between goals and strategies. Varying degrees of goal congruence between conflicting parties are paired with specific action models to provide a good "fit."

Holloway and Brager identify three major types of organizational change—alterations in behavior, technology, and structure—and explore the respective impact of each. The difficulties in assessing the significance of a change idea are noted, and some criteria are suggested by which such an assessment can be made. Practice implications stemming from an understanding of different types of change and their significance for those organizational participants with limited formal power are noted.

Patti focuses on the efforts of lower participants in organizations to initiate and sustain change where resistance is likely to come from organization members located in higher positions in the hierarchy. This is the obverse of the problem where those invested with organizational authority find resistance from below to their initiatives for innovation and change. While not specifically dealing with the question, Patti implies that varying obstacles stand in the way of planned change depending on the point of entry of change-directed activities. Change action can originate externally to the organization, say, from funding sources or public interest groups, or internally, from lower, middle, or higher participants. In each instance, tactics and strategies for effective implementation differ. Patti makes the point that where lower participants engage in change efforts, a set of variables determines the nature of the resistance they can expect from above. These analytical elements provide clues to the identification of various response patterns likely to be effective. Organizational resistance to change may be a universal institutional characteristic. The extent of that resistance and its organizational location will, however, tend to vary depending upon the specific relation of forces in time and space. Intervention strategy depends on such an assessment if it is to be appropriately responsive to the specific tasks at hand.

22

Concepts of Social Conflict: Use in Social Work Curriculum

SIMON SLAVIN

The current social turbulence in the nation, affecting, as it does, some of its most central institutions, and not least of all the universities, underscores the significance of conflict processes for the development of social practice and social policies. Few aspects of social work practice unfold without evidence of conflict, competition, or rivalry between individuals, groups, organizations, and/or institutions. Such conflict is pervasive in community life. Its very universality suggests that conflict is a property of social organization.[1] Quincy Wright, a careful student of the subject, suggests that "conflict in some form . . . is probably an essential and desirable element of human society. A society cannot exist without competition and conflict."[2]

While little empirical evidence is recorded on the subject, one has the impression that social workers frequently find themselves involved in interpersonal and intraorganizational disputes, that social agencies are frequently in competition and conflict with one another, and that social agency participants and adherents are frequently pitted against other institutions in the community, competing for scarce resources and attempting, through a variety of patterns of organization and action, to affect changes in their modes of operation and service delivery. One might have expected that this general circumstance would have led the profession to a careful study of the processes of social conflict and, consequently, to the development of insight and skill in dealing with them.

This paper was originally presented at the CSWE Seventeenth Annual Program Meeting held in Cleveland, Ohio, January 21–24, 1969.

In fact, little has been done in this field. This paper is a modest contribution to this lacuna in professional development. It will suggest a number of concepts central to an understanding of social conflict and to its management, and will review briefly a suggested typology of conflict strategy. The underlying assumption here is that some range of conflict concepts is essential for a well-designed conflict work curriculum, and, while most of these ideas seem especially relevant for community organizing work, its very pervasiveness in organizations suggests similar relevance for all aspects of social work practice.

The current study of conflict is advanced by the realization that "all conflicts have common elements and general patterns."[3] Considerable effort has recently gone into conflict analysis as a consequence of the imperative need to deal with problems growing out of the international threat of nuclear war. The conjunction in time of the civil rights revolution and the weaponry revolution has raised the interest in conflict and conflict control or management to a new high level.

SOCIAL CHANGE AND CONFLICT

Perhaps no relationship is more central to conflict than that of change. According to LaPiere, "Any change always involves considerable stress both individual and collective . . . in the process of being accomplished, the change produces its own stress and strains—discontents, frustrations, discussions and disappointments."[4] The extent to which change touches deeply felt values or interests is the extent to which it is likely to lead to overt conflict. The rate of change also has its consequences for conflict. The more rapid the rate of change, the more likely it is to upset existing social relationships and the more likely it is that conflict will result.

Social change implies a movement away from the status quo, a shift in the norms and relationships that compose the social equilibrium at any specific point in time. Such an equilibrium in a social system satisfies certain interest groups and, conversely, has a negative impact on other groups and individuals. Those who benefit from the existing arrangements resent change and tend to resist its manifestations. Thus, change tends to breed conflict between interest groups because it challenges the conventional basis of reward distribution. Under certain conditions, these strivings lead to organized conflict. The greater the disparity, the greater the likelihood that individual dissatisfaction and perception of inequality will assume collective forms.

Conflict and change have a reciprocal relationship—each is both source and product of the other. Change leads to conflict and conflict to change. These are natural processes characteristic of social systems.[5]

Within certain limits, some aspects of these processes can be moulded and directed through deliberate social action.

The central purpose for focusing on conflict is to develop diagnostic insight into conflict elements and processes and to provide principles that can serve as a guide to change agent activities. These should make it possible to plan ways of maximizing the creative and productive function of conflict.

THE NATURE OF CONFLICT

Kurt Singer has defined conflict as "a critical state of tension occasioned by the presence of mutually incompatible tendencies within an organismic whole, the functional continuity or structural integrity of which is thereby threatened."[6] In a similar vein, Boulding suggests that "conflict may be defined as a situation of competition in which the parties are aware of the incompatibility of the potential future positions and in which each party wishes to occupy a position that is incompatible with the wishes of the other."[7] It is the perception of the existence of the incompatible preferences, the mutual desire to achieve these preferences, and the behavior expended in the direction of gaining such positions that essentially characterize a state of conflict. The sheer existence of contradictory positions and preferences may constitute competition, rivalry, or hostility, but not necessarily conflict. Competition is a concurrent striving by social entities for scarce objects, while conflict implies antagonistic struggle directed against one another. The chief objective in competition is the scarce object. In conflict it is injury, destruction, or defeat of an opponent.[8]

THE POSITIVE FUNCTIONS OF CONFLICT

That conflict can be destructive is part of conventional wisdom and common sense. It is increasingly recognized, however, that conflict can also be functional for individual, group, and societal welfare. A fairly substantial literature has now appeared that points to the ways in which conflict has integrative and beneficent consequences for group and community life.[9]

Perhaps the most thoroughgoing significance of conflict grows out of the ways in which it places issues and problems on the community's agenda, calling attention in dramatic and often irresistible ways to social circumstances that require change action. When the normal procedures of community decision making are nonresponsive to imperative social need, conflict forces a facing of social issues and, in so doing, makes possible their attempted resolution. The absence of conflict under conditions of social disadvantage is often expressive of inertia, complacency, or deliberate inaction that permits the continuation of exploitative social relations in the community. Even the threat of conflict often results in responsive action.

Once conflict has broken out, the very process whereby parties contend with one another has the effect of sharpening interest and compelling thought about the issues at stake, of advancing and defending alternatives,[10] of distinguishing divergent points of view,[11] and of deepening analysis. Mutual challenge requires probing into the implications of opposing viewpoints. What appears simple and uncomplicated may, in fact, assume multiple and complex dimensions calling for further examination and clarification. Implicit in social conflict behavior is a form of reality testing not unlike that which takes place in therapy groups where, according to Frank, "the occasion of conflict is seen as a means of evoking and clarifying the distortions and neurotic attitudes which are highlighted by the struggle, whether it is resolved or not."[12]

Conflict is essentially an expression of a relationship between social entities that often mirrors unequal access to scarce objects that are socially valued. Such relationships often represent differential status positions. Conflict can have the effect of restructuring relations between groups,[13] without conflict, group accommodation can result in subordination.[14] Intergroup struggle compels recognition of group interest and group integrity, and, if pursued with strength and persistence, of group demands. Minorities find a place in the arena of competing interests and decision making when they assert their collective will in opposition to those they perceive as responsible for maintaining the status quo. In this process, the locus of power is laid bare, making possible a real confrontation between true contenders. Much community power is latent and camouflaged and operates through intermediary agents, formal and informal. When conflict is sufficiently intense, the real wielders of power are likely to be revealed. Negotiation can then take place with people in a position to make real commitments.

Neighborhood residents perceived as alienated and apathetic move into action whenever there is a threat of displacement as a result of urban renewal, highway construction, slum clearance, and the like. Their engagement in the conflict to keep their homes mobilizes energies and creates group identity and collective awareness that effectively dispels isolation and anomie. Negroes involved in the civil rights movement and in struggles for local control give evidence of community participation and involvement that defy stereotypes of apathy and detachment.

The role of conflict in moving organizations to creative effort has been frequently noted. Thus Katz suggests that "organizations without internal conflict are on their way to dissolution. A system with differentiated substructures has conflict built into it by virtue of its differentiated subsystems. If it moves toward complete harmony, it moves toward homogeneity and random distribution of all its elements. Entropy takes over."[15] Conflict, on the other hand, both "within and between bureaucratic structures provides means for avoiding the ossification and ritualism which threaten their form of organization."[16] Challenge engenders response and stimulates the search for new and better ways of doing things. Its absence tends to lead to complacency and acceptance of inbred habits of thought and action.

Finally, there is some recognition that conflict leading to violence may also be functional for society. While violence, with its destructive potentials, is generally considered to be antithetical to democratic processes, under certain conditions it serves to mobilize indifferent or callous authority in the direction of positive social change that modifies oppressive or exploitative social practices. Thus, prison riots often lead to institutional reforms; violent racial conflicts can lead to legislative reform and social policy development. There is, of course, always the possibility that violence may bring more repressive counterviolence. The context and environment of violence, the nature of predisposing issues and events, the strength, political and otherwise, of the parties involved, the degree, nature, and intensity of the violence behavior, all define whether one or another consequence is likely to be forthcoming. A clue to the diagnostic value of violence is suggested by Nieburg: "Demonstrations of domestic violence serve to establish the intensity of commitment of members of the political system."[17] Low commitments either in scope or intensity have less meaning for challenge to the status quo. High commitments may be ultimately irrepressible. Violence tends to point to weaknesses in a social or organizational system, and hence suggests modifications that may help establish new equilibria. "The risk of violence," Nieburg states, "is necessary and useful in preserving natural societies."[18]

KEY CONCEPTS IN CONFLICT

There are a number of elements that inhere in any conflict situation and that provide a conceptual basis for conflict analysis. They include parties, issues, power, goals, boundaries, alliances, equity, and strategies of conflict management. Each is reviewed briefly in the next section.

Parties

Conflict, which depends upon incompatible preferences, implies at least two polar aggregates, each seeking to achieve its preferences in the face of a challenge by the other. Parties to a conflict can be individuals, groups, and/or organizations, theoretically suggesting nine possible types of conflict. At one end there are conflicts between individuals and at the other, between organizations.

Conflicts between individuals may have their sources in incompatible personality needs, in differing reference group identity, or in contrasting ideological beliefs and sentiments. Planned actions to deal with individual conflict will inevitably be influenced by diagnostic judgments thus made. Individual conflict is often expressive of group or organizational conflict, and may become an important source of collective conflict as others rally to an individual's cause in controversy and as existing organizations recognize their inherent interest in the fate of individuals mobilized by such interest.

Conflicts that grow out of group differences, such as are characterized by ethnic minorities, labor, religious adherents, and the like, tend to heighten group consciousness and to assume organizational forms.[19]

Perhaps the most significant conflicts in community life are those in which organizations are the parties involved. Such conflicts take place both within and between organizations. The larger an organization, the greater the likelihood of differing sentiments and values among its members. Lines of communication and control tend to be more tenuous as distance increases between rank-and-file participants and successive levels of authority, making organizational compliance more difficult. Subgroups, cliques, and friendship clusters tend to form and become potential sources of organizational deviance. When subgroup sentiments are perceived to be violated by the organization's policies and practices, intraorganizational conflict tends to occur.

Another source of internal conflict grows out of the organizational structure that differentiates member roles. Such differentiation tends to establish conflicting interests on the part of members who occupy diverse organizational roles. Higher participants who constitute the organization's leadership do not necessarily have the same structural interests as lower participants, even if they share the same ideals, goals, sentiments, and values. For example, rank-and-file trade union members are chiefly concerned with the benefits they derive from union membership, such as wages, hours, fringe benefits, and the like. Union leaders may be more interested in considerations of union security and stability, as well as *their* benefits, which take the form of salaries, perquisites, and power. Higher salaries for union executives may require higher dues payments from members. In this connection, one might note that unions frequently discourage, and even actively oppose, unionizing efforts among their own employees.

The more successful an organization becomes, the more it tends to establish a system of vested interests among its higher participants. Organizations tend to be preoccupied with their own maintenance needs as they deal with the problem of organizational survival and growth. For members of an organization's secretariat, such maintenance concerns tend to have a direct personal reference. For them, the organization may mean employment, status, and power, in addition to ideology or sentiment. The possibility of organization becoming an end in itself for such role incumbents potentially places them in opposition to other role participants. Thus, organizations frequently are the arenas for disaffection and revolt of members against leaders, stockholders against corporation executives, young Turks against entrenched bureaucrats.

Conflicts between organizations grow out of competition for like or scarce resources. These may be finances, leadership, friends, adherents, public attention, etc. Such conflicts are greatest where resources are relatively fixed, so that competing moves take on the character of a zero-sum-game—what one organization gets diminishes the "take" of the other. For example, welfare organizations frequently tend to appeal to the same set of voluntary foundations for funds, to the pool of community leaders for their attachments, and to the same central source of distribution of centrally gathered funds.

Interorganizational conflicts often take on intraorganizational forms simultaneously. This is a consequence of either differing values or divergent interests between higher and lower participants. The goals promulgated by constituent parts of an organization may not only differ, but may also find points of linkage with similar segments of competing organizations. Thus, the common structural characteristics of the leadership core of two organizations in conflict may lead to common aims that override their differences. Collective bargaining negotiations between the union officialdom and the employer representatives frequently lead to implicit understandings that take precedence over the common strivings of union members and their official representatives. At a certain point, particularly where stalemate appears, in achieving a settlement the interests of the higher participants of one party (union officials) frequently are more congruent with the interests of their counterparts of the second party (employer representatives) than with those of their lower participants (union members). Situations such as these lead to charges by lower participants of "selling out" to the enemy or of "betraying the members." They tend characteristically to lead to the employment of secret negotiations prior to or at the same time that official talks are being held.

Such secret dealings frequently involve third or fourth parties who are free to reformulate positions taken by the competing organizations or to develop entirely new lines of inquiry. Secret dealings tend also to lead to the use of "spies" to ferret out secrecy moves, to the public issuance of rumors concerning parallel moves made by the parties, or reports of secret "deals" made.

Issues. Parties are generally joined in conflict with respect to some substantive matter that has significance and meaning to the contestants.
The degree to which there is a potential investment of feeling or an attachment of significance to these issues has an important bearing on how
intense a particular conflict is likely to be and the ways in which it can be
effectively handled. Conflict issues involve events that have divergent
consequences for people affected by them. These frequently arise out of
divergent interests among social units located in a competitive or conflict
field. Interests are goals and objects that have salience for individuals,
groups, or organizations and, when perceived and understood, tend to
provide direction to their actions. Such interests may be material (they
have economic or political value), psychological (they confer status or
grant control and power), or structural (they grow out of different loca-
tions in social structures or organizations). Assessing the interests that
motivate members of opposing parties can be a difficult task, since actions that promote interests are not always expressive of them on the
surface. Much of the rhetoric of conflict is carefully designed to hide the
underlying motivations and to demonstrate ways in which stated positions accord with conventional and idealistic sentiments. The task of the
practitioner often is to help reveal the latent content of observed behavior of opponents and, at the same time, make manifest the actual, if un-
perceived, interest of members of his own system.

Among the most difficult and intractable conflicts are those that
grow out of differing and conflicting values and beliefs. Groups with
strong ideological roots tend to develop attachments of intensity on the
part of their adherents. They tend also to be uncompromising as a way
of insuring their purity, continuity, or growth. Maintenance of rigid
group boundaries and the administration of more or less rigid criteria of
belief commitments tend to characterize such groups. Most, if not all, social conflict contains an element of value incompatibility. The extent to
which such differences lie at the base of a particular conflict depends in
part on value ordering. Strong value orderings inhere in organizations
whose goals are defined by strong ideological or religious commitments.
Political organizations that are ideologically rooted similarly have strong
value orderings and tend to be involved in sharp conflicts with opposing
groups professing contradictory or competing values.

Whether an organization with strong value orderings will tend to be
more or less uncompromising in a conflict situation will depend on:

1. the degree of internal cohesion,
2. the degree of centralization of internal organizational control, and
3. the degree and exclusiveness of commitments to group or organizational values.[20]

Where these elements are positive and extensive, organizations will be ready for conflict that is intense and of substantial duration. They will respond to challenge quickly and will tend to initiate conflict where they perceive possible invasion of their rights or preserves.

The social work practitioner works in a complex value field where the values of his profession, his employing agency, his client system, the community at large, and his own value preferences frequently diverge, even if they do not assume outright conflict forms. In his contact with other professionals and other agencies, he frequently comes up against the same value barriers.

It is highly likely that some aspect of value or interest divergence can be identified in all conflict situations.[21] The more strong value elements conflicts have, the greater the difficulty one can expect in dealing with them. Similarly, the greater the vested interest at stake, the more tenacious and uncompromising parties tend to be.

Power Relations

There is general consensus in the literature that power and its distribution is a concept that is central to an understanding of conflict. To some it is *the* core concept that helps explain both the genesis and course of conflict, and it plays a crucial role in defining strategies to be used in its management. Thus North et al. state: "It is evident . . . that a conflict is always concerned with a distribution of power. Indeed, an exertion of power is prerequisite to the retention of a share in the determination of future relations—as well as for the acquiring or retaining of other benefits perceived as the 'reasons' for conflict."[22]

In what is perhaps the most ambitious attempt to develop a theory of social conflict, Dahrendorf places central emphasis on the relationship of dominance and subordination that characterizes the structure of authority in associations such as industry, the state, and the church.[23] Authority is defined as legitimate power. For him, the distribution of authority in associations is the ultimate "cause" of the formation of conflict groups.

The power dimension is a variable quantity in conflict relationships. The more fundamental the issue at stake, the more significant power becomes and the higher one reaches into the power hierarchy in the course of struggle. The relative distribution of power not only has an impact on the course of conflict, but becomes itself a value and an interest. In this sense, it is both an instrument and a cause of conflict. The exclusion of some segments of the population from the structure of power creates conditions for collective redress. Their bid to play a part in the processes of community decision making that affect their circumstances of living

serves as a rallying point in the contest that attempts to effect a redistribution of power. The values they assert are democratic insofar as a
broader sharing of power advances democratic goals. A restructuring of
power is also an interest in the sense that enhanced power, on the part of
those who have little, leads to a greater capacity to achieve both latent
and manifest interests.

The uses of power in the course of conflict is largely determined by
the extent to which contending parties have access to power resources.
While power is a property of social systems, it is manifested through persons located in certain segments of the social structure. Where access to
such persons and, through them, to organizations in which they wield
influence is open, conflict strategy is based in part on reaching them and
attempting to attach them to the cause at hand, a phenomenon I call
power steering. Differentiation within any strata of power frequently
leads to competitive bidding for such support by the parties in conflict.
Where, however, access is closed or limited, conflict parties tend to build
their own bases of power. This they do through the recruitment of large
numbers to the cause and the imaginative use of tactics that mobilize
support and release social energy.

Goals

Parties are drawn into conflict with one another because they compete
for a limited supply of goods, objects, values, or positions. It is the scarcity of these resources that creates conditions of conflict.

In each conflict there is a potential payoff to the parties. These constitute the conflict goals that bring the parties into contact with one another. It is the very commonality of interest that defines the nature of
the conflict. It is important to identify specifically what the conflict goals
are and how realistic and salient they are to the involved party. Planned
conflict is goal directed. The goals have an important bearing on the significance of the conflict and the ways in which it is conducted.

There is a significant relationship between intensity and scope on
the one hand, and the expected payoff in planned conflict on the other.
Practitioners and participants need to make judgments as to whether
there is enough to be gained to warrant the amount of social energy expended in any particular conflict campaign. Small effort for major gains
may be totally unrealistic and result in a waste of collective energy. Major
effort expenditure that yields little in desired directions can, similarly,
have a negative effect on group morale. In general, the more substantial
the goals and the greater the stakes, the more intensive mu.t be the planning that goes into developing a conflict effort.

Boundaries

Conflict takes place within a particular field where moves of one party can be made that result in its aggrandizement at the same time that another party is diminished. Thus, there is an "area" occupied by conflict that has a quasi-spacial dimension. The parameters of this conflict space can be determined by the specific resources possession of which is at issue, by the physical area occupied by the parties, by the extent of organizational membership, by claimed jurisdiction, or by the kinds and number of issues that engage the contending parties. Where the boundaries defining the claims, interests, or values of different parties are in dispute, conflict may result. Those who claim rights and responsibilities within their perceived boundaries tend to resist invasion.

The boundary concept is important to the practitioner in helping him match organizational resources to organizational goals in planned conflict. Conflict can become dysfunctional when too much "ground" is covered or when the organizational effort attempts to accomplish too much. To a considerable extent, the intensity of conflict may be indicative of the strength of the mechanisms that maintain the equilibrium of the status quo. On the other hand, a conflict can go beyond the boundaries of maximum intensity to the disadvantage of the concerned party. This is as true of intraorganizational conflict as it is of interorganizational or community conflict. While conflict within an organization helps maintain its viability and creativity, too much internal conflict can lead to its dismemberment. The stronger an organization and the greater the attachments of its members, the more conflict it can tolerate. There are, however, limits beyond which no organization can contain conflicting elements and survive. Much the same is true of conflict in the community. Conflict tends to create a reactive response. The extent of the response is determined by the nature of the challenge and by the strength and will of the opposing parties. Too much planned conflict can stimulate overwhelming counterreaction and result in negative rather than positive consequences. One of the persistent problems in planned conflict grows out of the unplanned and often undisciplined attachment of segments of the community that can result in unanticipated mass behavior.

Alliances

Social conflicts frequently involve more than two prime parties. Other individuals, groups, or organizations may feel a stake in the issues under contention. There is a tendency for multiple party conflicts to polarize around one or the other of the major contenders. This is clearly seen in politics and in wars. Political alliances and coalitions are traditionally a part of the political process. This is true in the two-party system as well as in those countries where multiple parties exist. The latter tend to join together several political organizations that are more or less stable and that shift with circumstances. In the former, single parties are themselves composed of coalitions of formal or informal interest groups. There may, in actuality, be a wider range of interests and beliefs *within* each of two opposing political parties than between them. Wars bring together different national states which share some common interests or values in two opposing camps. Effectiveness in conflict in both war and politics often depends on the nature and strength of the alliances formed to do battle.

Conflict groups in the community have a similar interest in knowing and cultivating potential allies and friends. In some instances, they strive to establish formal coalitions. Informal alliances without organizational ties play, perhaps, an even more important role. The ability to sustain a conflict position and to resist attack frequently depends on the extent to which allies are recruited and their support maintained. However, the greater the reliance on coalition members, the more the pressure develops to release part of the objectives of the conflict.

Coalitions and alliances are, in the long run, frequently unstable. Their capacity to sustain cooperative effort depends largely on the degree of perceived congruence of goals. Where goal linkage has short-run dimensions, alliances fall apart when the proximate goals are achieved, or when defeat is apparent. Victory brings into focus the long-range intragroup differences, and sets a new stage for conflict in which new and divisive interests or values appear. Thus the united effort in World War II produced an effective coalition until the point of surrender. Having achieved the immediate common goal—defeat of the Axis powers—the longer-run differences in national aims, interests, and philosophies asserted themselves in new national policies that pitted former enemies against former allies. Victory seems to sow the seeds of its own destruction.

After defeat, coalitions tend also to splinter, each group blaming the other, while frustration and disillusionment tend to reduce group cohesion and the attachments of members to the cause.

Equity

Social conflicts have their own dynamics, form, and structure, irrespective of the nature of the issues that brought them about. They do, however, also deal with substantive matters that have greater or lesser significance for people they involve or affect. Except for unrealistic conflicts that deal with sheer ventilation, there is often an underlying ethical and humanistic base that motivates the constituents of the parties opposing one another. In wars as in social life, a small determined nucleus of high morale and dedication often oppose even seemingly overwhelming forces with considerable effectiveness.

Part of the task of the practitioner is his assessment of where equity lies in the conflict between parties. Most indigenous social movements engage in conflict with forces of superior power and resources. The collective action directed toward constructive social change in the community often takes the form of conflict between power and equity.

Strategies of Conflict Management

Once conflicts have gotten underway they have their own life cycle—beginning, middle, and end. Even the most acrimonious and heated conflict comes to an end with some new circumstance and relationship between the parties. Wars end in treaties, strikes in settlements, unhappy marriages in separation or divorce. The task of the social practitioner—union organizer, civil rights leader, or community organizer—is to help conduct his side of the battle in such a way that positive consequences are maximized and costs minimized.

There are a variety of ways in which conflicts are conducted and brought to some more or less stabilized conclusion. Such modes of resolution bear a relationship to the nature, sources, types, and intensity of specific conflicts. Some lend themselves to certain approaches that would be totally inappropriate in other situations. The use of an inappropriate strategy may well lead to an intensification of hostility and prolonged conflict or to early defeat of one of the parties. A needed area of research lies in the empirical study of conflict types and the strategies of conflict management that are useful and productive in each type. Even the best intention and motivation can lead to a sequence of negative and unanticipated events because the "wrong" strategy was applied, or because it was planned poorly.

Where the dominant element in conflict concerns the struggle for power and control, the use of persuasion and dissemination of information in the hope of developing better human relations can hardly be expected to lead to effective settlement. On the other hand, where the differences between parties are narrow and the common interest readily perceived, severe forms of action—such as attempted suppression of one party by the other—will more likely result in exacerbating the conflict and a disruption of settlement rather than in speedy resolution.

A simplified classification of conflict strategies suggests itself. There are at least four major groupings of approaches to conflict management, within each of which there are a variety of adaptations. At one extreme are orientations that are intended to prevent the outbreak of overt intergroup hostility or to remove the negative consequences of interparty conflict. They attempt to apply rational methods of a problem-solving character to a situation that might otherwise deteriorate. At the other end of the spectrum lie orientations based on the avowed opposition and hostility of the parties that lead to "declarations of war." Here parties lack a common perception of goals, and at least one of the parties thinks it can compel the other to concede or disappear. The situation is one of win-lose confrontation. A middle range of conflict approaches aims at some accommodation or blunting of the demands or positions of the parties. There is no likelihood that the issues can be ignored and no proximate wish to destroy the opposing side. Differences are negotiated and bargaining processes organized. These strategies are based on some minimal degree of common goal perception or community of interests. Here, both parties "win," in a sense, in contrast to the circumstance where one party wins and the other loses.

The general strategies and their adaptations are shown in Table 22–1.

Integrative Strategies. The classic demonstration of integrative problem solving is found in the intergroup experiments of Sherif and his associates. After creating intense hostility between two groups of boys in a camp setting, Sherif set about the task of dispelling the hostility and antagonistic behavior. The key was found in introducing *superordinate goals* into the relationship between the parties—"goals that are compelling for the groups involved, but cannot be achieved by a single group through its own efforts and resources."[25] This strategy is contingent on the possibility of locating potentialities for such goal linkages and of finding creative ways of directing action toward common ends.

Utilitarian Strategies. A variety of approaches are included in the strategies that I have labeled utilitarian. The *fait accompli*, as described by Gordon Allport, suggests that unpopular or highly controversial changes should be initiated directly, firmly, and without equivocation. "Official policies once established are hard to revoke. They set models that, once

TABLE 22–1. Strategies of Conflict Management

Integrative	Utilitarian	Negotiative	Coercive
Superordinate solution	Fait accompli	Direct bargaining	Suppression
	Co-optation	Third party	Radical protest
	Persuasion and	negotiation:	Nonviolent protest
	dissemination	Conciliation·	Violent protest
	of information	Mediation	
	Early containment	Arbitration	

accepted, create habits and conditions favorable to their maintenance.
. . . Clear cut administrative decisions that brook no further argument
are accepted when such decisions are in keeping with the voice of conscience."[26] Where feelings run deep and issues indicate sharp controversy, the fait accompli attempts to set action in a potential conflict field
before opposing forces have time to mobilize their resources and develop momentum for counterattack.

Much has been written about *co-optation* as a mechanism for dealing
with external threat and securing organizational survival. Selznick, who
developed the concept out of his analysis of the TVA, concluded that the
"absorption of nucleuses of power into the administrative structure of
an organization makes possible the elimination or appeasement of potential sources of opposition."[27] There may, however, be unintended
and unanticipated consequences that follow upon the introduction of
opposing elements into an organization's decision-making structure.
Goals may be muted or modified, as in the case of the TVA, or, if the opposition is powerful enough, it may lead to organizational takeover, resulting in a form of counter-co-optation.

The utility of a strategem of *early containment* of conflict grows out of
Coleman's study of a wide variety of community conflicts. "Social controversy," he concluded, "sets in motion its own dynamics."[28] Once begun,
conflicts become elaborated, moving from specific to general issues,
then to new and different issues, and, finally, from disagreement to an-
tagonism and personal vilification. Dealing with potential differences at
relatively early stages can have the effect of limiting hostile escalation.

In the American ethos of consensus, a natural approach to the management of conflict lies in the attempt to deal with differences through
persuasion and dissemination of information. Where differences reflect deep
attachments to values or interests, persuasion may, however, have little
impact. It works best where the level of conflict intensity is low, and
where the basis of difference is faulty or blocked communication, or misunderstanding. Persuasive and educational devices can correct misperceptions and distortions, but rarely can they deal effectively with realistic
and deeply felt differences.

Negotiative Strategies. The strategic approaches to conflict discussed so
far all involve circumstances in which an overall common goal and identity of interest can be built into the conflict field, or where some pattern
of action can be organized that has the effect of "sidetracking" or freez-
ing potentially explosive hostility while maintaining the viability of the
system in which divergence appears. Another set of procedures lend
themselves to situations where these potentials are absent but where
some degree of commonality as well as difference can be brought into
the perceptual field of the parties to the conflict.

Situations calling for negotiation through bargaining are characterized by a mixture of conflict and mutual dependence that bind parties to
one another, yet compel each to contend for a division of resources in
accordance with their differing interests. Most "ultimately involve some
range of possible outcomes within which each party would rather make a
concession than fail to reach agreement at all."[29] In the bargaining process, each party's actions are guided not only by what they think will advance their own position or maximize their payoff, but by what they di-
vine the opposing party's choices and actions to be. Party A's behavior
depends in substantial part on his expectations of what Party B will do if
Party A moves in direction X. But these are reciprocal expectations,
where "one must try to guess what the second guesses, the first will guess
the second to guess and so on."[30]

Negotiation and bargaining tend to be appropriate stratagems
when power relations are relatively equal. In the words of Kirsh: "If collective bargaining is to be a process of private decision making by the
parties, free choice would necessarily presuppose equal power on each
side of the bargaining table."[31]

Bargaining works best when it takes place berween organized and
solidary groups whose leaders reflect the views of their constituents,[32]
when a minimum of covert intent can be read into moves made by opposing parties, when parties perceive the importance of coexistence
"and act without threatening the survival of the other."[33] The essential
mechanism at work is the perception that continued disagreement, an-
tagonism, and overt conflict is more costly to both parties than an agreement that provides for some gain for each.[34]

Coercive Strategies. The final set of strategies in our typology of conflict management deals with situations in which coercion tends to be
functionally appropriate. Up to this point we have discussed conflict patterns where a variety of procedures could be employed that relied in
some way on a sharing or mutuality of goals even in the face of certain
divergent or incompatible expectations. Where parties lack a degree of
common reference and goals are mutually exclusive, the resolution of
difference depends on an assertion of force or compulsion to gain ends
not otherwise achievable. Coercive strategies come into play when other
mechanisms have little hope of achieving change. The greater the disparity between projected group images and aspiration and the prevailing state of affairs, the more likely that force will enter the conflict
arena. Coercion challenges the status quo and threatens interests enhanced by the existing social arrangements. It invariably calls forth
counteraction and pressure to destroy or modify protest effectiveness.
Thus, coercive approaches are characterized by open confrontation between parties, by more or less intense emotional or ideological invest-

ment in group goals, by strong group identity, and by sharp cleavage between organized entities.

A crucial consideration in analyzing such conflicts concerns the extent to which parties are either invested with power, have access to power resources, or are able to locate channels that permit maneuvering within relevant power systems. The presence or absence of accepted and legitimatized power resources predispose parties to the use of variants of coercive strategies. Consideration of the use of coercion in collective action turns on the relationships of conflict parties to goals, power, and commitment.

Coercive action, from one point of view, has as its purpose the creation of a new circumstance in the conflict where other, less drastic approaches become feasible. Aside from suppression and surrender, it serves to bring parties together as a consequence of contestual pressure where they formerly failed to find common cause for settlement. When coercion is effective, it leads to some pattern of accommodation or negotiated agreement, or to some indicated action, such as legislative or administrative enactment, that is responsive to the question at issue. Coercion does not necessarily solve problems, but it can create the conditions under which competing parties can develop shared goals that supercede, in part, the basis for preexisting hostility. Thus strikes lead to the collective bargaining table, demonstrations to intercommunication and legislative action, school boycotts to new forms of intergroup decision making, and rent strikes to conferences that propose remedies.

While there are many ways of identifying coercive approaches in community organization and social action, it may be useful to think of the following four types of activity: suppression, radical protest, nonviolent protest, and violent protest. These are not necessarily mutually exclusive categories, but are suggestive, and represent differing traditions on the American scene.

A TYPOLOGY OF MODES OF CONFLICT MANAGEMENT

The selection of appropriate strategies in any specific conflict situation is largely based on the degree to which the goals or objectives of the parties are linked. Such goal relationships vary from total convergence to total divergence. The location of goals in this spectrum determines the aptness of particular strategies. Four sets of goal relationships parallel the four strategies suggested above.

When there is mutual identity of goals, they are said to be *superordinate*. Such goal identity can either be implicit in the relationship between the parties, awaiting only a new perception or consciousness, or it can be invented or created through deliberate manipulation of the situation that calls forth creative effort at restructuring the relationship.[35] Where goal differences can be submerged so that the discordant influences of goal conflict can be deflected, inhibited, or suppressed, at least overtly, one can speak of goal *sublimation*. There are many situations in which goal differences and subgoal mutuality are both operative simultaneously. Parties may seek differing objectives, yet find a common need for identifying shared outcomes so that normative relationships can be established or reestablished. Such a mixed goal circumstance indicates some degree of goal *convergence*. Finally, when parties are motivated by clearly opposed goals and seek the imposition of one for the other, we have goal *divergence*.

The combination of four strategies and four sets of goal relationships yields 16 possible relationships between goals and strategies, as shown in Table 22–2.

In practice, the utility of a particular strategy will generally depend on the degree to which it is congruent with the goal circumstance that inheres in the conflict. In the table, these tend to be located in boxes 1, 6, 11, and 16.

Because the power phenomenon is so central to conflict, it may be useful to speculate about its relationship to the four congruent conflict modes suggested above. In type 1, power may be a negligible ingredient. The identity of ends and the rationality implicit in the methodology of conflict management can override power differences. Problem solving is likely to be less destructive and to require less energy expenditure than other approaches. In the case of type 6, it is likely that power differences will be modest. Unequal power will tend to seek more assertive methods and be unprepared to pursue anything other than the full fruits of combat. Overwhelming power will tend to lead to coercive strategies and will characterize type 16. When winner can take all, why settle for anything less than total victory? Power weakness on the other hand, which tends to be met by nonrecognition or suppression on the part of those in authority, may present few alternatives to coercive action in circumstances

TABLE 22–2. Goals and Strategies of Conflict Management

Goal Relationships	Integrative	Utilitarian	Negotiative	Coercive
Identity	1	2	3	4
Sublimation	5	6	7	8
Convergence	9	10	11	12
Divergence	13	14	15	16

where divergent goals have strong salience. Type 11 is best indicated when there is a relative parity of power. Negotiation proceeds most productively when the power of the parties is roughly equal. Parties with superior power tend to ignore or overwhelm the weaker foe rather than cohabit the conference table.

CONCLUSION

This discussion has underscored the importance of social conflict processes for an understanding of planned action for social change. It stressed the positive and creative functions of conflict and suggested a set of concepts that are useful for analyzing conflict situations and in planning conflict action. A proposed typology of conflict management strategies suggests routes for subsequent research that can shed further light on appropriate practitioner and client system response to potential or actual threat or disruption growing out of conflict potential inherent in social and organizational relationships.

NOTES

1. Raymond W. Mack, "The Components of Social Conflict," *Social Problems* Vol. 12, No. 4 (Spring, 1965). "Wherever human beings are found (1) social organization exists, (2) social conflict ensues, and (3) social conflict is, at least to some extent, deprecated" (p. 388). *See also* Ralf Dahrendorf, *Class and Class Conflict in Industrial Society* (Stanford, Calif.: Stanford University Press, 1959), p. 208; and E. E. Schattschneider, *The Semi-Sovereign People* (New York: Rinehart and Winston, 1960), p. 71, "All politics, all leadership and all organization involves the management of conflict."
2. Quincy Wright, "The Nature of Conflict," *The Western Political Quarterly*, Vol. IV (June, 1951), pp. 197–198, 200.
3. Kenneth E. Boulding, *Conflict and Defense* (New York: Harper and Row, 1962), p. 189.
4. Richard T. LaPiere, *Social Change* (New York: McGraw-Hill Book Co., 1965), p. 478.
5. Alvin L. Bertrand, "The Stress Strain Element of Social Systems: A Micro Theory of Conflict and Change," *Social Forces*, Vol. 42, No. 2 (October, 1963).
6. Kurt Singer, "The Resolution of Conflict," *Social Research*, Vol. XVI (1949), p. 230.
7. Boulding, *op. cit.*, p. 5.
8. Raymond W. Mack and Richard C. Snyder, "The Analysis of Social Conflict—Toward an Overview and Synthesis," *The Journal of Conflict Resolution*, Vol. I (June, 1957), p. 218.

9. George Simmel, *Conflict and the Web of Group-Affiliation* (Glencoe, Ill.: The Free Press of Glencoe, 1955); Lewis A. Coser, *The Functions of Social Conflict* (Glencoe, Ill.: The Free Press of Glencoe, 1956); Robert C. North, Howard E. Koch, Jr., and Dina A. Zinnes, "The Integrative Functions of Conflict," *The Journal of Conflict Resolution*, Vol. IV, No. 3 (September, 1969); H. L. Nieburg, "The Uses of Violence," *The Journal of Conflict Resolution*, Vol. VII, No. 1 (March, 1963); Joseph S. Himes, "The Functions of Racial Conflict," *Social Forces*, Vol. 45, No. 1 (September, 1966).

10. Gary W. King, Walter E. Freeman, and Christopher Sower, *Conflict over Schools* (East Lansing, Mich.: Institute for Community Development, Michigan State University, 1963), p. 35.

11. Lyle E. Schaller, *Community Organization: Conflict and Reconciliation* (New York: Abingdon Press, 1966), p. 77.

12. Jerome D. Frank, "Training and Therapy," in *T-Group Theory and Laboratory Method: Innovation in Re-Education*, Leland P. Bradford, J. R. Gibb, and Kenneth D. Benne, eds. (New York: Wiley and Sons, 1964), p. 450.

13. Dan W. Doddson, "The Creative Role of Conflict in Intergroup Relations," Mimeo, undated, p. 4.

14. Robert C. Sorensen, "The Concept of Conflict in Industrial Sociology," *Social Forces*, Vol. 29, No. 7 (March, 1951), p. 266.

15. Daniel Katz, "Approaches to Managing Conflict," in Robert L. Kahn and Elise Boulding, *Power and Conflict in Organizations* (New York: Basic Books, 1964), p. 114.

16. Lewis A. Coser, "Social Conflict and the Theory of Social Change," *The British Journal of Sociology*, Vol. VIII (September, 1957), p. 200.

17. Nieburg, *op. cit.*, p. 54.

18. *Ibid.*, p. 43.

19. Dahrendorf, *op. cit.*, distinguishes between "*quasi-groups*," which are "aggregates of incumbents of positions with identical role interests," and interest groups, which have "common modes of behavior" (p. 180). Thus, quasi-groups are the recruiting ground for interest groups. Industrial workers constitute a quasi-group; trade unions, an interest group.

20. Mack and Snyder, *op. cit.*, p. 234.

21. Vilhelm Aubert, "Competition and Dissensus: Two Types of Conflict and Conflict Resolution," *The Journal of Conflict Resolution*, Vol. VII, No. 1 (March, 1963), p. 29.

22. North *et al.*, *op. cit.*, p. 370.

23. Ralf Dahrendorf, "Toward a Theory of Social Conflict," *The Journal of Conflict Resolution*, Vol. II, No. 2 (June, 1958), pp. 177–178.

24. For a somewhat similar general classification, see Herbert A. Shepard, "Responses to Situations of Competition and Conflict," in Robert L. Kahn and Elise Boulding, eds., *Power and Conflict in Organizations* (New York: Basic Books, 1964), p. 33. See also Robert C. North, *et al.*, p. 368; and J. David Singer, "The Political Science of Human Conflict," in Elton B. McNeil, ed., *The Nature of Human Conflict* (Englewood Cliffs, N.J.: Prentice-Hall, 1965), p. 141

25. Muzafer Sherif, *In Common Predicament* (New York: Houghton Mifflin Co., 1966), p. 88. See also Muzafer Sherif, O. J. Harvey, B. Jack White, William

R. Hood, and Carolyn W. Sherif, *Intergroup Conflict and Cooperation: The Robbers Cave Experiment* (Norman, Oklahoma: University of Oklahoma Book Exchange, 1961); Muzafer Sherif, "Superordinate Goals in the Reduction of Intergroup Conflict," *American Journal of Sociology*, Vol. 63 (1958); Muzafer Sherif and Carolyn W. Sherif, *Groups in Harmony and Tension* (New York: Harper and Bros., 1953).

26. Gordon W. Allport, *The Nature of Prejudice* (New York: Doubleday and Co., Anchor Edition, 1958), p. 471.

27. Philip Selznick, *The TVA and the Grass Roots* (New York: Harper and Row, 1966). Cooptation is defined as "the process of absorbing new elements into the leadership or policy-determining structure of an organization as a means of averting threats to its stability or existence" (p. 13).

28. James S. Coleman, *Community Conflict* (Glencoe, Ill.: The Free Press of Glencoe, 1957), p. 17.

29. Thomas C. Shelling, *The Strategy of Conflict* (Cambridge, Mass.: Harvard University Press, 1960), p. 70.

30. *Ibid.*, p. 87.

31. Benjamin S. Kirsh, *Automation and Collective Bargaining* (New York Central Book Co., 1964), p. xi.

32. John A. Fitch, *Social Responsibilities of Organized Labor* (New York: Harper and Row, 1957), p. 40.

33. Herman Lazarus and Joseph P. Goldberg, *The Role of Collective Bargaining in a Democracy* (Washington, D.C.: The Public Affairs Institute, 1949), p. 21.

34. Robert P. Blake, Herbert A. Shepard, and Jane S. Mouton, *Managing Intergroup Conflict in Industry* (Houston, Texas: Gulf Publishing Co., 1964), pp. 76–77.

35. Richard E. Walton, "Two Strategies of Social Change and Their Dilemmas," *The Journal of Applied Behavioral Change*, Vol. 1, No. 2 (April-May-June, 1965), p. 171.

23

Some Considerations in Planning Organizational Change

STEPHEN HOLLOWAY
GEORGE BRAGER

The literature on organizational change has two major emphases. The first is on how managers can induce compliance from lower ranking members to gain acceptance of administratively inspired innovation. The second, stemming from the organizational development field, highlights the process by which third-party consultants can, with managerial support, create a more open organizational system. Both view change as a process that is initiated at the top of an organizational hierarchy and then disseminated downward, and both pay scant attention to the special case of the human services organization.

The literature thus tends to be less useful to professionals in the human services than might otherwise be the case. For one thing, "top-down" change ignores the fact that most social agency administrators, not to mention middle-level and line workers, are responsible to superordinates—and thus are "bosses" in relative terms only. Furthermore, neglecting the special case of the human services agency ignores a primary difference between it and other organizations—namely, its commitment to client service. One may question the utility of principles about change divorced from the specification of *what* is to be changed. Only as the parameters of specific changes are defined and their impact

This chapter is a partial and revised version of chapter 1 of *Changing Human Services Organizations: Politics and Practice* by George Brager and Stephen Holloway (New York: Free Press, 1978).

appraised will change theory be maximally useful to professionals at whatever hierarchical level.

Although this paper was written with middle-level and line workers in mind, we believe that it is applicable to upper ranking administrators as well. It identifies three major types of organizational change: alterations in behavior, technology, and structure. The interdependence of the three types is discussed, and some criteria for assessing the significance of change are suggested. The paper concludes by noting some practice implications stemming from an understanding of the types of change and their significance.

The professional's interest in change typically grows out of struggling with a problem or limitation in organizational functioning. As an alternate state of affairs is envisioned that eliminates the problem or limitation, the change idea is born. Unlike the academic who will be preoccupied with a precise definition of "change" in the organizational context, the human services professional is more concerned with the *impact* of the proposed change on the problem that initially led to its conception. He will view the organization as altered or not depending on the extent that operations after the change more fully represent his commitments than did operations before the change. Such a notion suggests that, if not the technical definition, surely the meaning of organizational change is buried in the values and perspective of the observer.

MODIFICATIONS IN PEOPLE, TECHNOLOGY, OR STRUCTURE

Organizational change or innovation ultimately entails modifying the actions and interactions of numbers of organizational participants.[1] These modifications in behavior result from alterations in the people themselves, in the organization's technology, or in its structure. Change may thus be defined as alteration in any of these three elements. Although the goal of all change is the behavior patterns of people, the primary focus of intervention varies among the three variables.

People-Focused Change

People-focused change assumes in some measure that the participants perform unsatisfactorily as the *direct* result of their own insufficiencies. In this view, it is not structural arrangements that are responsible for inadequate performance (e.g., confused role definitions or a maldistribution of organizational rewards), nor is the problem seen to be caused by the agency's activities. Rather, the activities are viewed as appropriate to the organization's mission, but staff are insufficiently skilled in providing them; or role definitions are seen as clear, but workers are uncertain about how to apply them.

Training and other forms of education are the primary modes of intervention that focus directly on people. These might include ongoing, elaborate, and formal devices or informal mechanisms such as discussion, appeals to conscience, and sensitivity sessions. A second method of people change is the replacement of present staff or the addition of persons with different competencies, experiences, or qualifications. (When upper level staff are replaced, or when there is a large influx of different types of people—e.g., placing poor people on boards—the change might as well be characterized as a structural change as a person-focused change.)

Although inadequate performance is sometimes a source of organizational difficulty, there is, we believe, a too ready disposition to define organizational problems in terms of the abilities or attitudes of incumbents and thus to overemphasize people change. The manifestation of a problem is more obvious than its source, and since most organizational problems are apparent in the behavior of members, other, less visible causes tend to be ignored. For example, a problem may be defined as "staff unwillingness to change with the times" when, in fact, the difficulty stems from the existence of subtle organizational penalties in the form of an increased work load or being labeled "troublemaker" for workers who introduce new ideas.

People change is the type of change most likely to garner the support of top hierarchies. It is implicitly critical of the organization's personnel rather than the organization's program and structure or its ideology, and is therefore far less controversial. Indeed, changes in people are often encouraged by powerful participants for political reasons, since it is often in their interests to give the appearance of dealing with a problem rather than to solve it. (As this comment suggests, many relatively minor changes in people, particularly as reflected in their attitudes rather than in their behavior, can be viewed as changes in an organization only by a broad stretching of the definition of the term.)

Technological Change

Technological change refers to alterations in the agency's services—the procedures and activities that contribute to organizational output. The range of examples is as large as there are varieties of services and methods of providing them, and the change may be directed to the type of service itself (e.g., a reorientation from individual to community intervention) or to alterations within a particular modality. The degree of magnitude of the change is ordinarily greater in the former instance, but variations in the magnitude of technological change occur in the lat-

ter case as well. The change may be as minor, for example, as the replacement of a brief intake interview by a self-administered questionnaire or as major as a basic overhaul of the interviewing process itself.

When the magnitude of the innovations is roughly equal, a technological change is more likely to impact on an organization than a change
in people. Slight modifications in the style or competence of the people
who comprise the organization may have little appreciable effect on
other aspects of the organization. On the other hand, slight changes in
agency policy can have far-reaching consequences for agency operations
(for example, a minor change in a service can result in many more or
different clients seeking the service).

Similarly, changes in technology are less subject to reversal than are
changes in people, since they tend to be categorical changes as opposed
to changes in degree. Compare, on the one hand, the change in an organizing effort from house-to-house solicitation to making contacts
through local community groups with, on the other hand, the change in
an administrator's way of conducting staff meetings from an authoritarian style to encouraging staff participation. With the person change, the
opportunity to backslide into the former authoritarian style is substantial. Although it may be significant, the change is a matter of degree. In
the case of the technological change, however, once it is implemented,
there is no context for reversal. The change is categorical and thus self-
stabilizing.

Structural Change

By structure we mean the ways in which the members of an organization
are arranged in relation to one another, the prescribed relationships and
rules, either formal or informal, that define organizational authority
and responsibility. Shifts in patterns of communication, the creation of
new roles or the redefinition of current roles, and redistributions of rewards and responsibilities—all constitute examples of structural change.
(For a more detailed discussion of structural change, see Mayer, 1972.)

The impact of organizational structure on the behavior of members
is often clear, as, for example, when the application of sanctions to compel a desired behavior directly induces the compliant response. Katz and
Kahn (1966, pp. 79–83) note, as a matter of fact, that the authority relations represented by structure are the chief organizational means of controlling human variability. But the effects of structure on behavior may
also be subtle and unrecognized. For example, conflicts that are defined
as clashes of personality may really be generated by structural arrangements (e.g., overlapping responsibilities set in motion a struggle for
"turf").

Changes in structure range on a continuum from slight to major in the same way as do innovations that focus on people or technology. The degree of change is theoretically limitless—from changing the supervisor to whom a single individual reports, to the total reorganization of the agency. Similarly, structural changes vary in the extent to which they are categorical or a matter of degree. A categorical change in structure, for example, might involve the decision to move the client eligibility unit of a public service agency from Department X to Department Y, which would make it a self-sustaining change. A structural change reflecting degree, on the other hand, might require the director of Department X to consult with colleagues in Department Y on certain types of eligibility cases, a change that is often subject to informal subversion over time. In any case, however, for reasons discussed below, the impact of changes in structure is typically most profound, somewhat less with changes in technology, and least significant with changes in people.

CHANGE IMPACT

Keeping in mind that the point of departure for consideration of change is the professional's perception of an organizational problem that compromises his interests and ideological commitments, change impact can be defined as the extent to which the innovation has the effect of more fully implementing those commitments. It is thus a relative concept. The impact of a change is "significant" or not depending on the expectations and assessments of the perceiver. There is a further complication as well. Not only is the significance of a change difficult to assess, per se, but the time frame of the assessment frequently affects one's determination of its significance.

A "minor" change may trigger a "major" one at some future time. Or minor changes may accumulate so that their full significance goes unobserved until late in the process. For example, the introduction of a new elective course in a university would ordinarily be viewed as an insignificant alteration of its curriculum. Assume, however, that over a period of time, the course increases in favor. More sections are offered. Subsequently, some faculty decide that the subject matter is sufficiently important to make it a required course. This position is ultimately adopted, and a large number of sections are now organized. Some instructors are retrained to teach the new subject matter, and as the university hires new faculty, one criterion becomes expertise in the hitherto uncovered area. By now a significant change has occurred, but at what point in the process was an observer to assess its significance?

The time dimension in assessing change impact may work in reverse as well. That is, a change may at one point in time appear to be useful or important but may be merely a short-term fluctuation within a longer term pattern of stability. So, for example, in response to pressure, an agency may decide to increase its representation of clients from the minority community, and assigns a worker to recruit minority clients—a significant change on its face. But if one were to examine the long-range experience of the agency, one might discover that the decision had been made before and would be made again as the pressure on it mounted or slackened.

Although the assessment of change impact is necessarily subjective and is complicated by considerations of time, there are three criteria that can serve as guidelines in assessing the significance of a change. Two have been referred to in the prior section of this paper: the magnitude of the change (the degree to which the people, technology, or structure of the organization is altered by the change attempt) and its permanence (the extent to which, once made, the change is subject to reversal). Both of these criteria are usually, though not always, related to a third: the number of organizational elements affected by the change, or its scope.

Organizations are systems composed of interdependent parts, each of which contributes to and receives something from the whole. Within each of these parts, or subsystems, there are further subdivisions that are similarly interdependent, down to the organization's smallest components. Thus, a modification of one component has the potential for modifying any number of other related elements.

Examples of the interdependence of organizational elements are boundless. We cite three organizational experiences for the sake of clarity:

1. A hitherto authoritarian administrator subsequently encourages worker participation in staff meetings. As a result, staff now generate proposals for program change. New programs are initiated that require in turn that staff responsibilities be shifted, informal relations revised, and resources reallocated.
2. A traditional mental health clinic opens an outreach program in an impoverished neighborhood to induce poor clients to use its service. New life problems and new behavior patterns must now be handled by staff. Some workers are more, some less, prepared to proffer help to the new clientele. The self-esteem of workers rises or falls, superordinate judgments regarding the competence of particular workers shift, and the patterns of relationships that existed earlier undergo marked transformation.
3. Following a self-evaluation study, the board of trustees of a traditional family-service agency reorganizes its departmental structure to include a large social-planning and public-policy unit. The unit is given ascendancy in the table of organization, and the agency's heavy investment in the provision of traditional social services gives way to an emphasis on demonstration programs intended to influence legis-

lation. Many of the staff flounder, some seek retraining, and others leave the agency.

In each of these examples, a change has occurred in all three major variables—people, technology, and structure. In the first, the case of the authoritarian administrator, the ripple effect was set off by a change in a person; the second set of changes was initiated by a technological innovation, the outreach program; and structural modification was responsible for the third.

Not all elements within an organization are so interdependent as our discussion has implied. Persons and units within organizations develop protective mechanisms that immure themselves from influence. Furthermore, if a change is small in magnitude or is more a matter of degree than a categorical change, it is both more subject to reversal and less likely to impact on other variables. The single most useful criterion to assess the significance of a change, then, is the interdependence of the changing element with other organizational variables. This is the case whether the change starts in one variable and sets in motion change in another or whether the change triggers movement within the subcomponents of any one of the three variables. It is also the reason that a change that is perceived to be self-contained is considerably less likely to be resisted than a change that is perceived to impact other organizational elements as well.

Since changes in people often occur without appreciable effect on other elements in the organization, when all other things are equal, people-focused change has the least impact. Changes in technology, on the other hand, are likely to affect a myriad of other factors: interpersonal relations, staff work load, authority arrangements, communication patterns, and the like. And since in one sense the structure *is* the organization, changes in one aspect of structure are potentially able to impact every other aspect of the organization.

PRACTICE IMPLICATIONS

Change is instigated by a "performance gap"—the perception of a discrepancy between what a human services agency could do and what it actually does (Zaltman et al., 1973, p. 2). Which one of the three variables is targeted to produce the change—people, technology, or structure—is determined in large measure by the change proponent's definition of the source of the trouble. But even when the source of the problem is correctly perceived (and, because of training and experience, social workers are overly quick to define organizational issues in personality terms), the feasibility of the change—or political factors—must also be taken into account.

The fact that modifications in one organizational component have potential for modifying related components is highly suggestive for practice purposes. Professionals with a sophisticated understanding of organizational dynamics and change may choose to approach an innovative attempt indirectly rather than head-on (e.g., as a person-oriented rather than a structural change). Furthermore, how the change goal is designed and defined is a factor of critical importance in this regard.

The more modest the goal, the greater the likelihood of its acceptance by those who are its targets or are affected by the change. This is not universally true, of course. Some board members, administrators, and workers respond to novel approaches, and some agencies are imbued with change-oriented values. But more often than the reverse, the uncertainty of change generates a tension that people and organizations avoid when they can. This being the case, our discussion of the three criteria by which to assess the significance of change is useful for developing change strategy as well, since it provides guidelines for determining the extent of resistance one is likely to encounter. Thus, the greater the magnitude of a change goal and the more it departs from current agency practice, the more difficult it will be to gain broad acceptance. Similarly, the more irreversible the goal, the more risk it engenders, and the more difficult it will be to obtain endorsement. This is, of course, why time-limited experiments and demonstration programs are so frequently proposed. Finally, the broader the scope of a change goal, the more widespread its impact on other organizational actors and the larger the number of levels or functional subgroupings that must be brought along. Hence, the more resistance one might anticipate.

It is beyond the scope of this paper to outline the various practice techniques that may be used to take into account the factors mentioned above. We cite two for illustrative purposes, one relating to the design of the change goal, the other to how it is defined.

Partializing a goal is an often effective means of minimizing its threat potential. A goal may be partialized by reducing its scope, thus reducing the number of people involved in or affected by its adoption. For example, an innovative idea may be proposed for only one department—the most receptive to the idea—before an attempt is made to diffuse it throughout the organization. Or the content of the goal may be partialized by dividing it into developmental components. Thus, a sequence of steps may be planned. Point A must be effected before moving to point B, and completing point B is a requirement of C. Not only does careful sequencing reduce the threat potentials of change, but actions taken in the early stages of a process (e.g., step A) can subsequently be invested with meaning that was not explicit in the initial action. A first step can thus be defined retrospectively as a commitment to fuller action—in this case, a commitment to B and C.

The apparent impact of a change on organizational participants may also be minimized by how one defines the change. Some change ideas lend themselves to a definition of limited scope, and indeed all changes, even highly significant ones, can be presented as less far-reaching than they in fact are. One technique is to minimize threat or uncertainty by presenting the proposal as involving little or no change on the ground that it is related to the traditional values of the agency or more closely conforms to current programmatic directions than the procedure or policy it is intended to replace. For example, in radically altering its program, Henry Street Settlement in New York City developed a policy statement that read in part as follows: "The statement is fully in accord with the history of Henry Street. It selects from that history a particular emphasis and highlights it as a central purpose" (NFSNC, 1968, p. 14). One may suspect that the words are as much a bid for the support of "old-timers" on the Henry Street Board as they are a reflection of historical fact.

Sometimes professionals may define their goal as a procedural rather than a policy change, for procedural modifications are less threatening than policy changes, and can be decided by staff without board approval. Another technique to minimize the impact of a change on participants is to allow a new idea time to percolate until it does not seem new at all.

These comments are intended to be suggestive only. The point to emphasize is that a focus on change that neglects how lower ranking participants influence upper ranking ones—whether it is the executive in relation to his board or workers in relation to the executive—falls short of offering a full understanding of how change occurs and how it may be pursued. Political factors, which are part of the fabric of all organizations, are overlooked by a top-down emphasis, since power is assumed and is thus not incorporated as a critical element. The mission and specific responsibility of professionals within human services agencies are also ignored by the top-down focus. To offer a high standard of service to clients, professionals at all hierarchical levels must be skilled in the uses of organizational influence. Further understanding of the types and significance of particular organizational changes and the development of practice technology to put this understanding to use are required. Its place ought to be high on the professional agenda.

NOTE

1. We use the terms *change* and *innovation* interchangeably, although some organizational theorists distinguish between the two. Our meaning relates to something that is new or different to the unit that adopts the change, rather than to a discovery or invention, per se.

REFERENCES

Katz, D., & Kahn, R. *The social psychology of organizations.* New York: John Wiley & Sons, 1966.

Mayer, R. *Social planning and social change.* Englewood Cliffs, N.J.: Prentice-Hall, 1972.

National Federation of Settlements and Neighborhood Centers. *Making democracy work.* New York: Author, 1968.

Zaltman, G., et al. *Innovations and organizations.* New York: John Wiley & Sons, 1973.

24

Organizational Resistance and Change: The View from Below

RINO J. PATTI

INTRODUCTION

Bureaucratic organizations have come to occupy a position of almost unique disfavor among human service professionals. Recognized by most as a necessary evil, such organizations tend in general to be characterized as sluggish, uncreative, and mired in rules and procedures which prevent the professional from offering the service he would otherwise be able to provide unfettered by these constraints. Bureaucracies are further criticized as being inherently preoccupied with maintenance and self-perpetuation, often to the extent that consumer welfare is sacrificed.[1] It is not my intent to elaborate on this critique except to point out that it has tended to obscure the necessity of analyzing each organization in terms of its receptivity or resistance to innovation. In too many instances, conventional wisdom about "the bureaucracy" has served as a substitute for careful differential assessments of organizations and their varying capacities for change.

In this paper I direct attention to four variables which can provide the internal change agent[2] with a partial framework for analyzing the magnitude and nature of the resistance he will likely encounter in efforts to effect organizational change. The four variables to be discussed are:

1. the nature of the change proposal;
2. the value orientation and decision-making style of the decision maker;

3. the administrative distance between the practitioner and the decision maker; and
4. "sunk costs," that is, the investment an organization, or some part thereof, has made in the arrangement the initiator of change intends to alter.

In presenting this analytic framework my intent is to provide a practitioner with a tool that may enable him to make a differential assessment of resistance. Such an assessment, as I suggest later in the paper, is crucial to making an informed choice of change objectives and interventional strategies.

In what follows, organizational resistance will be viewed from the perspective of the administrative subordinate who, in a given instance, must obtain the approval of his superior for changes he is proposing. Thus, in this context, the subordinate is any employee, be he administrator, supervisor, direct-service worker, researcher, or program analyst, who is actively attempting to influence decision makers at some point further up in the administrative hierarchy to adopt his plan of action.

For the most part, discussions of organizational resistance tend to view the agency from the top down or, more specifically, from the vantage point of high-level administrators who generally have the authority to institute changes they consider desirable.[3] This is to be expected since these actors carry a major responsibility for initiating and managing change. At the same time this perspective has, at best, limited value for the low-power practitioner because his interest, his information, his experience, and, most certainly, his authority are likely to be distinctly different from those of his counterpart in higher administrative circles.

DEFINITIONS AND ASSUMPTIONS

Before proceeding with an analysis of those variables which have some bearing on resistance to change, it is first necessary to define some terms and state the major assumptions that will be central to the following discussion.

Change will refer to the formal acceptance of a proposed addition, modification, or deletion in administrative policy, program, or procedure by a person, or persons, with authorization to do so. I will not be concerned here with other kinds of changes, often just as important, that occur in the informal system (e.g., interpersonal relationships, communication, distribution of power) and for which no formal decision is required. Nor will I be concerned with modifications in policy, program, or procedure that fall within the authority domain of the practitioner himself. For example, if a caseworker decides to initiate group treatment for certain of his clients, or to modify his own record-keeping system, and has the authority to do so without gaining the formal approval of someone in the hierarchy, we will not consider this a change for our purposes.

Resistance refers to those forces or conditions within the organization that tend to decrease the likelihood that decision makers will accept or act favorably upon a proposal for change initiated by an administrative subordinate. No effort will be made to address the resistance that may arise from a decision maker's judgment that a proposed innovation is not sound or beneficial to the agency or the clientele it serves. Innovations are not inherently desirable, and in any given instance a supervisor may simply reject a new course of action out of a conviction that it will not add to, or may detract from, an agency's service capability. Resistance arising from this source will not be dealt with here.

In what follows, it will be assumed that the practitioner is attempting in good faith to effect change in the organization's policies, programs, or procedures in order that it may be a more effective instrument for the delivery of social services. I will further assume that the change agent is competent and responsible in the performance of his professional role and that his involvement in the change effort is not intended to divert attention from or displace responsibility for his own personal or professional inadequacies. Finally, I will proceed on the assumption that he has conscientiously attempted to formulate his proposal on the basis of the best and most complete information available to him. It is necessary at this point to observe that unless these conditions have been met, the resistance the administrative subordinate encounters may be attributable more to him than to the organization he seeks to change.

THE CHANGE PROPOSAL

Since the range of change proposals made by practitioners may be as diverse as the activities that occur in the field of social welfare, I will attempt to focus this discussion by conceptualizing such efforts in terms of two dimensions: *generality* and *depth*. These dimensions are selected because on the face of it they seem to be critically related to organizational resistance.

Generality refers to the scope or pervasiveness of the proposal; in simple terms, the size of the organizational unit that will be affected by the changes sought. Three levels of generality are proposed here:

1. *Component*—those change efforts that seek modifications in organizational arrangements or operations which have relevance primarily

for the change agent or for a small group with whom he interacts on a day-to-day basis (e.g., supervisory unit).

2. *Subsystem*—those change efforts that seek to alter the arrangements or operations of an entire unit or class of organizational participants (e.g., a department, district office, all caseworkers).

3. *System*—those efforts aimed at changing some aspect of the organization that will have operational implications for its entire membership.

In reality, changes at either of the first two levels of generality are likely to affect the third, but our concern here is not with the eventual ramifications of the change but with its intended, first-order consequences.

The second dimension concerns the *depth* of change that is sought.[4] Again, three levels are suggested:

1. *Procedural*—those proposed changes that seek to alter the rules and procedures guiding the day-to-day behavior of employees who are carrying out the policies or programs of the agency. The goal here is to facilitate the flow of work activities or to utilize resources more efficiently, not to alter the substance or purpose of the services provided. Examples might be improved methods of interdepartmental referral, the development of mechanisms for increased communication and coordination among staff (e.g., interdisciplinary team conferences), or the introduction of new statistical forms to enable an agency to monitor its workload better.

2. *Programmatic*—those innovations aimed at modifying the operating policies or programs carried out by an organization in order to implement its basic purposes and objectives. The focal concern is to substantively alter the services that an agency provides so that it can more effectively accomplish its mission. Changes at this level may take the form of new treatment modalities (e.g., family therapy, behavior modification) or the addition of programs such as day care, job placement, or homemaker services.

3. *Basic*—those efforts that are aimed at changing the core objectives of an agency. The intent is to effect a fundamental shift in the organization's mission so that it will address itself to a different set of problems and outcomes. Examples here might be transforming a character-building agency into one that seeks to correct emotional disturbances in children, or changing a custodial institution into one that is committed to rehabilitation.

When these variables of generality and depth are related to one another a ninefold classification of change proposals emerges. It is my premise that as either the generality or the depth of a proposal increases, the resistance to be expected from organizational decision makers is, all other things being equal, also likely to increase. This is to be anticipated since the more fundamental and far-reaching the proposal, the greater the costs of innovation and the potential for instability are likely to be. Not only must the agency devote a greater than usual share of its resources to establishing new arrangements and behavior patterns, but the period of transition is almost certain to be accompanied by a lessening of the decision maker's ability to predict and control employee behavior and the reactions of external support groups.

VALUE ORIENTATIONS OF DECISION MAKERS

Practitioners in the lower reaches of social welfare bureaucracies may often assume that organizational decision makers will be resistant to proposals emanating from below. Unfortunately, this assumption often serves to deter administrative subordinates who would otherwise promote their ideas for change. A more useful perspective would be to proceed on the premise that superiors vary considerably in their receptivity to innovation, and thus in how they react to proposals for change.[5]

One approach to making such a differential assessment involves an analysis of a decision maker's value orientations. *Values* are defined here as the personal goals held by an official that serve to guide his organizational behavior, especially how he decides issues. They are a reflection of those conditions he believes will produce a sense of self-fulfillment, satisfaction, or accomplishment. The assumption here is that, notwithstanding limits to rationality,[6] a decision maker consciously attempts to choose those courses of action for the organization which are most likely to maximize the prospect of attaining the goals he holds most important. Personal goals are not necessarily self-aggrandizing or selfish in the conventional sense. They may include values that the decision maker perceives as altruistic or in the public good.

The following list of personal goals[7] indicates something of the range of values that may influence decision-making behavior. While all of these goals may be perceived as important, the decision maker is likely to arrange them in a hierarchy so that some are more important in influencing his behavior than others. Thus the attention of the practitioner should be directed not toward the presence or absence of certain values but toward their relative position in the decision maker's goal hierarchy. In other words, while all goals may be operative in some degree, it is likely that some are more consistently salient than others. The goals include:

1. *Power*—authority and control over organizational behavior.
2. *Money*—increases in income or income substitutes.

3. *Prestige*—respect and approval from those who are responsible for funding the agency, determining promotions, hiring and firing, etc.
4. *Convenience*—avoidance of conditions that will require additional personal efforts.
5. *Security*—protection against losses of personal power, prestige, or income.
6. *Professional competence*—respect from peers for knowledge, technical proficiency, or professionally ethical behavior.
7. *Client service*—achieving maximum program effectiveness and efficiency in the interest of better service to clientele.
8. *Ideological commitment*—maintenance of the agency as an instrument of an ideology or philosophical stance.[8]

This scheme does not exhaust the range of values that may motivate decision-making behavior, nor does it account for the fact that each proposed innovation may well call into play a somewhat different constellation of personal values from a superior. For example, under ordinary circumstances, if a decision maker places high value on the retention of power but a particular proposal has no implications for his ability to achieve this goal, then another value (e.g., convenience) may become a dominant factor in his consideration. Nevertheless, despite its limitations, the scheme provides the change agent with a point of departure for assessing those goals that are likely to influence the superior's decision on his proposal at a given point in time.

An analysis of literature further suggests that these personal goals are not randomly distributed among decision makers but rather tend to cluster characteristically in certain organizational role types. Brief profiles of each of three modal types—the conserver, the climber, and the professional advocate—are presented to illustrate the relationship between goals and decision-making behavior.[9]

The *conserver* is, as the name implies, largely concerned with maintaining his place and routine in the organization. His primary preoccupation is with security and convenience, that is, with maintaining whatever power, prestige, privilege, and income he now possesses. As one might expect, decision makers who are conservers tend to consider any significant change in the status quo, especially if it affects their domain, anathema. Such officials are often fearful, cautious, and lacking in self-confidence. They are likely to be alienated from the organization and its mission and secretly somewhat pessimistic about the effects of its programs. Cynicism about new efforts or ideas tends to be expressed in terms of failures associated with past similar ventures. Conservers frequently divorce job and social life, concentrating most of their creative energies in the latter arena. Although some administrators may be conservers by personality predisposition, such an orientation tends more often to be a product of longevity in the organization, advanced age, lack of promotional opportunities, and a declining sense of personal efficacy produced by years of frustration and disappointment while fighting the good fight.[10] This is not meant to imply that all officials approaching retirement are conservers but merely that there is a considerable tendency for those who have been in the bureaucracy a long time to develop this orientation.

The decision-making behavior of the conserver, as the preceding profile suggests, will tend to approximate what Gawthrop refers to as a "consolidative" orientation. He defines consolidation as "a deliberate and conscious effort to resolve demands for change regardless of source solely in the context of existing organizational structures, if at all possible."[11]

In contrast to consolidation, innovation (at the other end of the decision-making continuum) represents "a deliberate effort on the part of executive officials to search for improved performance programs, to diagnose organizational weaknesses in advance, and to predict as accurately as possible the consequences of innovative change."[12]

The consolidative bias of the conserver does not mean that such decision makers indiscriminately reject all proposals for change, because to do so would obviously be to court disaster. Rather, consolidative behavior is more likely to be manifested by a failure to search for, or identify, emergent problems and issues. The conserver tends to be relatively impervious to informational inputs regarding program gaps or deficiencies until such information, through the sheer weight of repetition or wide popular acceptance, takes on the nature of conventional knowledge. Finally, when conditions requiring change are upon the organization and some response is imperative, the change implemented is likely to be incremental and modest.

The *climber*, the second modal type of decision maker, is primarily concerned with acquiring power, position, and prestige.[13] He does this in a number of ways, including assiduously cultivating those in authority who have the power to affect his personal fortunes, taking on responsibilities or functions not previously associated with his job in order to increase the scope of his office, and moving opportunistically from one job to the next in search of more money and status. The climber's apparent commitment to the goals and programs of an organization is, in fact, likely to be an allegiance to the regime in power, whether this regime be the board, legislature, or chief executive. He thus systematically avoids dissenting from or criticizing organizational policies as well as interpersonal conflicts with superiors or important constituents. The climber is not excessively burdened with moral ambiguity or ethical conflicts and tends to resolve such matters as they arise, quickly and decisively. He values action, efficiency, and "getting things done." In short, his concern is with the "how" rather than the "why." It goes without saying that the climber is ambitious, but it is also true that he tends to be energetic and hardworking. The boundaries between work and personal life are extremely permeable, and frequently these dimensions become undifferentiated parts of his existence. The climber tends to become involved in a variety of community activities that bring him high visibility and contact with elites. It is these involvements that frequently provide opportunities for upward mobility.

It is probably most difficult to anticipate the decision-making style of the climber and thus his reaction to a specific proposal for change. In terms of Gawthrop's consolidative-innovative continuum, the climber's decision-making behavior would probably be characterized mainly by its inconsistency. That is, since he relates to his job opportunistically, one would expect him to act similarly regarding change. Accordingly, changes in public sentiment, funding patterns, or the views of important constituents are likely to be reflected in his decision-making behavior almost immediately. The climber's goal hierarchy makes him no more inherently disposed toward one style of decision making than another. If stability and continuity are the currency of the time, then he is most likely to take a consolidative approach. If experimentation is fashionable, then he is likely to encourage and support proposals for change.

There are, however, two factors which over time would seem to constrain the climber's decision-making inconsistency. The first is that the climber, concerned as he is with upward mobility, must establish some kind of track record, a history of accomplishments. Since this is more likely to occur if he is *doing* rather than *not doing* something, we would expect him to be inclined to innovation. It is also probably true that the climber cannot afford an extreme image. He can afford to be tagged neither as timid or unimaginative on the one hand nor as brash and revolutionary on the other. This being the case, one might expect the climber to operate in the middle ranges of the consolidative-innovative continuum but seldom, if ever, and certainly not for long, at one end or the other.

The *professional advocate*[14] does not deny the goals that are characteristic of the climber, particularly with regard to power and prestige. The distinction lies in what each considers instrumental as apart from ultimate values. The climber considers the acquisition of power and prestige of paramount importance; the substance of what he is engaged in, the social goals of the enterprise, are his vehicle. The professional advocate, on the other hand, may acquire prestige, status, and power and may indeed actively seek such resources; their acquisition, however, is likely either to follow from or be used in the service of achieving some organizational objective.

The professional advocate is committed to his organization as an instrument of service. This commitment is more often to an image of what the organization can be and do rather than to what it is and is doing. He is likely to be identified with its goals and policies not because, as is true with conservers and climbers, this protects or advances some personal interest, but rather because it most closely approximates his professional ideals. The word "approximates" is crucial here because the advocate is seldom satisfied with what his organization is accomplishing and is likely to be its most severe critic. However, his displeasure does not ordinarily take the form of cynicism but is rather more likely to be expressed as a continual search for new approaches, personnel with fresh ideas, additional funds, enlarged jurisdiction, etc. His dissatisfaction with what is leads him to experiment. Critical, ambitious, and sometimes even imperialistic, the advocate often finds himself in conflict not only with members of his own staff but with executives of other agencies and even, on occasion, his own board. His relations with those in authority stand in sharp contrast to the climber's. While the latter is likely to celebrate authority figures and defer to them on substantive issues, the advocate sees them as resources to be persuaded and enlisted in the cause of enhancing his organization's effectiveness.

Given this portrait of the professional advocate, one would expect his decision-making behavior to be strongly oriented toward innovation. This is likely to be reflected in a relatively high investment in searching the environment (both internal and external) for incipient or emerging trends, issues and problems, feedback regarding current program operations, and proposals for change. Since the professional advocate places considerable emphasis on informational input, his capacity to receive unorthodox or unpopular recommendations will probably be somewhat greater than that of either the conserver or the climber, as will be his ability to tolerate the uncertainty and tension involved in receiving and processing such a wide range of stimuli. Concerned as he is with problem solving and goal attainment, the advocate tends not to avoid rather considerable departures from existing policy and program directions, when such departures are in the interest of increased effectiveness. He is prepared, in short, to adopt fundamental and far-reaching changes and to bear the costs of instability and conflict that frequently accrue, if these changes promise an improved capacity for goal attainment.

While the professional advocate has a bias toward innovation, he can also be a staunch defender of the status quo if the changes suggested are contrary to the ideological or philosophical stance he espouses.

In summary, I have suggested in this section that administrative superiors, indeed all organizational actors, tend to behave in ways that will maximize certain personal goals that they consider most important. I have further suggested that a superior's goal hierarchy tends to be reflected in certain modal role orientations, most particularly in approaches to decision making when change is called for. These modal types are seldom observed in their pure form, but my contention is that the practitioner who is attempting to promote an innovation can utilize this typology as a point of departure for analyzing the resistance that he is likely to encounter from decision makers.

ORGANIZATIONAL DISTANCE

Another variable which appears to be crucial in assessing the potential resistance that may be encountered in efforts to change is what might be called *organizational distance*. In this context, organizational distance refers to the number of administrative levels between a subordinate who is making a proposal and the administrative superior who must ultimately decide upon it. All other things being equal, it is suggested that the greater the distance a proposal must traverse, the greater the likelihood that it will meet with resistance at the point of decision. Thus, if this premise is correct, one would expect to have greater success in gaining approval from an immediate superior than from, for instance, an agency executive who is three or four levels higher in the administrative hierarchy.

At the outset it is important to note that my concern is with those processes (forces and conditions) that are natural concomitants of organizational distance. These processes can be augmented or neutralized by the actors in a change scenario, that is, they can be consciously manipulated by subordinates and decision makers to affect the outcome of the change proposal. In the discussion that follows, however, I will focus only on ways in which distance itself can generate resistance to changes initiated by subordinates. Two major aspects are considered here: the processes that affect the substance and relevance of a proposal as it is communicated through one or more intermediaries; and the conditions under which the proposal is considered and decided upon.

The greater the number of intermediaries through which a proposal for change must be communicated, the more vulnerable it becomes to information loss, distortion, and delay.[15] One or more of these may have the effect of altering a proposal's substance or diminishing its timeliness.

First, it is in the nature of multilevel organizations that every subordinate must condense the information he conveys to his superior. Were this not the case, the sheer bulk of information emanating from below would soon grow to unmanageable proportions. The caseworker communicates only a portion (indeed, a small portion) of what he considers relevant information to his superior, who in turn further collapses the information for presentation to his superior. This "winnowing process"[16] occurs at each level and inevitably entails a certain amount of information loss. While proposals (suggestions, recommendations) are less subject to condensation than information bits, here too the pressures of time frequently require that they be simplified or abbreviated in the course of passing through the communication network. As a consequence, it is not at all unusual for a proposal initiated several levels down to be only a skeleton of itself when presented to the decision maker. That this occurs is evidenced by the frequency with which change agents can be heard to complain that their proposal was oversimplified or inadequately represented in the decision-making forum.

In addition to information loss, a proposal for change often becomes distorted as each intermediary inevitably filters it through his own perceptual screen. Values, vested interests, past experiences, feelings toward the practitioner—all these influence the intermediary's perception of what will be favorably or unfavorably received in the upper echelon. A proposal that may incur disfavor from superiors, for example, is often presented with somewhat less enthusiasm and vigor.

There is finally the matter of time. Since the timeliness of the proposal is often as crucial as its substance, delays that occur in the process of communicating across several administrative levels can have a determinate influence on the outcome. Such delays need not be motivated by opposition, although the popularity of phrases like "pigeonholing" and "sitting on" is testimony to the fact that they often are. More pertinent here is that intermediaries often delay transmitting a proposal because their superiors are preoccupied with other matters or overloaded.

Singly or in combination, these processes can have the effect of making a proposal for change less acceptable to decision makers. This need not occur inevitably, but it seems fair to conclude that the greater the number of intermediaries, the greater the likelihood that information loss, distortion, or delay will take its toll on a proposal for change.

Organizational distance would also seem to be important to an assessment of potential resistance insofar as it is related to the conditions under which change proposals are considered and decided upon. First, the further removed a practitioner is from the ultimate decision maker, the more likely it is that their respective organizational perspectives and criteria for decision will differ. The needs, interests, and priorities of incumbents in various echelons do differ, and these differences tend to become more sharply delineated as organizational distance grows. While these varying perspectives need not be in conflict, it frequently happens that they are.

Second, and not unrelated to the point just made, the more distance there is between the change agent and the decision maker, the less opportunity there will be for sustained face-to-face interaction between them. In very practical terms this means less opportunity for the change agent to elaborate, argue, persuade, and compromise. This is perhaps best illustrated by the not unusual experience of being given fifteen minutes on the crowded agenda of an executive staff or board meeting to present a proposal. The constraints of time, unfamiliarity, and differences in language become formidable barriers to a persuasive presentation. Under these circumstances, it is not unusual for the subordinate to feel that he has not adequately represented his recommendations. Contrast this with a proposal made to an immediate supervisor with whom the practitioner has day-to-day interaction: this context permits the actors to explore their respective points of view, probe motivations, develop common referents, and negotiate differences. The obvious point is that the context in which a proposal is made and a decision arrived at is itself an important determinant of the outcome.

Finally, the higher a change agent must go in the administrative hierarchy for decision, the more likely his proposal is to come into competition with the interests of other groups. At each successive level in the administrative hierarchy, the decision maker is confronted with an increasingly complex array of contending interests that must somehow be mediated. For the practitioner, this fact has important ramifications because it means, in effect, that as the array of competing interests becomes more varied and complex, his proposal will be weighed against a set of criteria that go beyond the merits of his proposal. The further removed the initiator of change is from the decision maker, the less likely he is to have the information needed to anticipate or counteract these competing interests.

In summary, then, I am suggesting that the distance between the initiator of change and the decision maker can itself be a crucial determinant of the amount of resistance that a proposal will encounter. There are, of course, ways to counteract or neutralize the consequences of distance, but before these can be developed, the change agent must be aware of their potential for generating resistance.

SUNK COSTS

The variable of *sunk costs*[17] may also constitute the source of resistance to change efforts initiated by administrative subordinates. Sunk costs refer to the investments that have been made by an organization (or its members) to develop and sustain any institutional arrangement or pattern of behavior that is currently in force. Investments are here defined broadly as inputs of money, time, energy, or personal commitment. They might include, for example, the staff time and energy that have been devoted to recruiting, developing, and maintaining foster homes over a period of time, or the funds that have been expended to train workers in a new mode of treatment (e.g., behavior modification). More specifically, sunk costs might be represented in the money that has been spent to remodel and furnish a building so that it can accommodate program activity. An equally important, if more subjective, element of sunk costs is the personal commitments made by members of an organization to an existing arrangement. It might be difficult, for instance, to attach a dollar figure to a social worker's effort to establish interdisciplinary team conferences on a surgical ward, but the worker will surely be able to attest to the energy costs that have been incurred in the process.

This latter aspect of sunk costs is frequently associated with length of employment in an organization.[18] That is, the longer a person has worked in an agency, the more likely he is to have a personal stake in its existent programs, procedures, and objectives. Since this dimension of sunk costs is subjective and often difficult to elicit (who would admit that he is opposed to change?), length of employment can sometimes be used to make an assessment of potential resistance. One way to gain an indication of resistance to innovation in a bureaucracy might be to sum the total number of years of employment for all persons in the department or unit that will be affected by the proposed change, and divide it by the number of employees. The dividend, when compared to those of other departments, may provide one measure of the relative opposition to be expected.[19]

Generally, it would appear that the greater the magnitude of an organization's investment in some arrangement or pattern of behavior, the more likely it is that a change in that arrangement will be resisted. Sunk costs, in other words, generate an organizational bias toward continuity. There are, of course, conditions that serve to counterbalance this bias. If, for example, the benefits gained from an investment have been less than anticipated, or existing arrangements have produced dysfunctional consequences (e.g., unfavorable community reaction, client dissatisfaction, loss of funding), an organization may be willing to write these costs off as a bad investment and strike out on a new course of action. External inducements that promise rewards greater than those currently received can also make it worthwhile for an agency to sacrifice its investments. Nevertheless, where sunk costs are large, organizations are not likely to make such judgments quickly. They are rather more likely to opt for continuity than for change.

IMPLICATIONS FOR CHANGE AGENTS

Assessing potential resistance to a proposal for change does not of necessity predict the fate of that proposal. Indeed, the purpose of being able to anticipate resistance is precisely that the change agent can mobilize resources and conduct interventions in a way that will decrease or neutralize opposition. Thus, it is my position that this kind of analysis is crucial preparation for a low-power subordinate who, with limited resources, wishes to maximize the effect of his efforts.

The action implications which flow from an analysis of resistance are manifold and cannot be fully explored here.[20] For illustrative purposes, however, I will suggest several ways in which the kind of analysis previously developed can inform a practitioner's interventions.

Feasibility

A change agent's ability to achieve a goal is very likely to depend upon whether he chooses a feasible goal in the first place. But how is feasibility assessed? Following Morris and Binstock, we would contend that "if the proposed innovations are resisted by the target organization, the *feasibility* [emphasis added] of the planner's goals is determined by his capacity for overcoming that resistance."[21] An analysis of organizational resistance can be useful in determining feasibility by putting into sharper perspective the resources the change agent will need to achieve approval and implementation of his goals. If the practitioner finds that one or more of the sources of resistance are likely to be operative in the change situation, he is then in a position to appraise whether it is possible to mobilize the resources that will be needed to overcome that opposition. Is it likely, for example, that he will be able to generate sufficient pressure to convince a "conserver" decision maker to adopt a change that requires a major redirection of organizational focus? Can he reasonably expect to convince such a decision maker that his interests (goals) are better served by anticipating change than by waiting until it is foisted upon the agency? If the conserver approves a proposal, can a staff that is heavily committed to the status quo be expected to implement it?

Answers to questions like these, even when one allows for the vagaries of prediction, can assist the change agent in deciding whether the resources he has, or can likely mobilize, are sufficient to the task at hand. If they are not, he may find it preferable to redefine his goals in terms that are more consistent with the resources he can muster.

Focus of Intervention

An assessment of resistance can also aid the practitioner in determining where to focus his interventions. If he finds, for instance, that the decision maker with a professional-advocate orientation is favorably disposed to a proposed change but declines to give approval because of anticipated adverse effects on the morale or efficiency of staff, then it may be a better use of the subordinate's time and energy to focus his attention on the staff. Efforts to persuade or influence them to accept a proposal may not only free the decision maker to give his approval but insure that the change, once authorized, will be effectively implemented.

In another situation, the change agent may find that the major obstacle to gaining approval for his recommendations is simply his failure to represent his ideas adequately to the decision maker. Here again, he may decide that it is not pressure upon the superior which is indicated so much as efforts to increase the likelihood that his proposal will be given a full hearing. This might be accomplished by cultivating the support of intermediaries in the communication network, dramatizing the proposal to draw the attention of the decision maker, going around the administrative hierarchy directly to the superior, etc. Finally, in those cases where the administrative superior's role orientation and decision-making style resemble those of the "climber," the practitioner may find that a most effective point of leverage is to achieve the support of some community influential who has access to the superior.

Type of Intervention

An assessment of resistance may also enable the practitioner to make a more informed choice of strategy. Let us assume for the moment that an administrative subordinate is proposing a change that is both high in generality and basic in character. Let us further assume that the worst possible combination of resistive forces is at work, that is, a conserver decision maker at some distant point high up in the hierarchy and a staff that has for many years worked at developing and maintaining the agency's programs. Under these circumstances, the change agent who would pursue a consensually oriented strategy, based solely on information giving and rational persuasion, is very probably doomed to fail. A more suitable strategy in this scenario is likely to be one that makes it costly for the organization to pursue its present course, one that assumes fundamental differences between the subordinate and the decision maker, in short, a strategy characterized by aggressiveness, stridency, and coercion. The practitioner may not be inclined to pay or impose the costs that are associated with this approach, but he should not assume that the kind of change he is seeking can be accomplished without this magnitude of commitment.

On the other hand, one who is seeking approval for a modest program or procedural change in a relatively new agency with a professional-advocate executive and a shallow hierarchy is equally misled if he adopts a conflictually oriented strategy. To do so under such circumstances may not only elicit spurious resistance to his proposal but use up personal credit the change agent might wish to call on in future endeavors.

CONCLUSION

This paper has been an effort to translate selected aspects of organizational theory into analytic concepts that can have some practical utility for administrative subordinates who are attempting to promote change in their agencies. The four variables discussed—the nature of the change proposal, the decision maker, organizational distance, and sunk costs—are suggested as analytic focal points for the practitioner who wishes to assess the resistance he is likely to encounter in seeking change. While a certain degree of resistance is to be expected in virtually any proposal for change, the contention of this paper is that it will vary significantly from one situation to another depending upon the particular configuration of variables that obtains. It is further argued that an assessment of the quality and quantity of resistance is crucial if the change agent is to make an informed choice of intervention strategy.

It is important to note that the four variables discussed in this paper are only some of those that will determine an organization's resistance to change. Others that could not be dealt with here, but which require attention, are the nature of an organization's external environment (including its sources of legitimation and funding), its stage of development, and its technology. All of these appear to have some bearing on resistance and should eventually be part of an analytic scheme employed by change agents.

It is my hope that this paper serves simultaneously to provide low-power change agents with a beginning framework for organizational analysis and to stimulate further inquiry into this crucial aspect of change methodology.

NOTES

1. See, e.g., Robert Presthus, *The Organizational Society* (New York: Random House, Vintage Books, 1962); and Warren G. Bennis, "Beyond Bureaucracy," in *American Bureaucracy*, ed. Warren G. Bennis (Chicago: Aldine Publishing Co., 1970), pp. 3–16. Critiques more specific to social welfare can be found in Irving Piliaven, "Restructuring the Provision of Social Services," *Social Work* 13 (1968):34–41; and Robert Pruger, "The Good Bureaucrat," *Social Work* 18 (1973):26–32.
2. Hereafter the terms "practitioner" and "administrative subordinate" are used interchangeably with "change agent."
3. See, e.g., Alvin Zander, "Resistance to Change: Its Analysis and Prevention," in *Social Work Administration*, ed. Harry Schatz (New York: Council on Social Work Education, 1970), pp. 253–57; and Paul Lawrence, "How to Deal with Resistance to Change," *Harvard Business Review* 47 (1969):4–13, 166–76.

4. This scheme for classifying depth of change is adopted from Anthony Downs, *Inside Bureaucracy* (Boston: Little, Brown & Co., 1967), pp. 167–68.
5. The empirical evidence on this point is scanty and somewhat inconsistent. Weinberger's analysis of agency executive behavior led him to the conclusion that administrators tend to resist making decisions that involve the reordering of goals or the reallocation of resources (Paul E. Weinberger, "Executive Inertia and the Absence of Program Modification," in *Perspectives on Social Welfare*, ed. Paul E. Weinberger [New York: Macmillan Co., 1969], pp. 387–94). Tangential but apparently supportive evidence is reported by both Epstein and Heffernan, who found agency executives to be conservative in their attitudes toward social change strategies that are likely to have a disequilibrating effect on agency behavior (Irwin Epstein, "Organizational Careers, Professionalization and Social Worker Radicalism," *Social Service Review* 44 [1970]:123–31; Joseph Heffernan, "Political Activity and Social Work Executives," *Social Work* 9 [1964]:18–23). A somewhat different profile of executives' reactions to change emerges from Hanlan's partial replication of Epstein's study. He concludes, e.g., "On the basis of these limited findings, these executives cannot be characterized as a group within the profession who are most resistant to social action strategies," and later, "The study findings reported here, while limited to a small selected sample, provide some challenge to the assumption that these social work executives are co-opted into conservative and non-social action directions by nature of their occupancy of hierarchical positions" (Archie Hanlan, "Social Work Executives. Recent Graduates, and Social Action Strategies," unpublished paper [n.d.], pp. 11, 13). One source of the inconsistency reported in these studies may be the fact that executives, as I suggest here, fall into subgroupings with distinctly different value orientations.
6. In the context of a single decision-making episode, insufficient information, emotional stress, inability to foresee consequences, etc., may prevent the decision maker from rationally choosing, from among the available courses of action, those that will maximize the potential for goal attainment.
7. This is a modification of a list suggested by Downs, pp. 84–85. Goals 6, 7, and 8 are different from those suggested by Downs. The modification is necessary to reflect some of the distinct features of the culture of social work.
8. This goal category refers to those decision makers whose primary goal is to preserve or maintain an agency because of their commitment to some broad principle like the maintenance of ethnic identity or the value of private or volunteer philanthropy. The preservation of the agency becomes a vehicle for promulgating a particular ideology which, in the administrator's view, serves the public interest.
9. This typology was constructed from an analysis of several classification schemes that attempt to relate goals and role orientation to the behavior of organizational officials. While these schemes conceptualize organizational behavior in rather different ways, there are notable areas of agreement and overlap among them (Downs, pp. 88–111; Presthus [n. 1 above], pp. 164–268; Alvin Gouldner, "Cosmopolitans and Locals: Toward an Analysis of Latent Social Roles," *Administrative Science Quarterly* 2 [1957]: 281–306,

444–80; and Leonard Reissman, "A Study of Role Conceptions in Bureaucracy," *Social Forces* 27 [1949]: 305–10). The designations "conserver" and "climber" are borrowed from Downs.

10. See Downs, pp. 96–99.

11. Louis C. Gawthrop, *Bureaucratic Behavior in the Executive Branch: An Analysis of Organizational Change* (New York: Free Press, 1969), p. 181.

12. *Ibid.*, p. 182.

13. Presthus (pp. 164–204) refers to these officials as upward mobiles.

14. The professional advocate shows characteristics of Presthus's "ambivalent" and Gouldner's "cosmopolitan," but differs from both because of his high commitment to the agency.

15. An elaboration of impediments to upward communication in bureaucracies can be found in Daniel Katz and Robert L. Kahn, *The Social Psychology of Organizations* (New York: John Wiley & Sons, 1966), pp. 245–47; and Gordon Tullock, *The Politics of Bureaucracy* (Washington, D.C.: Public Affairs Press, 1965), pp. 137–41.

16. Downs, p. 117.

17. See James G. March and Herbert A. Simon, *Organizations* (New York: John Wiley & Sons, 1966), p. 173; and Downs, pp. 195–96.

18. Jerald Hage and Michael Aiken, *Social Change in Complex Organizations* (New York: Random House, 1970), p. 97. Some functional aspects of personal commitment to organizational arrangements are discussed in Donald Klein, "Some Notes on the Dynamics of Resistance to Change: The Defender Role," in *Concepts for Social Change*, ed. Goodwin Watson (Washington, D.C.: National Training Laboratories, 1967), pp. 26–36.

19. Victor Thompson, *Bureaucracy and Innovation* (University: University of Alabama Press, 1969), pp. 61–88. See this source for suggested approaches to measuring resistance to innovation in complex organizations.

20. A further discussion of factors that should be considered in choosing and planning change strategies can be found in Rino Patti and Herman Resnick, "Changing the Agency from Within," *Social Work* 17 (1972):48–57.

21. Robert Morris and Robert H. Binstock, *Feasible Planning for Social Change* (New York: Columbia University Press, 1966), p. 94.

PART V

Trends and Context in Administering Human Services

Editor's Introduction

Like social work generally, social administration tends to reflect the social, economic, and political ethos in which it is nurtured. The relative preoccupation with the management of social organizations fluctuates with the demands made upon it. This is particularly true with respect to the availability or unavailability of resources. An expansive economy generates growth and emphasizes creativity for program development, discovery of new needs, and the broadening of existing efforts. An economy of scarcity restricts resources, engenders cutbacks, and places greater stress on efficiency and accountability.

With its promise of continued economic growth and expansion, the post-World War II period of the fifties and sixties placed great stress on innovation and change in the nation's struggle to contain the social problems that seemed endemic. A burgeoning economy could assure social planners that new theories and insights into pervasive social malaise would find ready support in national policy and governmental largesse. Grants from federal and regional agencies as well as national and local voluntary foundations were eagerly promoted and as eagerly sought by universities, other social institutions, and community action groups.

These grants focused largely on programmatic concerns—new ways of doing things—and on testing the theories that underlie these efforts. Vast numbers of new and innovative programs got underway with relatively little attention paid to the availability of people trained to manage and direct them.

With time, the explosive growth in government-financed social programs came into conflict with a narrowed base of financial resources. This had the effect of shifting attention to the ways in which managerial skill could, through tighter control and more efficient operation, help contain the growing drain on the national economy. More and more one heard about cost containment, cost-benefit ratios, and cutback management. New patterns of budgeting and financial accounting became prominent.

Striking developments in computer technology and information systems provided a new base for exploiting these developments. As computer hardware became affordable by the general run of social service agencies, new skills in management became highlighted.

In the social and related human services, administration and management began to assume a significance in the seventies and eighties far beyond anything previously noted. A spate of books appeared with increasing frequency during the past decade. Schools of social work more frequently incorporated programs for training administrators. The periodical literature expanded exponentially, and included a new journal devoted entirely to the subject.

Heightened economic austerity in the eighties, with its concomitant regressive social policies, has further sharpened the push for competent, efficient, tough-minded management of social programs. In response, concern has arisen for the integrity of service objectives and meeting the needs of people increasingly affected by social dislocation and unemployment, given the reduction in public and private resources for social programs. This conflict is evident in the stress on efficiency versus effectiveness, on professional versus bureaucratic goals, on instrumental versus terminal values.

In the current social climate of conservatism and negativism toward the achievement of the welfare state, social work has been buffeted from many sides. Not only have public resources for development, education, and research been reduced to a trickle, but new challenges have simultaneously appeared from the professional community. Schools of business administration and public administration institutes and programs have more and more staked their claims to competence in a field that has largely been the domain of social work. Additionally, in the last decade, claims have been made for a new profession of human services, with a national organization, increasing numbers of college concentrations, and accreditation of degree programs. At the same time, more and more attention is given to the field of nonprofit organizations, of which the social services are seen as a part. These developments are largely stimulated by special institutes and the offshoots of schools of business. These and other professional strains see the huge welfare "industry" as a new opportunity for their graduates and trainees.

The selections in this section examine the issues, future trends, and contexts that will attend the practice of administration in the human services in the decade ahead. Sarri points to some of the problems in social policy that will demand the attention of social administrators. In particular, she deals with the declassification of social work positions in public services and the continuing, pervasive problems associated with institutional racism and sexism. Issues of ethical practice, of worker accountability to clients and others, of declining resources, and of organizational effectiveness are likely to be prominent in the coming period. Sarri touches briefly on other trends she feels will occupy administrators. They concern public-private relationships and increasing reliance on private sector involvement in providing social services; the centralization-decentralization dilemmas; pressures for participation in management decision making; the increasing reliance on computerized information systems; the greater stress on budget and fiscal management skill. These and other developments present managers with clearly labeled challenges. Social workers increasingly trained in managerial skill hold promise for greater competence in the direction of service organizations, a competence that will be all the more necessary if the values of service to clients in need are to be enhanced.

The changing economy and concomitant ideological crises confronting the welfare state underlie Hasenfeld's analysis of the developing environmental context for the human services. He sees an economy of scarcity and the privatization of services foreshadowing changes in the patterns of social agency management in the period ahead. Although decline and retrenchment can be expected to be widespread, there may be hope for a revitalized effort to create a base for survival and renewal, accompanied by political action on behalf of the welfare state. Implicitly, Hasenfeld suggests an historical sense of ebb and flow in social policy. At the moment, the ethos is regressive, with a drive to curtail services and compel cutback management. But in a different environment, the ethos may change. Lessons learned now about organizational management and the professional preparation of administrators may, in time, bring about opportunity for growth and creativity in the interest of essential client service.

25

Management Trends in the Human Services in the 1980s

ROSEMARY C. SARRI

INTRODUCTION

It is obvious that we have entered a new era in which all who are concerned about social welfare and the social work profession must think, plan, and implement innovations that will enable us to meet a growing demand for human services with stable or perhaps declining resources. Rather than attempt to outline strategies from a 1980 baseline, I prefer to begin this examination of the problems within a historical perspective. I will confine myself to the past quarter century. One can characterize the late 1940s and 1950s as a time of gradual rebuilding and reaction to World War II and the significant social policy changes of the 1930s. Toward the end of the 1950s there were numerous proposals for new policies and programs to alleviate racial discrimination, dependency and neglect, crime and delinquency, and mental illness. Many of these proposals were accepted and rapidly expanded during the social reform period of the 1960s. In fact, several were integrated into major social movements that sought to eliminate poverty, insure civil liberties, enhance educational opportunity, reduce crime, and acknowledge the right of all citizens to treatment and service. The Advisory Council on Public Welfare in 1966 entitled its statement of recommendations, "Having the Power, We Have the Duty—to Strike Away the Barriers to Full Participation in Our Society." Then, the tragic events associated with the long Vietnam War quickly put an end to that optimistic goal. Moreover, some even questioned the validity of the goals of elimination of poverty, racism, and so forth. Throughout the 1970s skepticism and pessimism continued despite the fact that income maintenance, health, criminal justice, and educational program expenditures all grew at unprecedented rates.

In 1950, the total federal, state, and local expenditures in the public welfare sector amounted to 12.7 billion dollars. That grew to 177.4 billion by 1975, an increase of 1300 percent (Skolnick & Dales, 1976). However, despite the growth in terms of expenditures and numbers of clients reached, we have few social indicators that suggest that the situation in 1980 is relatively improved over 1970—perhaps because structural unemployment, substance abuse, housing and school integration, and problems of youth have become more chronic and complex. We all recognize the tremendous growth in the size, diversity, and complexity of the welfare enterprise, but far less evidence is available about increases in effectiveness or efficiency in service delivery to clientele, or about the impact of services that are received.

Unfortunately, the growth in size and scope was not accompanied by a comparable growth in the legitimacy of these programs in the minds of the public. If anything, there has been a diminution in support for traditional social welfare intervention and for professional social work in sectors where social problems are the most severe and where individuals are at the greatest risk.

Other critics assert that the social welfare establishment has not been effective in solving social problems such as poverty because that has never been the "real" goal. Instead, the argument goes as follows: the welfare system is an institution of formal social control to keep the working classes subordinate and healthy so that they will be able to contribute to the attainment of the goals laid down by those in power. But even this proposition now seems questionable when one examines the policies and programs for youth and young adults in our society. They seem to be preparing them for a life of dependency and inability to participate fully in the society.

Social work as a profession has reflected the societal swings from social reform to political conservatism and pattern maintenance. Thus, in the past several years we have witnessed greater concern with professionalizing activity. If, however, the society shifts again to mandate new social policies and programs that require active advocacy by the professional, it is probable that we will see a trend in that direction. We can also hope that individual social workers and the profession collectively will take a more active role in initiating that change as Chauncey Alexander (1979) has suggested.

It is, therefore, within this broad scenario that we will consider the issues and opportunities faced by those concerned with management of human services in the 1980s. Although we are less likely to be naively optimistic about what can be accomplished in the next decade to resolve or impact social problems, many suggest that more effective and humane management of human services is critical if there is to be a genuine and serious attempt to meet the challenging demands.

MANAGEMENT ISSUES CONFRONTING HUMAN SERVICE ORGANIZATIONS

One of the first issues that must be addressed is identification of the preferred conceptual model of the human service organization for the development of strategies, principles, and directions for management. Administration in these organizations has long resisted straightforward description, analysis, or prescription in terms of the major theoretical perspectives on formal organizations. Street (1978) notes that many of the studies of these organizations have focused attention only on those that maintain or expand problems rather than on management and other technologies that reduce or solve problems. As a consequence, administrators and practitioners are rightly skeptical about the utility of social science contributions for their tasks.

Initially one must consider how the management of the human services is alike or different from management of other complex organizations. Cyert (1975) argues that there are more similarities than differences, but he also acknowledges profound differences with respect to means for defining and increasing productivity, controlling resources and budgeting, and performance evaluation. On the other hand, the noted business management consultant Peter Drucker (1973) emphasizes the differences:

> The one basic difference between a service institution and a business is the way the service institution is paid. Businesses (other than monopolies) are paid for satisfying customers. . . . Service institutions, by contrast, are typically paid out of a budget allocation. Their revenues are allocated from a general revenue stream that is not tied to what they are doing. . . . [pp. 49–50]

Human service organizations are mandated and supported by external bodies to achieve certain goals for the society's well-being. Their substantive goals are to process and change people in socially approved ways. Moreover, people who are served are both the major input and output of the organization. Problems arise because their goals are usually ambiguous, indeterminate, and precarious in the environing society. In addition, the persons served are self-activating and capable of frustrating organizational efforts. These organizations pursue multiple goals and this experience is problematic because priorities must be established among potentially contradictory objectives such as control, rehabilitation, custody, protection, and the provision of opportunity. Because of all these attributes, plus the fact that they are dependent for resources on external bodies, it is imperative that the human service administrator be fully cognizant of the opportunities and constraints so that he or she can act as "expert-advocate" of the program managed rather than merely as a functionary for those who provide fiscal resources (Gummer, 1979).

It is also argued that managers of human service organizations must be knowledgeable about social service technologies as well as needs of clientele. They must be prepared to engage in political exchange to support those service technologies that will promote societal well-being (Titmuss, 1969). Selznick (1957) argues that it is of critical importance that executives exert leadership in the promotion and protection of critical values.

Although I have highlighted what appear to be critical differences between the human service organization and organizations that pursue profit and individual goals, there are many management technologies useful in all formal organizations—goal setting, resource allocation, personnel selection and control, assessment and evaluation, staff training and development. However, I do assert that what is of critical importance is employment of these technologies in ways that do not damage the substantive goals of the organization nor inhibit fair, humane, and just interactions with clients and citizens. Those who have studied administration in human service organizations adopt varied models to serve their respective purposes. These can be ordered in a continuum from wholehearted acceptance of a highly rational closed-system approach based on scientific management principles (Task Force, 1976; Shapira, 1971) to a mid-continuum perspective such as that of Patti (1978), Vinter (1963), and Hasenfeld and English (1974). The model at the opposite end of the continuum can be termed the "political economy" model as proposed by Zald (1971) and further explicated by Perrow (1978), Street, Martin, and Gordon (1979), and March and Olsen (1976).

The scientific management approach of the Task Force of the National Conference on Social Welfare (1976) emphasizes management to enhance front-line worker performance—"a human resources model of management." Among its critical elements are clearly articulated and operational goals, a case-management strategy of service delivery with explicit requirements for worker accountability, objective evaluation, simplification of bureaucratic procedures, and continual attention to problem solving and innovation. Patti, Vinter, and Hasenfeld and English argue for use of rational procedures and tested technologies, but they recognize the open system nature of the human service organization and the critical influence of the external environment in shaping and changing the agency. Those who advocate the political economy model start with the assumption that the organization is embedded in a larger social system in which the allocation of power and resources determines the goals of the organization. These goals are shaped by various interest groups within and outside the organization. Because of the "weak coupling" within the network that comprises social welfare, this approach is said to be more useful because it recognizes the disjointed features and processes. This approach also directs attention to the critical role of organizational resources and the impact that struggles for their control have on the organization.

Selection of one of these approaches as an organizing construct for the management of a particular organization should be made on the basis of an assessment of the external environment as well as the internal attributes. We lack an adequate framework regarding the management of human service organizations, but a critical first step in the delineation of principles is awareness of the organizational model that underlies administration.

DECLINING RESOURCES AND CRITERIA FOR THEIR ALLOCATION

A second issue concerns the decline in resources perceived as being available for social welfare. Social services and human service organizations depend for their continued existence on some form of economic surplus that is available for redistribution. Whether the redistribution takes place depends on political value decisions. What is deemed legitimate is ultimately a value question. Thus, questions are raised today about the capacity of our economic system to meet the legitimate demands placed upon it, and the situation is further confounded by the inability of the political system to aid the society in redefining and reallocating these claims '(Rein, 1977). As a result there is pressure for stringent controls on expenditures, for zero-based budgeting procedures, reliance on voluntary and private sector provision of social services, and rigorous program evaluation. Any one of these procedures, if applied properly, has the potential for enhancing organizational performance. But when they are covertly utilized only to reduce resource ·expenditure without respect to need, it is not surprising that social work practitioners show little enthusiasm for them. Managers must develop mechanisms for resolving these differences among contending parties.

ORGANIZATIONAL EFFECTIVENESS
AND PROGRAM EVALUATION

Interest in organizational effectiveness and program evaluation is likely to be emphasized in the next decade as much as it has been in the past several years. These two concepts are interrelated theoretically as well as in practice. Organizational effectiveness has a broader theoretical base than evaluation, but our knowledge of the former can be enhanced by application of evaluation procedures and knowledge. Similarly, theories of organizational effectiveness can be utilized to call attention to subsystems and their interrelationships. Evaluators thus can gain a more balanced view of performance throughout the organization, and such knowledge may be particularly useful in middle-level management.

Social workers have often greatly overpromised what they could deliver with respect to the impact and outcomes from their services. Evaluation findings generally indicate that few startling results can be achieved. As a result administrators need to be cautious about the quality of service that can be routinely delivered and about the utility of arbitrary standards set by external bodies on the basis of some consensus about desired values.

WORKER ACCOUNTABILITY
AND CONSUMER SATISFACTION

Closely linked to the issues that point to the need for evaluation to enhance effectiveness and resource allocation are the demands for evaluation that are being increasingly made by consumers of our services—the clients. They are concerned about obtaining more effective and prompt service and about insuring worker accountability. Moreover, court decisions increasingly emphasize the consumers' right to service, to use of the least restrictive alternative when custody is required, and so forth. Implementation of court directives also necessitates systematic evaluation. The issue then becomes one of determining whose interests will have priority and how each can be served.

Research findings indicate that when client consumers actually participate in meaningful decision making, they are more positive and satisfied about the agency and its program, *and* they are more highly motivated to comply with treatment or service requirements (Cooper, 1979). Similarly, findings from research on staff participation in management decision making also indicates that in decentralized organizations, the quality of service delivery will have a higher priority for staff. Moreover, staff then are more satisfied about the nature and conditions of their work. These latter factors are noted in several studies in a variety of human service organizations as being more highly valued than salary increases or security (Cooper, 1979). Obviously the resolution of problems associated with decentralized vs. centralized decision-making structures are difficult, as Glisson and Martin (1978) note. Their studies confirm those of others: that for organizational survival, resource procurement, expansion, and growth, centralized decision structures are preferable because productivity and efficiency are emphasized. On the other hand, to achieve greater client and staff satisfaction, quality and effectiveness factors are more important and these fare best under decentralized structures. Thus human service administrators are forced into the political arena in their attempts to resolve these dilemmas.

THE DECLINE OF SOCIAL WORK POSITIONS IN THE PUBLIC SECTOR ORGANIZATIONS

It is widely noted that there has been an absolute and relative decline in the numbers of professionally trained social workers in management roles in the public social services (Gummer, 1979). Pressures for declassification of social work positions are heard throughout the country, but social work professionals and educators have been unable or unwilling to adapt to the changing needs in the public welfare sectors. Some now assert that they have lost control of key administrative decision-making positions at the federal and state levels because of the lack of formal training in scientific approaches to management. Those who offer this observation also suggest that social work should move closer to the business and industrial community by maximizing rationality and scientific management. Strangely enough, this is happening at the time where there is a growing realization in the business-industrial sectors that the latter procedures are no longer the definitive answer to the problems they face. The revolution effected in the mid-seventies by changes in the cost of energy indicate to managers in the private profit sector that uncontrolled external factors have profound effects to which management can only respond.

We have argued in this paper that professional social work knowledge is necessary and desirable for the effective management of the human service organization. However, greater concern must be shown for program development, control, delivery, and evaluation rather than with maintenance of the status quo. Gummer (1979) asserts that professional social work training is no longer the preferred preparation for managerial responsibility in public welfare, and he chastises professional schools for their lethargy in responding to the need for more effective training. He suggests:

> Models of managerial practice in social welfare must be created that will enable social workers to use the new technologies of management within the normative framework of their field. . . . While new curricula must be designed such that a change will produce results only if ways can be found to bring the necessary kinds of expertise into schools of social work. . . . The one function of social work that has the strongest claim to legitimacy in the public domain is the care of the dependent, deprived, debilitated, and demoralized citizens of this society. [pp. 16–18]

INSTITUTIONALIZED RACISM AND SEXISM REMAIN PROBLEMATIC IN SOCIAL AGENCIES

Despite the fact that social work is directed toward the reduction and elimination of racism and sexism, the implementation of effective affirmative action programs is still lacking and poses a serious issue for the 1980s. Although information is far less adequate than one would desire, the evidence remains overwhelming that key administrative and policy positions in human service organizations are filled by white, male, middle-class persons, while minorities and women occupy subordinate and direct service positions (Kerson & Alexander, 1979; McDonough, 1979; Mahaffey, 1976; Belon & Gould, 1977; Perlmutter & Alexander, 1978). What is even more disturbing is that, as with other professions, there has been a substantial deterioration of the status of women in administrative positions in the last quarter century. The NASW survey in 1976 indicated that only 16 percent of the responding agencies were directed by women that year, whereas in 1950 44 percent of those agencies had female executives. In both cases approximately two-thirds of the line staff were female. Overall 37 percent of male, professionally trained social workers occupy administrative positions, while only 18 percent of the females have such responsibility. Similar patterns can be observed for minorities, for the constituency least represented in decision-making roles are black and Hispanic females.

Data with respect to minority representation on boards indicate that minorities and the poor are greatly underrepresented despite the fact that most agencies in the voluntary sector now receive substantial public tax dollars for services provided. Obviously these findings are of particular import for minority and female staff who are thereby jeopardized, but this situation also has negative consequences for client consumers as Rausch (1979), Dinerman (1977), and Kanter (1978) indicate. Rausch

(1979) and Davenport and Reims (1978) provide information on distorted perceptions of client behavior because of gender-linked ideologies and beliefs. Kanter (1978) argues that low achievement orientation reflects adaptive responses to situations of low status, power, and mobility. Women and blacks predominate in such positions. McDonough (1979) notes that while social work administrators as a whole are committed to fight discrimination, they lack awareness of structural constraints that operate to undermine their efforts, and they have not responded to the problem at the organizational managerial level. Needed are thorough reviews of job ladders and mobility patterns; joint performance appraisal systems; and systems for job rotation, flex time, job sharing, and job redesign. All of these areas can be researched and changed even if few additional resources are made available to the organizations.

ETHICAL ISSUES IN THE MANAGEMENT OF HUMAN SERVICES DESERVE MORE SERIOUS CONSIDERATION

Ethical issues pervade every function and position in the human service organization (Levy, 1979). Issues concerning organizational loyalty, expediting of services to clients, conflicts of interest between staff, and clients re professional practice are but a few examples of such issues. A study by Finch (1978) of twelve agencies produced some fascinating findings with respect to organizational priorities. He observed that accountability to funding sources was acknowledged as the highest priority, with the following alternatives of lesser importance to the respondents: improve the quality of services, expand the number of clients, increase staff morale, minimize cost, or innovate new services.

We Americans pride ourselves on concern about human rights and assert that our society was founded on principles of fairness, humaneness, and justice. However, these principles are honored more in the breach than in reality. There is growing concern about social responsibility with respect to the rights of clients and consumers, affirmative action, and participatory management. Some, such as Savas (1978), suggest that equity must be considered as a criterion in evaluating organizational performance along with effectiveness and efficiency.

Society in general and clients in particular are no longer satisfied with "good intentions." The morality of service delivery and administrative processes require more attention than they have received. Lewis (1977) suggested that clients deserve compensation when they suffer deprivations as a result of the way in which services are organized and delivered. Those who have had experiences in the criminal justice, mental health, or public welfare systems in the past decade can point to numerous examples of deprivations of this type (Cooper, 1976). Lewis further argues that agencies must adopt the ethical principles to guide the development of their service programs to insure that the most disadvantaged among the eligible recipients of their services are not further disadvantaged by the service itself and the manner in which it is provided.

TRENDS—A BRIEFER LOOK

The issues identified thus far appear to be the most critical ones that demand immediate attention in the management of human services. But there are several other trends that can be linked to or follow from these issues. In concluding this chapter, I wish to identify several of these briefly, with the suggestion that this set is more illustrative than comprehensive.

Private-Public Sector Interactions

The magnitude of involvement of private/voluntary agencies in delivering social services funded by public tax dollars is likely to continue and may even expand further, although the rate of growth will not be as great as it has been in the past five years (Kramer, 1979; Smith, 1975). Under provisions of Title XX, CETA, LEAA, mental health, and other federally funded social service programs there has been strong encouragement for contracting services from the private sector. In fact, some titles of this legislation require that services be purchased from the private sector. Only now are we becoming aware of some of the problems that may be associated with substantial reliance on the private sector for major categories of services. Preliminary findings from evaluation of Title XX, for example, indicate that the middle class and those with minor, rather than serious and chronic problems, have received a disproportionate share of services under Title XX.

Centralization-Decentralization

Simultaneous pressures for both centralization and decentralization of organizational structure are likely to continue to be observed. This pattern reflects developmental requirements of organizations, and as Kaufman (1971) suggested, they are likely to be present most of the time. The critical task for management is to assess what strategy of centralization is required to enhance performance toward goal attainment at a specific time in organizational development.

Participation in Management Decision Making

Closely linked to concerns about centralization are those involving the levels of participation in decision making by staff and clients. It appears likely that pressures for participation will continue to grow in many agencies as a consequence of external and internal pressures for participation. Moreover, research evidence appears substantial that job dissatisfaction and strain can be reduced by increasing participation in organizational decision making (Karasek, 1979). Participation is also positively related to reduced turnover and—given the significance of the latter problem in protective services for adults and children, in criminal justice programs, and in programs for the chronically ill and handicapped—such conditions urgently need improvement. Participatory management may also facilitate the achievement of affirmative action goals and the development of management strategies that will facilitate enhanced performance by all staff and clients.

Information Systems

Information systems to facilitate management decision making, practitioner problem solving, and program evaluation will continue to proliferate in complexity and magnitude in most human service organizations for several years to come. It is certainly possible that by the end of this decade, the vast majority of social agencies will have fully automated information systems that enhance the potential for efficient and rapid responses to clients while providing the basis for effective evaluation of output and impact. Microcomputer technology is already sufficiently developed that it can be used on a cost effective basis by most social agencies today (Schoech, 1979). These relatively inexpensive systems are "in-house" and "on-line" interactive systems capable of being utilized by most agency personnel with a minimal amount of training. Obviously any information system if it is to be truly effective must be designed with reference to the service technologies utilized by the agency.

Budgetary and Fiscal Management

Requirements for budgetary constraint are likely to continue to increase for the foreseeable future and demands for fiscal accountability will become more and more stringent. Even under the most optimistic view of the next decade fiscal control will be a priority problem for managers. Continual training of human service management in fiscal planning and control is urgently needed because these responsibilities cannot be delegated to accountants or other staff who are unfamiliar with client or agency characteristics.

In the past there has been a tendency to assert that programs need to find ways in which almost every program can be improved without additional resources. Obviously many programs have always received insufficient resources, but nonetheless we will need to concern ourselves with efficiency in service delivery more than we have.

Research-Based Practice Models

The growth of models for research-based social work practice can be expected to accelerate and should be welcomed by managers of human service organizations. These models will facilitate program evaluation and provide the basis for rationalizing the delivery of interpersonal technologies that often have been difficult to describe and defend. The utility of this approach is illustrated by Sundel and Homan (1979) in their model for management of a preventive child welfare service program. They emphasized how and why careful consideration must be given to problem assessment and the search for alternative solutions if one is to be able to measure program impact.

Social Work in Industrial Settings

Expanded development and delivery of social services in industrial settings can be expected in the next decade. This growth will be manifested in the volume of service delivery, in the areas and types of technologies included, and in the range of interorganizational structures that will be utilized. This growth will provide a challenge and an opportunity to design new collaborative arrangements between the public and private sectors. It would be most regrettable if this development were ignored or opposed, as some have suggested.

CONCLUSION

Thus, it seems that our expectations for the management of human services in the 1980s are high and provide all with substantial challenge. But the strategies and tasks are such that they can be analyzed and ordered on a priority scale to determine what is most appropriate for each organization. The problems facing the human service organization in the decade ahead require nothing less than excellence in their management, as well as in any other area of organizational endeavor. To date, our evidence suggests that it is more belief and hearsay that professionally trained social workers with competence in management are not as capable as persons trained in business or public administration. The goals of these organizations are multiple, often contradictory, and involve precarious social values. Thus there are no panaceas for the administration of such organizations—and let us hope that during the 1980s this fallacy will be recognized as such.

There have been deficits in the management of social agencies in the past, but these deficits can be identified and corrected. Social work managers must come to view themselves as properly responsible for the delivery of social services in accord with values and principles accepted by the profession since its founding.

REFERENCES

Belon, C., & Katayun, G. Not even equals: Sex related salary inequities. *Social Work*, November 1977, *22*, 466–471.

Cooper, T. Untoward outcomes of health care—who is liable? *Public Health Reports*, November 1976.

Cyert, R. *The management of non-profit organizations: With emphasis on universities.* Lexington, MA: Lexington Books, 1975.

Davenport, J., & Reims, N. Theoretical orientations and attitudes toward women. *Social Work*, July 1978, *23*, 306–310.

Dinerman, M. Catch 23: Women, work and welfare. *Social Work*, November 1977, *22*, 472–477.

Drucker, P. On managing the human service organization. *Public Interest*, Fall 1973, *33*, 43–60.

Figueira-McDonough, J. Discrimination in social work: Evidence, myth and ignorance. *Social Work*, April 1979, *24*, 243–254.

Finch, W. Administrative priorities: The impact of employee perception on agency functioning and worker satisfaction. *Administration in Social Work*, Winter 1978, *2*, 391–400.

Glisson, C., & Martin, P. Productivity and efficiency in human service organizations and related to structure, size, and age. Unpublished paper, School of Social Work, University of Hawaii, 1978.

Gummer, B. A framework for curriculum planning in social welfare administration. *Administration in Social Work*, Winter 1979, *3*, 385–395.

Gummer, B. Is the social worker in public welfare an endangered species? *Public Welfare*, Fall 1979, *37*, 12–21.

Hasenfeld, Y., & English, R. *Human service organizations.* Ann Arbor: University of Michigan Press, 1974.

Kanter, R. Powerlessness corrupts: The effects of structural variables on organizational behavior. Paper presented at the American Sociological Association Meetings, San Francisco, September, 1978.

Karasek, R. A. Job demands, job decision latitude and mental strain: Implications for the job design. *Administrative Science Quarterly*, 1978, *24*, 285–308.

Kaufman, H. *The limits of organizational change.* University, AL: University of Alabama Press, 1971.

Kerson, T., & Alexander, L. Strategies for success: Women in social service administration. *Administration in Social Work*, Fall 1979, *3*, 313–326.

Kramer, R. M. Public fiscal policies and voluntary agencies in welfare states. *Social Service Review*, March 1979, *53*, 1–14.

Levy, C. The ethics of management. *Administration in Social Work*, Fall 1979, *3*, 277–288.

Lewis, H. Ethics and planning in the public services. Unpublished paper presented at Symposium on Issues in Planning for the Public Services, April 28–29, 1977.

Lewis, H. The future role of the social service administrator. *Administration in Social Work*, Summer 1977, *1*, 115–122.

Mahaffey, M. Sexism and social work. *Social Work*, November 1976, *21*, 419.

March, J., & Alsen, J. *Ambiguity and choice in organizations*. Oslo, Norway: Universitetsfordget, 1979.

National Conference in Social Welfare. Task force on expanding management technology and professional accountability in social service programs, Washington, DC, 103rd Annual Forum, June 14, 1976.

Patti, R. Toward a paradigm of middle-management practice in social welfare programs. In R. Sarri & Y. Hasenfeld (Eds.), *The management of human services*. New York: Columbia University Press, 1978.

Perlmutter, F., & Alexander, L. Exposing the coercive consensus: Racism and sexism in social work. In R. Sarri & Y. Hasenfeld (Eds.), *The management of human services*. New York: Columbia University Press, 1978.

Perrow, C. Demystifying organizations. In R. Sarri & Y. Hasenfeld (Eds.), *The management of human services*. New York: Columbia University Press, 1978.

Rausch, J.B. Gender as a factor in practice. *Social Work*, September 1978, *23*, 388–396.

Rein, M. Barriers to the employment of the disadvantaged. In *Social policy*. New York: Random House, 1970.

Rizzo, A. Perceptions of membership and women in administration: Implications for public organizations. *Administration and Society*, 1978.

Rossi, P., Freeman, H., & Wright, S. *Program evaluation: A systematic approach*. Beverly Hills: Sage, 1979.

Sarri, R., & Hasenfeld, Y. (Eds.). *The management of human services*. New York: Columbia University Press, 1978.

Savas, E.S. On equity in providing public services. *Management Science*, April 1978, *11*, 804–808.

Schoech, D. A microcomputer-based human service information system. *Administration in Social Work*, Winter 1978, *3*, 423–440.

Selznick, H. *Leaderships in administration*. New York: Harper & Row, 1957.

Shapira, M. Reflection on the preparation of social workers for executive positions. *Journal of Education for Social Work*, January 1971, *7*, 55–68.

Skolnick, A., & Dales, S. Social welfare expenditures 1950–1975. *Social Security Bulletin*, 1976, *39*(1).

Smith, B.L.R. (ed.). *The new political economy: The public use of the private sector*. New York: John Wiley & Sons, 1975.

Street, D., Martin, G.T., & Gordon, L. *Functionaries and recipients: The ambiguity of roles and reforms in public aid*. Beverly Hills: Sage, 1979.

Sundel, M., & Homan, C. Prevention in child welfare: A framework for management and practice. *Child Welfare*, September-October 1979, *LVIII*, 63, 510–521.

Vinter, R.D. Analysis of treatment organizations. *Social Work*, July 1963, *8*, 3–15.

Zald, M. Political economy: A framework for comparative analysis. In M.N. Zald (Ed.), *Power in organizations*. Nashville, TN: Vanderbilt University Press, 1970.

26

The Changing Context of Human Services Administration: Implications for the Future

YEHESKEL HASENFELD

The context of human services administration is exceedingly complex, and is changing rather rapidly. To forecast its future is at best a hazardous task and at worst a foolish undertaking. It may be more appropriate, therefore, to focus on a few key issues and identify some future scenarios. This chapter begins by reviewing the changing economy and the ideological crisis facing the welfare state. It then suggests that these two forces have created a different environmental context for human services, characterized by an economy of scarcity and the degovernmentalization of human services. The effects of these developments on human service organizations are explored. There follows a brief discussion of the effects of cutback management on the internal structure of human service organizations. The chapter concludes with a speculation about the future.

THE CHANGING ECONOMY OF HUMAN SERVICES

It has become fashionable to describe the current state of the human services in the context of "the crisis of the welfare state." The human services are said to be a declining industry, victims of the fiscal crisis of the state. A measure of such decline can be clearly discerned from the federal outlays for social programs. As noted in Table 26–1, projected federal outlays for the major income security programs from 1981 through 1987 are showing a steadily declining growth, and for some programs such as AFDC and Foodstamps the projections are for an absolute reduction in outlays. In social service programs, where many innovative social work practices have been developed, real spending levels have been cut by 20 percent between FY 1981 and FY 1983 (see Table 26–1).

These trends are not confined to the United States alone. Other advanced welfare states, such as the OECD countries, are similarly caught in a set of socioeconomic conditions that seem to jeopardize the fiscal foundations of their welfare state programs. These conditions include a declining economic growth fueled by low productivity and investment, high unemployment, large budgetary deficits, and an aging population with an ever-increasing demand for human services (OECD, 1981).

Most projections suggest that the fiscal crisis of the welfare state

TABLE 26–1. Federal Funding for Major Social Services Programs (FY 1975–FY 1981)

Program	Federal Obligations (1981 dollars, in millions)						
	FY 1975	FY 1976	FY 1977	FY 1978	FY 1979	FY 1980	FY 1981
Title XX Social Services	3,259	3,297	3,468	3,868	3,672	2,887	2,490
Child Welfare[a]	246	278	288	318	293	341	524
Head Start	684	636	651	804	810	806	814
Administration on Aging[b]	386	398	612	656	684	788	749
Rehabilitation services	1,182	1,174	1,166	1,115	1,069	1,023	924
Community services	645	728	1,096	1,029	884	605[c]	527
Other services[d]	328	384	474	621	672	667	623
Total	6,730	6,895	7,756	8,412	8,084	7,118	6,651
Percentage change from previous year		+2.5	+12.5	+8.5	−3.8	−12.0	−6.6

[a] Includes other programs funded by the Department of Health and Human Services, Administration for Children, Youth, and Families, such as child abuse and runaway youth. Does not include Title XX funds for the same purposes.
[b] Includes Department of Agriculture Support for Nutrition Program.
[c] Does not include energy crisis assistance program.
[d] Includes developmental disabilities, legal services, domestic volunteer (ACTION), juvenile justice and delinquency prevention.
Source: Office of Management and Budget, *Budget of the United States Government, FY 1977–FY 1983* (Washington, D.C.: GPO).

could last into the next decade. On the one hand, this is due to a projected slow economic growth, limiting the resources available to welfare programs; on the other hand, it is due to the aging of the population, which increases the demands for welfare services. The pessimistic view of economic growth is based on the recognition that fundamental changes in the structure and organization of the economy must occur before significant improvements can be realized (Thurow, 1980). Even if substantial economic recovery is materialized, the hopes for a comparable expansion of the welfare state are dim. Two factors account for this. First, the expenditures for meeting already-obligated social welfare benefits are expected to rise dramatically, given the projected demographic characteristics of the populations, as can be noted in the case of Social Security and Medicare. Second, the concern for reducing budgetary deficits and promoting industrial growth is likely to overwhelm arguments in favor of further expansion of the welfare state. Consequently, human services will continue to function in an economy of scarcity. This is not to imply that all social welfare programs will experience a decline or stagnation. Some are likely to grow just by virtue of demographic pressures and changing social patterns, such as services for the elderly (Zald, 1977). Others are likely to grow in response to major economic transformation, such as services to the unemployed. However, such growth is likely to be at the expense of other human services. Thus, the overall trend is clearly toward the fiscal containment and contraction of the human services.

THE LEGITIMATION CRISIS

The fiscal crisis of the welfare state is also accompanied by a legitimation crisis. As political elites blame the welfare state and its programs for the economic malaise of the advanced industrialized state, a crisis of legitimation has been generated. The old, liberal ideological justifications of the welfare state are no longer in vogue. Indeed, new ideological strands transversing the political spectrum are beginning to emerge in response to the difficulties experienced by the welfare state, and are likely to have profound implications to the future administration of human services. These ideologies, although in general supportive of the welfare state, advocate distinct limits on its range and scope by redefining the obligations of government to its citizens, and vice versa. Although they are in their formative stages, several ideological themes can be discerned.

First, there is a strong acknowledgment that the strength of the welfare state hinges on economic growth. Consequently, when necessary, welfare state activities that jeopardize economic growth should be curtailed. It is recognized on both the right and the left that large governmental deficits produced by welfare state programs hamper economic growth, ultimately risking the foundations of the welfare state. Hence, such programs as Social Security and Medicare are viewed as requiring major fiscal and organizational transformations in order to reduce their burden on the economy. In addition, it is argued that the tax burden of the welfare state must be curbed in order to minimize individual and corporate disincentives to save and invest.

Second, there are growing sentiments that the establishment of priorities for the welfare state and the political decision-making processes underlying them must be based on the principle of corporatism (Rohatyn, 1981). As noted by Wilensky (1976), corporatist democracies are characterized by strongly organized national interest groups representing labor, employers, and professional associations and by a centralized government that is obliged by law or informal arrangements to seek their advice in the formulation of national policies. This tri-partnership between labor, business, and government implies that government plays an active role in stimulating industrial expansion, with labor and business cooperating with each other in the trade-offs between welfare state benefits and control over production costs. Trade unions may agree to moderate wage benefits, but they insist that they be distributed equally. Businesses may demand that wages be closely tied to productivity, but they accept in return corporate obligation for job security. And government undertakes to assume some of the costs of the "social wages" in return for increased taxation.

Third, there is a redefinition of citizenship rights and obligations vis-à-vis the welfare state. Although the commitment of the state to provide basic income protection to its citizens is unwavering, the new ideologies obligate citizens to a quid pro quo with the state. Citizens, whenever able, must make long-range personal investments in their own welfare and must utilize personal resources before seeking state protection. That is, citizens must make earnest efforts to reduce their dependence on the welfare state, relying on it only as a "safety net."

In this context, there is a redefinition of the social contract between citizens and the welfare state. In return for the benefits they receive, citizens should, in a direct way, be obligated to shoulder the responsibility of maintaining the fiscal viability of the state. This obligation may take numerous forms. For example, income security benefits should be viewed as taxable income, thus obligating citizens in higher income brackets to pay additional taxes on the benefits they receive. Similarly, able-bodied citizens receiving public assistance should be obligated to participate in public work. To quote Mead (1982, p. 23) "programs should try to assure recipients the same balance of rights *and* obligations that non-dependent people face in their daily lives. The needy should be supported, but they should be expected to work if employable, to stay in school if young, to obey the law, and so on."

Fourth, the changing relationship between citizens and the welfare state is coupled with a conception emphasizing the circumscribed role of the welfare state. It suggests that many of the relations between citizens and the welfare state should be mediated by nongovernmental organizations, both profit and nonprofit. These organizations will assume many of the functions of the welfare state currently discharged by governmental agencies (Kerrine & Neuhause, 1979). The justification for the need for these institutional intermediaries rests not only in their presumed efficiency and effectiveness but also in their broadening citizen choices (e.g., educational vouchers, health maintenance organizations).

Finally, the new ideologies emphasize the decentralization and localization of welfare state programs. Local control and management of welfare programs is said to accomplish several aims (Berger & Neuhause, 1977):

1. It tailors programs to the needs of the community.
2. It fosters greater reliance on local resources.
3. It gives citizens greater voice in the allocation of welfare resources and enhances local accountability and responsibility.
4. It reduces the excessive bureaucratization of the service delivery system.

The economy of scarcity and the changing welfare state ideologies will affect the future administration of human services in several key ways. First, they will alter the environment in which human service organizations function. Second, they will lead to significant changes in the financing and delivery of services. Third, they will force major internal changes in the structure and design of human services. The following sections explore each of these trends and suggest some potential organizational responses.

ENVIRONMENTAL SCARCITY, INSTABILITY, AND UNCERTAINTY

Human services as a class of organizations depend on donors for a steady flow of resources and support. As a result, they are particularly vulnerable to external influences and to the potential loss of autonomy (Hasenfeld, 1983). Moreover, in the absence of market mechanisms as a key determinant of organizational domain, the attainment of domain consensus in an environment dominated by competing normative interest groups is especially problematic. An economy of scarcity coupled with shifting ideologies will, therefore, undermine the already-precarious domain consensus and organization-environment relations for many of the human services. Following Aldrich (1979) we can predict that human service organizations will encounter an environment characterized by the following attributes:

1. paucity of resources,
2. concentration of the resources in a few elements,
3. turbulence, and
4. instability.

Organizations operating in such an environment encounter fierce competition for limited resources, conflict and lack of domain consensus, loss of autonomy, and inability to form stable external relations. As Whetten (1980a) points out, these conditions increase the risk that the organization will encounter environmental entropy, political vulnerability, and loss of legitimacy, all of which lead to decline and a high mortality rate of organizations.

Under these conditions, power is likely to shift to those external units in which the fiscal resources are concentrated. The political ramifications of such a shift can already be noted, for example, in the changing character of the Community Development Block Grants, whereby state governments have superseded direct federal-local relationships. According to Peterson (1982, p. 171), state governments "replace a wide variety of other local authorities, including county governments, community health centers, and local education agencies, as original recipients of funding." Although there are specific federal limitations on how states can allocate these funds, the power relations between state and local agencies have been significantly altered in favor of the former.

To survive in such an environment, many human service organizations will become captives of large donors, doing their political and ideological bidding. This pattern can already be noted in the ideological shifts that programs undertake in order to bid successfully for diminishing federal funds. The trade-off between procurement of resources and organizational autonomy will force organizations to abandon programs and services that are not consonant with the interests of the dominant donors.

The fierce competition for resources is likely to squeeze out small organizations or lead to their absorption by their larger competitors. More ominous, however, is the impact of such competition on interorganizational relations and cooperation. A rational service delivery system is based on agreements and cooperative arrangements among members of the organizational network. Scarcity and unpredictability of resources jeopardize the bonds that maintain such a network. Service agencies will attempt to shift some of the cost of services to other organizations, for example, through a tactic known as "dumping clients." At the same time there will be competition to control services and clients that enhance the organization's ability to mobilize resources. Both forces tend to undermine the stability of the service delivery system, leading to segmentation and fragmentation of services. Long-range planning in such an environment is exceedingly difficult, because of the instability and uncertainty of the resources. To paraphrase Gresham's law, short-term interests will drive out long-term visions and solutions.

DEGOVERNMENTALIZATION AND PRIVATIZATION OF HUMAN SERVICES

Significant changes are already underway in the financing and distribution of human services. Declining revenues and the changing ideologies combine to shift both the financing and delivery of human services to both the profit and nonprofit private sector (Danzinger & Ring, 1982). There is a long-standing tradition of the federal government's reliance on third parties to carry out many of its domestic functions, often described as the "third party government" (Salamon, 1981). Since the 1962 amendment to the Social Security Act and the subsequent enactment of Title XX, there has been a steady increase in the purchase of social services from the private sector. It is estimated that in several jurisdictions more than half of the federal and state social services funds are contracted to the private sector (Benson et al., 1978; Terrell & Kramer, 1982).

Shifting the service delivery system to the private sector is justified on the basis of greater economy and efficiency, reduced bureaucratization, increased responsiveness to client needs, and innovativeness (Terrell & Kramer, 1982). At least in theory, contracting services to the private sector enables government to set specific limits on the cost of services and to introduce incentives for the private sector to be cost-efficient.

However, the privatization of human services provides several latent functions to government. First, it creates a political climate that both enables and justifies cutbacks in government programs. Second, it sets the stage for shifting some of the costs of services directly to the consumer through user's fees. Third, government can undertake these policies while being buffered from the public; the private sector increasingly serves as the institutional intermediary between the citizens and the state. Accountability for accessibility to services and quality of care shifts away from government to the private sector.

The rising importance of the private sector in the provision of human services under conditions of declining governmental support will result in significant transformations in the organization of human services. First, the privatization of services is accompanied by increasing bifurcation of services by social class. With the introduction of contracting and user's fees, the consumer population is segregated more explicitly not only by its need but more so by its ability to pay. Certain government-operated services and designated, contracted private agencies will be targeted to serve the most destitute clients, while fee-charging agencies or programs will limit their services to clients who have personal resources or insurance. The segregation of services by social class is also accompanied by an inevitable differentation of quality. Although access to services may remain equitable and even improve, there are indications that the quality of care may actually become more inequitable, as in the case of medical care (Wyszewianski & Donabedian, 1981).

Second, the commercialization of human services makes them attractive to private sector entrepreneurial initiatives. There is money to be made from the human services by shrewd investment and management, as can be seen from the rise of the proprietary nursing homes industry. Because the demand for human services in certain areas such as health and custodial care remains very strong and is indeed rising, these become potentially profitable markets to be exploited. The entry of profit-making organizations into these arenas is increasingly evident. Starr (1982), for example, notes that over 30 percent of all community hospital beds are owned by multi-institutional corporations, and similar trends can be seen in nursing homes, day care, and chore services. In social work, there is evidence to suggest a steady increase in the number of professionals engaged in private practice either part time or full time (Wallace, 1982).

The implications of such a trend on the delivery of human services and quality of care are unclear at the present time. As Gilbert (1981) suggests, "welfare capitalism" is fraught with ambiguities and unpredictable consequences. It may increase consumer choice and improve efficiency. There is, however, concern that the commercialization of human services will inevitably substitute the profit motive for concern about quality of care and about the client's welfare. Organizations may select treatment technologies and establish service modalities that enhance their profitability but are not necessarily the most appropriate or most responsive to the service needs of the population. Moreover, professional autonomy over practice may be seriously eroded, as professional decisions become subject to corporate control. Finally, although the privatization of services increases consumer choice, "the major beneficiaries of greater choice would not be the traditional clientele of the welfare state, but consumers from middle and working classes to whom social welfare entitlements have been extended in recent years" (Gilbert, 1981, p. 36).

CUTBACK MANAGEMENT

How do human service organizations survive and adapt to an economy of scarcity and to an unstable and uncertain environment? Management theories are generally silent in considering organizational decline or zero growth. The underlying assumption of normative models of administration is organizational growth and expansion. Specifically, theories of organizational change underscore the importance of slack resources for successful implementation of innovations (Hasenfeld, 1980). Whetten (1980a) suggests that the growth bias may be due to:

1. the prevalence of a long period of continuous economic growth and
2. a broader social ideology that puts high premium on success and growth.

From a political economy perspective this is quite understandable: abundance of resources permits the organizational elite to assume a munificent posture, thus neutralizing conflicting interest groups and buying internal consensus (Scott, 1974). Much less is known about organizational survival and adaptation under conditions of cutbacks. Levine, Rubin, and Wolohojian (1982) have proposed that preconditions for effective redirection of resources include:

1. authority of the executive leadership,
2. continuity of the top management,
3. rapid feedback system from the operating system,
4. budgetary flexibility,
5. incentives to conserve resources, and
6. capacity to target resources to specific organizational activities.

They go on to suggest that human service organizations, particularly in the public sector, typically lack these preconditions. The authority of the executive leadership is constrained by external monitoring units; executive turnover is fairly high; there is lack of an effective management information system; reliance on multiple sources of funding limits budgetary flexibility; deficit spending discourages conservation of resources; and existing commitments to various interest groups hamper the retargeting of resources.

There are several critical dilemmas that human service organizations encounter under cutback management (Levine, 1979), the most serious of which is the exit of talent. Because personnel represent the largest fiscal outlay for the organization, conservation and adaptation to declining resources necessitates workforce reduction. Yet, under conditions of decline and limited rewards and incentives, the most talented and skillful personnel are likely to exit, while those who are less talented and less capable of assuming new roles are likely to stay (Hirschman, 1970). Strategies such as across-the-board layoffs and last-hired-first-fired may actually hasten the exit of talent. Planned attrition, although an effective and less costly strategy (Greenhalgh, 1982), is not always feasible. Thus, to protect its valuable human resources, the organization is often forced into inequitable distribution of rewards and abandonment of participative management, all of which increase internal conflict and foster discrimination and dissension. In the same vein, recruitment of talent to declining human services is likely to become increasingly more difficult, and one can expect that the quality of the workforce in the human services is likely to decline.

Organizational decline generates a great deal of pressure on the human services to deprofessionalize in order to conserve resources. The process of deprofessionalization is particularly prominent in those organizations where:

1. the service technologies cannot unequivocally demonstrate the need for professionals, and
2. the client population is powerless.

Both conditions give the organization greater liberty to reduce professional services. It is not surprising, therefore, that the declassification of social work positions occurs mostly in public social service bureaucracies responsible for the care of the most vulnerable populations, such as the chronically mentally ill, welfare recipients, neglected children, and the disabled elderly.

Cutback management forces human service organizations to consider strategies stressing efficiency and cost-effectiveness and to adopt the rhetoric of the business corporation, even though these may be in direct conflict with the mandate, domain, and service technology of the organization (Glassberg, 1978). Efficiency measures such as increased caseload per worker, elimination of support services, and reduction in services with relatively high cost per unit of service, may, of course, conserve resources. They may also, however, displace emphasis on effectiveness and responsiveness to client needs (Lipsky, 1980). In particular, these measures tend to drive out nonroutine service technologies that tailor services to the individual needs and circumstances of clients.

Accompanying the trend toward efficiency is the increasing concentration and centralization of power in the hands of the executive administrators. The organizational structure will become more formalized and rigid, characterized by hierarchical decision-making processes that increasingly rely on computerized management information systems (Bozeman & Slusher, 1979). Such a structure, however, is incompatible with nonroutine service technologies and will further reinforce their replacement by routine technologies. Centralization of power makes the future survival of the organization much more dependent on the leadership qualities of the executive cadre. At times of crisis, when strategic decisions about the future of the organization have to be made, the concentration of power enables executives to make and implement critical decisions (Hage, 1980). The chief characteristic of these decisions is their relative irreversibility, at least in the short run. Thus, they have profound impact on the future survival of the organization.

The concentration of power will be further enhanced by the technological revolution in information processing. The introduction of computerized management information systems into the human services provides the executives with access to and control over information about the activities of most units and staff in the organization. The implementation of a management information system is seen as a key organizational control mechanism to improve accountability and productivity. As such, it is likely to generate important transformations in the behavior of staff and in the organization of the service delivery system. Staff behavior will increasingly become controlled by the informational demands of the management information system and by the criteria used to evaluate performance. Similarly, services will be structured and organized so that they are in conformity with the system's requirements. In the short run, the introduction of a management information system will significantly constrain the behavior of staff and discourage innovation and experimentation in the delivery of services. In the long run, however, as human service workers become proficient in the use of computerized information systems, the technology can actually promote decentralization of operations and facilitate the development of empirically based practice.

CONCLUSION

In some respects, human services are victims of their own success. Through a period of rapid growth and expansion, the human services have broadened their domain, reaching the vast majority of the population. They have raised public expectations about the quality and outcomes of their services. Yet the expansion of the services created a condition of newness, in which lack of experience, lack of proficiency, and lack of mastery of the service technologies leads to uneven and unpredictable performance and results. These difficulties inevitably generate consumer disappointment. Hirschman (1982, p. 41) puts it eloquently when he proposes, "It is therefore precisely when a society makes a determined effort to widen access to certain services that the quality of these services will decline, with obvious negative effects on the morale of both new and old consumers." Therefore, the difficulties of the welfare state may be "quite possibly temporary growing pains. These pains may well cause considerable trouble when first encountered, but can eventually be brought under control as a result of various learning experiences and mutual adjustments" (Hirschman, 1982, p. 43).

Put differently, this period of decline and retrenchment can bring in its wake the seeds of renewal. Despite the negative consequences of the decline, it also forces human service organizations to take stock and to evaluate their performance and structure. From a population ecology perspective (Aldrich, 1979), the organizations that will adapt and survive will be those with superior performance and structure befitting the new environmental exigencies. Marginal programs, ineffective service technologies, and inappropriate organizational forms will be discarded. This period will force human services to sift through the knowledge and experience that has been accumulated and to select those which promise to offer superior performance and effective results. The process, while painful, should result in the reemergence of stronger organizations that can meet the expectations of the public for quality services.

Moreover, we should also anticipate a resurgence of political action on behalf of the welfare state from two quarters. First, although the initial decline of human services results in the exit of talent, subsequent recruitment will be based more on moral and value commitments to social welfare and social justice than on future personal gains. Hence, the future leaders in the human services are likely to demonstrate greater dedication and commitment to the welfare state and its success. Second, the public retreat from the welfare state will ultimately generate its own disappointments, and will activate renewed political interest in improving and enhancing social welfare institutions. Citizens, disenchanted with an ideology of individualism and personal gain, will turn toward ideologies that champion the cause of collective good, and will become motivated to mobilize political action on their behalf (Hirschman, 1982).

REFERENCES

Aldrich, H. *Organizations and environment.* Englewood Cliffs, N.J.: Prentice-Hall, 1969.

Benson, B., et al. *Social services: Federal legislation vs. state implementation.* Washington, D.C.: The Urban Institute, 1978.

Berger, P. L., & Neuhause, R. J. *To empower people: The role of mediating structures in public policy.* Washington, D.C.: American Enterprise Institute, 1977.

Bozeman, B. & Slusher, E. A. Scarcity and environmental stress in public organizations. *Administration and Society,* 11 (1979):335–355.

Danzinger, J. N. & Ring, P. S. Fiscal Limitations: A selective review of recent research. *Public Administration Review,* 42 (1982):47–55.

Gilbert, N. The future of welfare capitalism. *Society* (Sept./Oct., 1981):28–37.

Glassberg, A. Organizational responses to municipal budget decreases. *Public Administration Review,* 38 (1978):325–332.

Greenhalgh, L. Maintaining organizational effectiveness during organizational retrenchment. *Journal of Applied Behavioral Science,* 18 (1982):155–170.

Hage, J. *Theories of organizations.* New York: John Wiley & Sons, 1980.

Hasenfeld, Y. *Human service organizations.* Englewood Cliffs, N.J.: Prentice Hall, 1983.

————. Implementation of change in human service organizations. *Social Service Review,* 54 (1980):508–20.

Hirschman, A. O. *Exit, voice, and loyalty.* Cambridge, Mass.: Harvard University Press, 1970.

————. *Shifting involvements.* Princeton, N.J.: Princeton University Press, 1982.

Kerrine, T. & Neuhause, R. J. Mediating structures: A paradigm for democratic pluralism. *The Annals of the American Academy of Political and Social Science.* 446 (1979):18.

Levine, C. Organizational decline and cutback management. *Public Administration Review,* 38 (1979):316–325.

Levine, C., Rubin, I. S. & Wolohojian, G. Managing organizational retrenchment. *Administration and Society,* 14 (1982):101–136.

Lipsky, M. *Street level bureaucracy.* New York: Russell Sage Foundation, 1980.

Mead, L. M. Social programs and social obligations. *The Public Interest,* 69 (Fall, 1982):17–32.

OECD, *The welfare state in crisis.* Paris: 1981.

Peterson, G. The state and local sector. J. L. Palmer and I. V. Sawhill (eds.) *The Reagan Experiment,* 157–218. Washington, D.C.: The Urban Institute Press, 1982.

Rohatyn, F. Reconstructing America, *New York Review of Books,* 5 (Feb., 1981).

Scott, W. J. Organizational theory: A Reassessment, *Academy of Management Journal,* (June) 1974:242–253.

Starr, P. *The social transformation of American medicine.* New York: Basic Books, 1982.

Terrell, P. & Kramer, R. M. Degovernmentalizing public services: The use of voluntary social agencies by local government. Paper presented at the Seminar on Local Government Organization and Economy, Sigtuna, Sweden, 1982.

Thurow, L. C. *The zero-sum society.* New York: Basic Books, 1980.

Salamon, L. M. Rethinking public management: Third party government and the changing forms of public action. *Public Policy* (Summer, 1981):255–275.

Wallace, M. E. Private practice: A nationwide study. *Social Work,* 27 (1982):262–267.

Whetten, D. Organizational decline: A neglected topic in organizational science. *Academy of Management,* 5 (1980a):577–588.

————. Sources, responses, and effects of organizational decline. J. R. Kimberly, et al., *The Organizational Life Cycle*. San Francisco: Jossey-Bass, 1980b, 342–374.

Wilensky, H. L. *The 'new corpratism,' centralization, and the welfare state*. Beverly Hills: CA., Sage, 1976.

Wyszewianski, L. & Donabedian, A. Equity in the distribution of quality of care. *Medical Care*, 19 (1981):28–56.

Zald, M. Demographics, politics, and the future of the welfare state. *Social Service Review*, 51 (1977):110–24.

Index